Myopia Manual

An impartial documentation of all the reasons, therapies and recommendations

Unbiased summary of the literature, some ideas about linkages between the various published results, and recommendations for shortsighted people and people who don't want to become shortsighted at all.

Dr. rer. nat. Klaus Schmid, Physicist

Copyright Notice

All rights reserved. No part of this publication may be reproduced, stored in a retrieval system, or transmitted in any form or by any means, electronic, mechanical or otherwise, without the written permission of Klaus Schmid.

Disclaimer

This book is intended as an informational guide to be used as a supplement, not a substitute for professional medical advice. While the information and advice in this book is believed true and accurate, the author cannot accept any legal responsibility.

Note

This book is based on a paper, which is published on the Internet at
http://www.myopia-manual.de
On this Internet page updated versions will be published when appropriate.

Acknowledgements

This book is an effort to put pieces of the myopia puzzle together. These pieces were found in numerous books and scientific publications, and therefore I am extremely grateful to all these professionals for their work and their sharing of their results.

Additionally, quite a number of readers of the Internet version of this book helped with very constructive, encouraging and competent comments.

Dr. Bob Rich has done a great job of editing the book to convert the German-English of the author into proper English language, and to make the writing more clear.

Finally, thanks to my son Bernhard Schmid who was very helpful by taking care of all the data processing problems, which had to be solved to complete this book.

*This book is dedicated to my wife Veronica
and my children Nadine and Bernhard,
whose shortsightedness caused me
to write this book.*

Hopefully it will be helpful not only for them.

Table of Contents

Introduction 1

1 What is Myopia? 4
    1.1   How does it Feel being Myopic? 4
    1.2   Basic Terminology of the Anatomy of the Eye 5
    1.3   Accommodation 5
        1.3.1   Myopia and Emmetropia 5
        1.3.2   The Classical Theory of Accommodation 7
        1.3.3   A Controversial Hypothesis 7
    1.4   Refractive Myopia 8
        1.4.1   Night Myopia and Tonic Accommodation 8
        1.4.2   Pseudomyopia 9
        1.4.3   Other Types of Myopia 10
    1.5   Axial Myopia 11
    1.6   "What Type of Myopia Do I Have?" 11
    1.7   Consequences and Risks of Higher Myopia 11
    1.8   Myopia and Age 15
    1.9   Accommodation and Age 15
    1.10   Some more Age Related Geometrical Changes of the Eye 17
    1.11   The Refraction 17

2 What Causes Myopia in General? 20
    2.1   Is Myopia Inherited? 20
    2.2   Connective Tissue Disorders 22
    2.3   Active Growth by Imaging Effects 22
    2.4   Mechanical Effects 23
    2.5   General Overview of the Causes of Myopia 23

3 Myopia – Observations and Experimental Results 24
    3.1   Distribution of Myopia by Region, Age, Gender and Ethnicity 24
    3.2   Accommodation and Near Work 27
        3.2.1   Experiences and Results 27
            3.2.1.1   General Experiences and Results 27
            3.2.1.2   The Strength of Accommodation 30
            3.2.1.3   Timing- and Hysteresis- Effects of Accommodation 31
            3.2.1.4   Is there a Connection between Blur Sensitivity and Accommodation Deficits? 32
            3.2.1.5   Accommodation and the Nervous System 33
            3.2.1.6   Summary of Results about Accommodation 33
        3.2.2   Proposed Therapies Based on the Accommodation Issue 34
            3.2.2.1   Relaxing and Exercising 34
            3.2.2.2   Biofeedback 36
            3.2.2.3   Undercorrection for Near Work, Plus-, Bifocal- and Progressive- Glasses 36
            3.2.2.4   Intermittent, Short Term Wearing of Plus Glasses 40

	3.2.2.5 Plus glasses - are they Effective via Reduced Accommodation or via Modified Vergence?....40	
	3.2.2.6 Comparison of the Various Optical Methods..41	
	3.2.2.7 Psychological Problems with Special Glasses for Near Work 42	
	3.2.2.8 Permanent Undercorrection instead of Undercorrection for Near Work only 43	
	3.2.2.9 Is the Accommodation System Getting too Lazy by the Plus Glasses? 43	
	3.2.2.10 Refraction with a Cycloplegic Agent 44	
	3.2.2.11 Summary of the Accommodation Based Therapies 45	
3.3	The Effects of Image Quality 46	
3.3.1	Basic Results 46	
3.3.2	Biochemical Results 48	
3.3.3	Connective Tissue Related Results...49	
3.3.4	Remarks on the Image Quality Model 51	
3.3.5	"Emmetropization" towards Myopia...52	
3.3.6	Contrast and Spatial Frequency 54	
3.3.7	Monochromatic Aberrations 54	
3.3.8	Summary of the Effects of the Image Quality 55	
3.4	Phoria, Convergence and Astigmatism 56	
3.4.1	Phoria 56	
3.4.2	The AC/A Ratio 57	
3.4.3	The CA/C Ratio, and some more Types of Vergence 59	
3.4.4	Hysteresis of Vergence 60	
3.4.5	Glasses, Contact Lenses and Vergence 61	
3.4.6	Astigmatism 61	
3.4.7	Summary of the Vergence Related Effects 62	
3.5	Saccades and Focusing..63	
3.6	Mechanical Stress, Strain and Pressure 64	
3.6.1	Impact of Mechanics on Biochemistry 64	
3.6.2	Intraocular Pressure (IOP) 64	
3.6.3	The Muscles 66	
3.6.4	The Lens 67	
3.6.5	The Ocular Shape 68	
3.6.6	The Zonular Fibers 69	
3.7	Illumination / Light / Day- and Night-Rhythm 69	
3.7.1	Day- and Night-Rhythm 69	
3.7.2	Level of Illumination 71	
3.7.3	Color of Illumination 73	
3.7.4	Flickering Light 74	
3.8	Vision Training..74	
3.9	Recommendations from Optical and Mechanical Results 75	
3.10	Temperature 75	
3.11	Blood Circulation..77	
3.12	Some Specific Biochemical Issues..78	
3.12.1	The Immune System 78	
3.12.2	Oxidative Damage and Antioxidant Defense in General 80	
3.12.3	Enzymes Glutathione, Glutathione Peroxidase, Superoxide Dismutase, G6PD.............81	

	3.12.4	The Blood-Retinal Barrier	82
	3.12.5	The Vitreous Body	82
	3.12.6	Nitric Oxide (NO)	83
	3.12.7	More Biochemical and Biomechanical Effects	84
3.13		Mental Issues	86
	3.13.1	Stress	86
	3.13.2	Personality and Mentality	88
3.14		Physical Exercises	89
3.15		Myopic Changes in Pregnancy	89
3.16		Impact of Nutritional Components	90
	3.16.1	Carbohydrates, Blood Sugar Level, Insulin Metabolism	90
	3.16.2	Is there a Connection between the Blood Sugar Level and Negative-Lens-Induced Myopia?	93
	3.16.3	Calcium and Vitamin D	94
	3.16.4	Magnesium	95
	3.16.5	Copper and Zinc	95
	3.16.6	Chromium	97
	3.16.7	Manganese	98
	3.16.8	Potassium	98
	3.16.9	Iodine / the Thyroid Gland	98
	3.16.10	Vitamin A	98
	3.16.11	B-Vitamins	99
	3.16.12	Some More Antioxidants	99
		3.16.12.1 Selenium	99
		3.16.12.2 Flavonoids and Related Compounds, and vitamin E	100
	3.16.13	Folic Acid and Homocysteine	101
		3.16.13.1 Observations	101
		3.16.13.2 An Explanation	102
	3.16.14	Other Components of the Diet	102
	3.16.15	Overall Nutritional Status and Myopia	103
3.17		Pharmaceuticals	104
3.18		Congenital Myopia, and Inherited Diseases which are related to Myopia	105
3.19		Other Means to Slow Down or Stop Progression of Myopia	108
	3.19.1	Contact Lenses	108
	3.19.2	Reinforcement of the Sclera	109
	3.19.3	Acupuncture	110
	3.19.4	Electrostimualtion	110
3.20		Means to Correct Myopia	110
	3.20.1	Manipulation of the Cornea	110
		3.20.1.1 Orthokeratology	110
		3.20.1.2 Radial Keratotomy RK	111
		3.20.1.3 Photorefractive Keratectomy (PRK)	111
		3.20.1.4 Laser In Situ Keratomileusis (LASIK), Laser Epithelial Keratomileusis (LASEK)	111
		3.20.1.5 Intrastromal Corneal Ring	112
		3.20.1.6 Artificial Cornea	112
	3.20.2	Manipulation of the Lens System inside the Eye	112

3.21		Summary: What Causes Myopia?	113
	3.21.1	School and Myopia	115
	3.21.2	Is Myopia Caused by Mechanical or by Biochemical Processes?	115
	3.21.3	Prevention of Progression of Myopia or Prevention of Myopia	116
	3.21.4	Working against Myopia or against the Consequences of Myopia?	116
	3.21.5	Inflammation towards Progressive and Pathologic Myopia	116
	3.21.6	Functional- versus Structural- Deficits	116
	3.21.7	Are the Published Results really Contradictory? Maybe not!	117
4	**A Synthesis – or how some Pieces might Fit together**		**122**
4.1		Some General Remarks about Nutrition and Environment	124
	4.1.1	Biochemistry versus Mechanical Effects versus Optical Effects?	124
	4.1.2	Nutrition and the Environment have Changed Dramatically	124
	4.1.3	There is a very Large Biochemical Individuality	127
	4.1.4	There are Biochemical Alterations before Clinical Symptoms Arise	128
	4.1.5	There can be Selective Nutrient Deficiency	128
	4.1.6	Summary – the Balance	128
4.2		Some Relevant Biochemical Key Issues	129
	4.2.1	The Connective Tissue	129
	4.2.1.1	Connective Tissue in General	130
	4.2.1.2	The Connective Tissues of the Eye	131
	4.2.2	The Immune System	132
	4.2.2.1	Natural (Innate) Immunity	132
	4.2.2.2	Acquired Immunity	133
	4.2.2.3	Pathologic Immune Responses	133
	4.2.2.4	Effects of the Immune System on the Tissue	134
	4.2.2.5	Turnover of Connective Tissue and the Immune System	134
	4.2.2.6	TH1/TH2 Balance	135
	4.2.2.7	Neurotransmitters and the Immune System	135
	4.2.2.8	Stress and the Immune System	136
	4.2.2.9	Acupuncture and the Immune System	137
	4.2.2.10	Melatonin and the Immune System	137
	4.2.2.11	The Eye and the Immune System	137
	4.2.2.12	Summary Immune System	138
	4.2.3	Miscellaneous issues	139
	4.2.3.1	The Metabolism of the Feedback Process Leading to Myopia via Degraded Image Quality	139
	4.2.3.2	Oxidative Processes and Antioxidant Defense	139
	4.2.3.3	Cortisol and other Hormones	140
	4.2.3.4	The Nitric Oxide (NO) Balance	140
	4.2.3.5	"The Nerves": Neurotransmitters, Stress and Personality	147
	4.2.3.6	Homocysteine	148
	4.2.3.7	The Day- / Night-Rhythm, Illumination, and Melatonin Metabolism	150
	4.2.3.8	Blood Sugar Level / Insulin Level	151
	4.2.3.9	The Sodium / Potassium Balance	153
	4.2.3.10	Hormones	154
	4.2.3.11	Physical Exercises	154

	4.2.3.12	G6PD (Glucose-6-Phospahate Dehydrogenase) Deficiency – an Example	155
	4.2.3.13	Is there an Analogy between Structural Heart Problems and Progressive Myopia?	158
	4.2.3.14	Is there an Analogy between Arthritis and Progressive Myopia?	158
4.3		The Impact of Nutritional Components	159
	4.3.1	Minerals	160
	4.3.1.1	Calcium	160
	4.3.1.2	Chromium	162
	4.3.1.3	Copper	163
	4.3.1.4	Magnesium	166
	4.3.1.5	Manganese	167
	4.3.1.6	Selenium	168
	4.3.1.7	Silicon	171
	4.3.1.8	Zinc	172
	4.3.2	Vitamins	173
	4.3.2.1	Vitamin A	173
	4.3.2.2	B-Vitamins	173
	4.3.2.2.1	Vitamin B2 (Riboflavin)	173
	4.3.2.2.2	Vitamin B5 (Pantothenic Acid)	174
	4.3.2.2.3	Vitamin B6 (Pyridoxine, but also Pyridoxal or Pyridoxamine)	175
	4.3.2.2.4	Vitamin B12 (Cobalamin)	177
	4.3.2.3	Folic acid (member of the family of B-vitamins)	177
	4.3.2.4	Interactions between B Vitamins	178
	4.3.2.5	Vitamin C	178
	4.3.2.6	Vitamin D – or Sunlight	179
	4.3.2.7	Vitamin E	180
	4.3.3	Other Components of Nutrition, and some Facts about Nutrition	181
	4.3.3.1	Flavonoids	181
	4.3.3.2	Carbohydrates	182
	4.3.3.3	Lipids and Fatty Acids	183
	4.3.3.4	Amino Acids	184
	4.3.3.5	Proteins	184
	4.3.3.6	Some Other Nutrients	185
4.4		Nutrition, some General Facts	186
4.5		Impact of Nutrition and Behavior– Summary	188
4.6		The "Right" Supply with Vitamins and Minerals, and the Supply Status	190
4.7		The Speed of Nutritional Effects	194
4.8		Overall Recommendations	194
5		**Additional Information**	**198**
5.1		Optical Correction	198
	5.1.1	Glasses	198
	5.1.2	The Material of the Glass	198
	5.1.3	The Coating of the Glass	199
5.2		Contact Lenses	199
	5.2.1	Basic Types of Lenses – Soft Lenses versus Hard Lenses	200
	5.2.2	How about Lenses for Permanent Wear?	203

	5.2.3	Potential Complications	204
	5.2.4	Parameters of the Material for Contact Lenses	204
		5.2.4.1 Oxygen Transmission	205
		5.2.4.2 Wettability and Resistance against Deposits	207
		5.2.4.3 Hardness and Stability	208
		5.2.4.4 Specific Weight and Refractive Index	208
		5.2.4.5 UV Blocking	209
	5.2.5	Parameters of the Geometry of Contact Lenses	209
	5.2.6	Surface and Edge Finishing	211
	5.2.7	The Fitting of Contact Lenses	211
	5.2.8	Determining the Refraction after Wearing Contact Lenses	212
	5.2.9	Maintenance of the Lenses	213
		5.2.9.1 Maintenance of Hard RGP Lenses	213
		5.2.9.2 Maintenance of Soft Lenses	214
	5.2.10	"I Cannot Wear Contact Lenses"	215
	5.2.11	Presbyopia	215
	5.2.12	Contact Lenses and Nutrition	216
5.3		Refractive Surgery	217
5.4		Useful Links	219
6		**References**	**221**

Introduction

The Situation - and the Target of this Book

Old-fashioned traditional medicine stated that myopia is an inherited condition and the only solution is to prescribe glasses. People who objected to this "therapy" (it's not really a therapy, but only a short term covering of symptoms) were treated as ignorant.

In many papers, however, it was reported that today very many people are becoming myopic even though their parents or grandparents were not. On the other hand, life today is very different from that of our ancestors – just to mention the changed working environment and changed nutrition. Therefore, it is rather obvious that these changes in the environment have an impact on the incidence of myopia. Definitely, some people are more sensitive to these changes than others – by heredity.

If we can map all these negative influences and understand how they are affecting myopia, then we have a chance at minimizing myopia in some, decreasing its progression in others and in some cases, preventing it altogether. At the very least, we may be able to minimize the very serious consequence of blindness.

The idea of finding just one mechanism for myopia and solving this problem once and forever is very tempting, and some authors give the impression that they are close to this goal, and that all the other researchers, optometrists and ophthalmologists are wrong. Strangely enough, these authors often disagree with each other. The conclusion is not that some researchers are right, and of the rest of the researchers are wrong – all of them are right in their specific view of their experiments and experiences. Clearly, various different mechanisms exist that can lead to myopia. It is more important to find commonalities in the results than the contradictions.

Unfortunately, it appears that it appears that too little financial resources are available for research in myopia, since the industry financially benefits from the existence and progression of myopia than from its prevention. Just one number: In 1993 the USA spent 3.4 billion $ US on optical correction of myopia[1]. Definitely, the number is substantially higher today – not counting the personal inconvenience, the inability to work in a planned profession, and the suffering because of the permanent progression of myopia: in some countries myopia is the first or second leading cause of blindness[2].

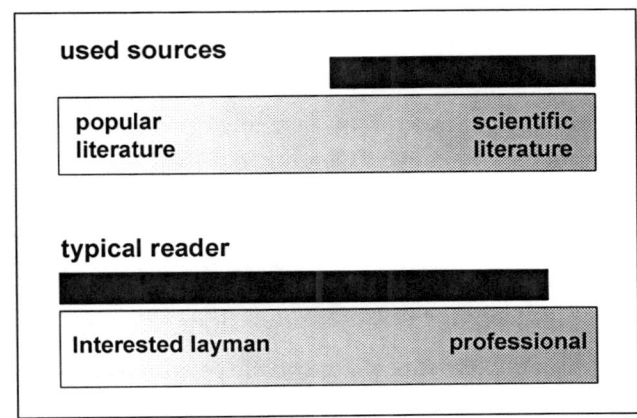

I will outline the main results reported by researchers and practitioners. Since I have no personal involvement, i.e. no personal results to promote, I am able to do this in an unbiased and neutral way. In a separate chapter I will try to find common patterns for the results.

The author of this book doesn't pretend to be a judge about whose myopia theory is right and whose theory is wrong – in the framework of their experimental conditions all of them can considered to be right in a way! Therefore, my personal views are generally clearly marked as "*Notes*".

The typical reader for whom this book was written is somebody who has myopia, or whose relative has myopia, and who is willing to take the tough route through a lot of scientific results. Maybe even some professionals in the area of myopia can benefit by getting a guide to numerous research results.

Some readers might be bored or frightened by these numerous scientific results given in this book. I decided, however, to include them to make all the recommendations and conclusions credible. There are already numerous books on the market that focus on mere recommendations without going into the details of the scientific background – I did not want to add another one to this category.

The purpose of this book is

(1) to increase the overall knowledge about myopia, particularly progressive myopia in an easy-to-read but scientifically correct format without skipping opinions and results which are still controversial
(2) to suggest the best ways to handle myopia.

The advice given in this book does not replace the treatment by a health professional, but it should enable the reader to enter detailed discussions with her/his personal optometrist, ophthalmologist or physician.

Do not expect simple "cook book" approaches to make your myopia disappear. The reader can expect to gain a better understanding of the various mechanisms and factors that produce myopia and to learn some of the means to treat its symptoms.

Do not expect to find an easy answer about the exact cause of your specific myopia. Obviously, myopia can be caused by a lot of different off-balanced processes in the human system. You will find, however, a lot of material that will enable you to consider which of your personal conditions might be part of the problem.

You will find that there are many controversies among the experts. Also, many of the cited references indicate the need for more research.

Additionally, most of the published results were collected data, which were found to be associated with myopia, and they are not definite proofs about what causes myopia. For most of these causes, however, there are potential scientific explanations given (e.g. in section 4). An example for the risk of misinterpreting associated facts as causes is as follows[3]: It can be said, e.g. that most of the children who run across the street and get hit by an automobile were wearing tennis shoes, so therefore, tennis shoes must have caused the accidents. Obviously, the tennis shoes were only a common association, not a related factor. This is the problem in sorting out causes from associations in the study of myopia.

Nevertheless, Research has already collected a tremendous amount of information, which can be very helpful to preserve your eyesight! It does not make sense simply to wait until research has solved the myopia problem – maybe this will be too late for you.

Chapters 1 to 3 detail the basic material about myopia, the remaining sections contain material which can help to create a link between the sometimes contradictory publications about myopia, and some background information which might be of interest for involved people.

Myopia is a result of more than what happens within the optical system. It is also affected by nutrition and other aspects of lifestyle. As Eaton et al. stated[4]:

"These diseases are the results of interaction between genetically controlled biochemical processes and a myriad of biocultural influences – lifestyle factors – that include nutrition, exercise, and exposure to noxious substances."

I strongly recommend that you read the book as a whole before choosing recommendations to try out. However, the final recommendations are listed in section 4.8. If you are too discouraged by all the detailed material, you should better jump to this section instead of stopping reading at all.

The author welcomes every kind of feedback – please send an email to klausschmid@onlinehome.de

1 What is Myopia?

1.1 How does it Feel being Myopic?

Most of the readers of this book don't have to read this, because they know how it feels being myopic. They are hoping to gain some improvement, or even to cure the condition.

Other people, however, are reading this book to get help for their child or a friend. They don't have personal experience with myopia.

Being myopic means you cannot focus on distant objects without an optical device like glasses or contact lenses. Without these devices distant objects are blur – the higher the myopia the more blurry they are.

Some people might consider glasses or contact lenses to be at the most a minor inconvenience. Children, however, often feel really handicapped, and people doing sports can feel the same. In any case, if there is a higher grade of myopia the loss of the optical device leaves the person feeling helpless.

As long as there is complete vision achieved with optical devices there might be a substantial psychological problem, but not a real medical problem. People with higher grades of myopia, however, are threatened by a permanent degradation of their vision or even blindness (see section 1.7).

At the least, then, myopia is inconvenient, and can be risky. This should be enough reason to find out about ways to minimize it. Like for every problem in life prevention is the best remedy – in spite of the fact that most often people will take action only when the damage is already happening. There is a German proverb saying "damage makes you wise" – but better get wise without too much damage. Therefore, please read the complete book.

1 WHAT IS MYOPIA?

1.2 Basic Terminology of the Anatomy of the Eye

For clarification of the terminology, a cross section of the eye is shown in Figure 1.

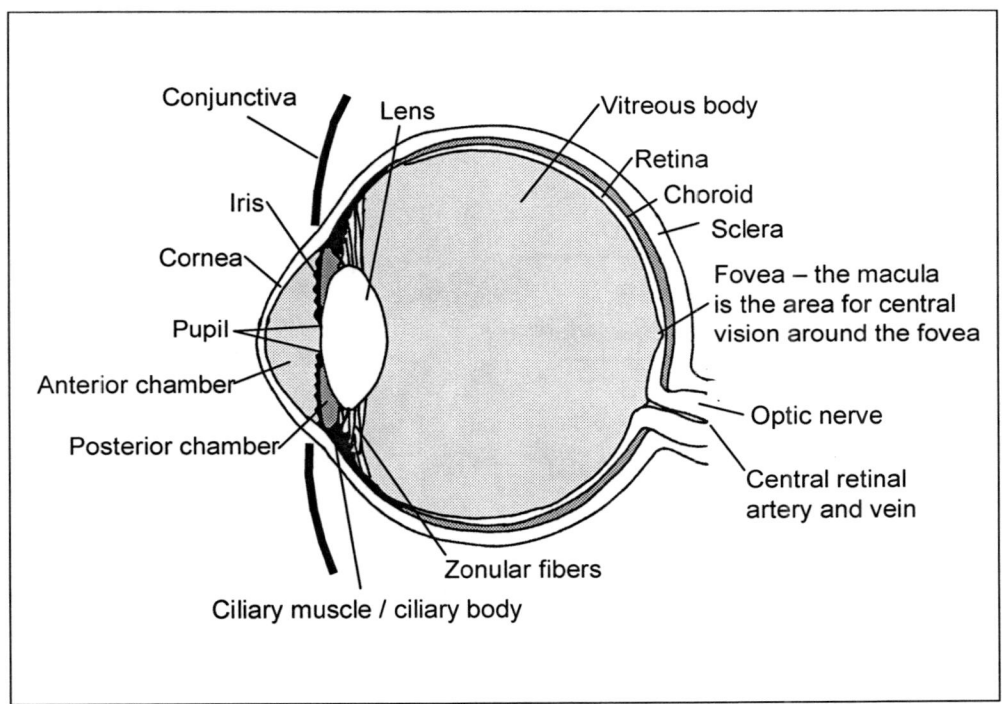

Figure 1 The anatomy of the eye

1.3 Accommodation

Accommodation is the adjustment of the refractive power of the lens of the eye to achieve an exact image of the object on the retina.

1.3.1 Myopia and Emmetropia

Myopia (or shortsightedness, or nearsightedness) is a condition in which distant objects are not displayed sharply on the retina by the optical system of the eye, because the rays converge already before they hit the retina.

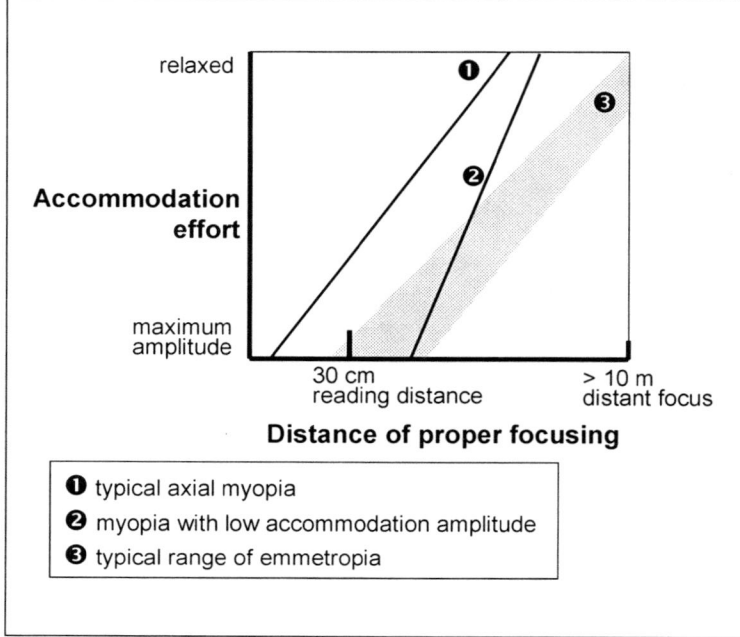

Figure 2
The accommodation effort of myopes and non-myopes

Figure 2 shows effective accommodation, when a proper focusing on the retina is achieved. E.g., in typical axial myopia even with relaxed accommodation proper focus of distant objects cannot be achieved. The emmetropic eye can adjust for all distances by an appropriate accommodation effort. Low accommodation amplitude results in an exact vision of a narrow range of distances only.

The states of myopia and emmetropia are defined according to the handling of parallel rays of light (i.e. far distance):

Emmetropia is most often defined as a state, where parallel rays of light can be focused properly on the retina. For **myopia** this focus point lies in front of the retina.

Obviously, **emmetropia** can be achieved not by one specific ocular model, but by **a range of ocular configurations**, which may all lead to a good vision at distant objects.

Emmetropia and hyperopia (farsightedness) blur into each other:

- Proper distant focus can be achieved without accommodation as well as with some residual accommodation.
- Near focus (e.g. for reading) is largely dependent on the person's ability to accommodate (i.e. the individual amplitude of accommodation), which decreases with age (see section 1.8).

The reasons for myopia can be (see Figure 3):

- The refractive power of the lens system is too high: **refractive myopia**. Parameters of the lens system are the curvature of the cornea, the curvature of the lens at the front as well at the back, and the refractive indices of the anterior chamber, the lens and the vitreous body

- The distance between the lens system and the retina is too large: **axial myopia.**

The critical reason is the second one, as it can lead to the dangerous progressive myopia by excessive stretching of the sclera.

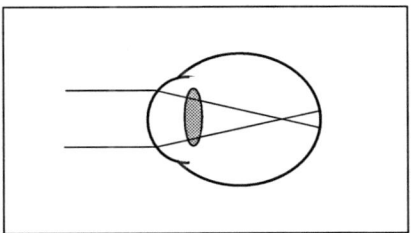

Figure 3 The focusing of the myopic eye

In the next sections the basics of accommodation, i.e. the adjustment of the eye to different distances of the objects, and some specific sub-categories of myopia will be discussed.

Literature-references to ophthalmology in general and to literature about myopia are given at the end of this book in chapter 6[5, 6, 7, 8, 9, 10, 11, 12, 13, 14, 15, 16].

1.3.2 The Classical Theory of Accommodation

The general view of ophthalmic science is:

- Due to its own original shape the lens would get into the shape of a round ball without a force on it. This shape corresponds to near focus.
- The pulling action of the zonular fibers, which connect the lens with the ring-shaped ciliary muscle, can flatten the lens. This shape corresponds to focus on a distant object.

Consequence:

- If the **ciliary muscle is relaxed**, there is a pulling tension on the lens via the zonule fibers, and therefore the focus is set to "**distant object**".
- If the **ciliary muscle is contracted**, the diameter of this ring-shaped muscle is decreased, and there is no more pulling action on the lens via the zonula fibers and therefore the focus is set to "**near object**".

1.3.3 A Controversial Hypothesis

Based on experiments, which he conducted on his own eyes, McCollim published the following model[17]:

- "Compression of the globe by the **extraocular muscles** [which move the axes of the eyeballs] can cause the lens to accommodate" ... "accommodation can be actuated **without the intervention of the ciliary muscle**".

- "... a single factor, external pressure on the globe, produces two separate effects, in opposite directions: anteriorly it **accommodates the lens [by forcing the vitreous against the lens]**, and posteriorly it **elongates the globe**."

    The fact that it was found by measurements that the eye is elongating during near accommodation[18, 19] supports aspects of this thesis.

As a consequence to these experimental results it was concluded by McCollim[17] that "with repeated periods of prolonged accommodation the lens would never have sufficient time to return completely to the unaccommodated state", i.e. there is a substantial **time lag for the reshaping of the lens**.

Conclusion: While the reshaping is taking place the refraction will diagnose myopia. After the reshaping the refraction will not find myopia.

Note:
This time lag for the reshaping of the lens was generally found in myopic eyes (see section 3.2.1). The model of a longer lasting time lag of the shape change of the lens could explain a progression of myopia: The fitted glasses would become inadequate, and could induce a further increase of myopia (see section 3.2.1.3). In fact, the progression would depend on how long the eye takes to return to shape. This effect of a time lag for readjustment is called **hysteresis**.

1.4 Refractive Myopia

Besides mere static geometrical anomalies of the lens system of the eye, there are two more dynamic refractive effects:

1.4.1 Night Myopia and Tonic Accommodation

Night myopia is when the eye adjusts in the dark or already in dim light, or due to a lack of image contrast **to near focus, even if all the objects are far off**. It is also called **dark focus of accommodation**, or **tonic accommodation, or resting state of accommodation**[16]. Consequently, a measurement of the refraction (i.e. the determination of appropriate optical glasses to obtain good vision on these distant objects) gives the result that the eye is myopic.

Night myopia can reach values of up to about $-4.0\,D$[20], more typical around $-1.0\,D$ (D stands for diopters, the measure for the degree of myopia; people with myopia of $-1.0\,D$ can see still clearly at a distance of 1 m, at $-4.0\,D$ the distance is 0.25 m. For more details about the definition of diopters see section 1.11). At presentations where projectors with poor brightness are used, this effect might be important as well. Some authors recommend some additional optical correction for night use only, e.g. for night driving[5].

The reason for this myopia is some basic residual accommodation[21], as stated by Leibowitz et al.[22]: "the focus of the eye tends to return passively to an individually characteristic intermediate resting position or dark-focus whenever the stimulus to accommodation is degraded or when the quality of the image is independent of focus."

Night myopia decreases with age[23] and therefore it can be of special importance for young drivers at night. In one experiment with people aged 16 to 25 years, 38% had night myopia of - 0.75 D or more, and 4% had – 2.50 D or more[24].

As mentioned above, the reduced distance vision at low light is caused mainly by residual accommodation, but some other effects have an impact as well:

- The optical effect of the larger pupil decreases the depth of focus – like a large aperture of a camera

- At low light levels there is a change of the biochemistry of imaging on the retina: in bright light the receptors in the retina are cones with higher image acuity, and imaging of colors, whereas in low light the receptors in the retina are rods with reduced image acuity, and imaging of black and white only. The transition between both states, i.e. to get maximum sensitivity when moving from the bright to the dark, doesn't happen immediately, but takes some minutes[25]. This is a problem e.g. when driving a car in sunlight and entering a tunnel.

- The low light imaging by rods in the retina can be further reduced by a lack of vitamin A and zinc.

There is conflicting evidence regarding a connection between tonic accommodation and myopia. Some studies associate higher tonic accommodation with myopia, while others indicate that lower tonic accommodation is associated with myopia[16].

1.4.2 Pseudomyopia

If there is a **transient spasm or excessive stress** in the ciliary muscle during excessive near work, the zonular fibers are relaxed (and the ciliary muscle is not relaxed) even at distant-focus, giving the impression of a myopic eye. It is said that this pseudomyopia frequently precedes axial myopia, and it is most frequently found with young people[5].

Another mechanism for pseudomyopia has been postulated: It was stated[6] *[reference was missing in the sample]* that as an automatic reaction to mental stress the axes of the two eyes are set parallel and the focus is set to "distant", and the pupils are opened wide. In a hunter-gatherer lifestyle, this has a survival advantage in that it may lead to the early detection of danger. However, if a child working at near focus - like during a test - will subject the eyes to competing forces:

- Between near focus and distant focus (ciliary muscle), and
- Between inward adjustment of the axes of the eyes (convergence for near work) and parallel adjustment.

This can lead to a spasm of the involved muscles and further to pseudomyopia (and maybe to permanent myopia).

Besides these effects of the ciliary muscle, transient myopia, which is caused by a hysteresis (i.e. a longer time necessary for readjustment) of accommodation, can be based on:

- **A transient ocular elongation** caused by accommodation (see section 3.6.5).
- **A hysteresis of the shape of the lens** as well (see sections 1.3.3 and 3.6.4).

1.4.3 Other Types of Myopia

There are some other types of myopia:

- **Keratoconus** is when the shape of the cornea is not uniform but more pointed; this can add additional refractive power of up to –20 D.
- With increasing age the **refractive index of the cornea** can be changed, to result in very moderate myopia.
- Beyond 40 to 50 years **presbyopia** appears, i.e. the lens loses some (and later all) of its flexibility due to structural changes. Generally this results in problems with near work and accommodation. If, however, the lens shape is "frozen" in a slightly accommodated state, problems with distant focusing may appear, which corresponds to myopia.
- **Diabetes** can change the refractive index of the lens, leading to myopia if the blood sugar is elevated, and to hyperopia (farsightedness) if the blood sugar is low[26] (see section 3.16.1).
- **Antibiotics** like sulfonamides, tetracyclines and corticosteroids can induce myopia[27].
- **Amblyopia** is when the visual acuity is reduced without visible pathologic defects. In most cases one eye only is affected. The affected eye is often **highly myopic**. This is named anisometropic amblyopia (see section 3.18).

1.5 Axial Myopia

Axial myopia occurs if the length of the eyeball is more than the average length of about 24 mm[28]. In this case the ratio of the length of the eye (anteroposterior dimension) to the height/width of the eye (transverse dimension) is larger than 1.0. Roughly 1 mm in length corresponds to - 3.0 D.

The increase in the length of the eye is said to happen only at daytime[29].

There are several forms of axial myopia:

- **Simple myopia** (sometimes called **school myopia**), which normally starts at age 10 – 12, stays normally under - 6 D and remains quite stable after the age of 20 years. No structural defects of the eye can be diagnosed in this case.
- **Benign progressive myopia** up to 12 D, which is often stabilized at an age of 30 years. Most likely structural / biochemical defects of the eye can be diagnosed.
- **Malign myopia,** which does not stop progressing at all. Up to – 30 D can be reached, with serious consequences, which may lead to blindness. Structural / biochemical defects of the eye can be diagnosed.
- **Pathological myopia**, if there are already pathological changes in the eye (see section 1.7), independent from the refractive error.

1.6 "What Type of Myopia Do I Have?"

The main and most worrying question is, whether it is a simple (not dangerous) myopia, or a myopia that can lead to a permanent damage of the vision (see section 1.7). This question can be answered only be an optometrist or an ophthalmologist, who will check the background of the eye for some signs of already appearing damage.

Note:
You may regret doing nothing if myopia appears at a young age, or if it is increasing. Even if there is no visible damage yet, follow the recommendations in section 4.8.

1.7 Consequences and Risks of Higher Myopia

Some numbers from the statistics about the consequences of higher myopia[5]:

- England, 1966: Myopia was responsible for 8.8% of blind registrations.
- England, 1972, age between 50 and 59: Myopia was responsible for 18.2% of blind registrations, only behind diabetic retinopathy.

- Bavaria/Germany, 1992, up to age 18: Myopia was responsible for 11.5% of blind registrations[30].
- Myopic macular degeneration is the seventh greatest cause of registered blindness in adults in Europe and in the United States, but has become the leading cause of blindness in Taiwan[31].
- Myopia accounted for 5% of the causes for blindness of people aged 20 to 59 years in Denmark[32].
- 2% of Americans have pathologic myopia[33].

As the rate of myopic people is still increasing significantly today, the problem of resulting blindness can also be expected to rise further.

By the way: My motivation in writing this book is to inform people of this risk.

> **It is not the intention to frighten you with these data, but to trigger you to do your very best to avoid these potential consequences of higher grades of myopia.**
> **Most of the readers of this book will never be affected by the potential risks of myopia, but I am very glad if some of the readers can avoid or reduce permanent eye damage by following advice given in this book.**

A basic effect of high myopia is that the posterior sclera shows substantial thinning by the elongation of the eye. The normal sclera has a thickness of about 1.35 mm on the back of the eye. A highly myopic eye has a typically reduced thickness of the sclera of about 0.2 to 0.5 mm [6] and a thinned choroid as well. It is, however, still an open question, whether the thinning of the sclera is due to:
- An **optically** regulated mechanism,
- An excessive **mechanical** stretching force,
- A **defective connective tissue** of the sclera.

Section 3 contains more information about these issues.

Basic reasons of most of the serious consequences of myopia are vitreochorioretinal dystrophies, i.e. **disturbed structures** of the layers of vitreous, choroid, and retina. It was found that 52.6% of people with weak myopia and 86.4% of people with high myopia had this disorder[34].

Some basic pathological consequences of high myopia can be[5, 35]:
- **Retinal detachment:**

    There is an elevated risk for retinal detachment, i.e. the retina is separated from the choroid and the sclera, often accompanied with tearing of the retina. Retinal lattice degeneration and retinal breaks are often early signs of later retinal detachment[36]. Some publications, however, are contradictory with respect to an increasing risk with the degree of myopia. Some people are saying that there is an increased risk for myopes, which is, however, not dependant on the degree of myopia[8]. Other sources state a risk for retinal detachment e.g. for 0 D to – 4.75 D a risk of 1/6662, for – 5.00 D to – 9.75 D a risk of 1/1,335, and for more than – 10.00 D a risk of 1/148[5]. In other words, an additional risk factor of 3 for low myopia, and up to 300 for high myopia[37] was reported.

- **Vitreous liquefaction and detachment:**

The vitreous body between lens and retina consists of 98% water and 2% fibers of collagen. It gradually becomes liquefied with age, and especially in myopic eyes[36, 38]. This is due to a loss in the regular arrangement of the fibers. In early stages, small objects can be seen when looking at bright and uniform backgrounds (called fleeting flies, or floaters). In later stages, the vitreous body can collapse and lose its connection to the retina. This separation is connected with the risk of retinal detachment and corresponding damage of the retina. Immediate medical examination is necessary if symptoms like flashing lights or a rain of soot can be seen. No treatment is available for vitreous detachment by itself. About 6% of "normal" people between age 54 to 65 and 65% of the people between age 65 to 85 have a vitreous detachment. The higher rate of vitreous detachment of myopic people is sometimes explained by the larger volume, which has to be filled by the vitreous body.

It was concluded that the liquefaction is caused by the functional disorder of the blood-retinal barrier in myopia[39].

- **Various Myopic maculopathies:**

There can be a thinning of the choroid and the retina and a **loss of capillary vessels** in eyes with high myopia[2] and as a consequence an atrophic **loss of retinal cells** (i.e. cells are dying), resulting in a loss of vision in this area[12] (visual field defect).

In pathological myopia the **death of retina cells (apoptosis)** can occur due to various biochemical processes, e.g. related to oxidative events (see section 3.12).

Furthermore, there can be **bleedings** in the retina and the choroid, leading to a partial loss of vision[12].

Choroidal neovascularization (CNV) / myopic macular degeneration is also a consequence of "normal" macular degeneration, and it is caused by **abnormal blood vessels that grow** under the center of the retina. It generally occurs among people over 30 and can result in a progressive loss of vision. The worldwide incidence of CNV due to pathologic myopia is estimated to be 50,000 new cases per year excluding Asia, where the rate may be even greater due to a higher prevalence of pathologic myopia[40] (see section 3.17 about a treatment for CNV).

Myopic macular degeneration is said to be the seventh greatest cause of blindness of adults in Europe and the USA, and has become the leading cause of blindness in Taiwan[31].

- **Posterior Staphyloma:**

    In pathologic myopia there can be a herniation-like deformation ("out-pouching") of a thinned sclera, which can hardly be corrected with lenses. It also leads to other complications.

- **Glaucoma:**

    The increased pressure within the eye that often accompanies myopia (see section 3.6.2), can damage the optic nerve. The results of older techniques for measuring the intraocular pressure of myopes were wrong: even when the pressure was high, the softer myopic tissue was interfering with the measuring process in a way that the result was a normal, i.e. lower pressure than in reality. Later a measurement called "applanation tonometry" was invented. This technique is claimed to be independent from the rigidity of the sclera. It is said that **open-angle glaucoma** occurs twice as often with the myopic eye as with the normal eye[5].

- **Cataract:**

    The lens is loses its transparency. It is reported that myopia induces an earlier onset of cataracts. Statistical data are lacking[37].

Soft contact lenses, and the complications of refractive surgery, can lead to infections, which may cause blindness[37].

Each myopic person is strongly advised to see an ophthalmologist at the slightest sign of visual abnormalities, and people with high grade of myopia should have the background of their eyes checked regularly!

Notes:

- *In many cases, a general systemic problem may cause one of these diseases, and also myopia. This then explains the noted association, without implying that myopia is the cause of the disease. In these cases the therapy should focus more on the systemic problem, and not primarily on the optical myopia problem only (which should be positively influenced by the therapy as well).*

- *As progressive, pathological myopia is based on defects of the connective tissue, the connective tissue related coronary problem mitral valve prolapse (MVP) might have an increased probability, which makes preemptive measures still more appropriate, as stated by Yeo et al.[41]: "Although most patients with MVP are asymptomatic or have minor symptoms, it is associated with significant morbidity."*

1.8 Myopia and Age

Myopia may be categorized according to the age of onset:[5]

- **Congenital myopia** exists already at birth and stays through the whole life. 1-2% of the population is in this category.

- **Youth-onset myopia** starts between ages 5 and 20. In the USA about 20% of the population is affected by this category.

- **Early adult-onset myopia** starts between ages 20 and 40. About 8% of the population is affected by this category.

- **Late adult-onset myopia** starts after age 40.

In general, the earlier the myopia appears, the higher are the D values it will reach[5]. But on the other hand, as stated by Goldschmidt[42] "myopia progression can stop at any time transiently or permanently". This statement, based on experience of optometrists and ophthalmologists, shows how shaky the overall knowledge of myopia development still is.

Independent of myopia, it was found that "There was a **significant correlation of scleral stiffness with age** ..."[43], which gives some hope to myopic people, because the increasing rigidity results in less axial growth or even in a standstill of growth.

1.9 Accommodation and Age

The average power of accommodation, of which the eye is capable, depends on age:

10 years:	about 12 D, i.e. an emmetropic person can see clearly from infinity to 0.08 meter
30 years:	about 8 D, i.e. an emmetropic person can see clearly from infinity to 0.13 meter
50 years:	about 2.5 D, i.e. an emmetropic person can see clearly from infinity to 0.4 meter
60 years:	about 0.6 D, i.e. an emmetropic person can see clearly from infinity to 1.7 meter

D stands for diopters. This dimension equals to the reciprocal value of the focal distance of a lens (see section 1.11).

This process of a diminishing of accommodation is called **presbyopia**.

Consequently, almost everybody has to wear glasses or contact lenses during a more or less extended period in life. An older person with moderate myopia can often read by simply taking the glasses off. And for wearers of contact lenses there is the chance to wear bifocal contact lenses. This is a reason to avoid corrective surgery.

The graphical presentation of this mechanism is shown in Figure 4.

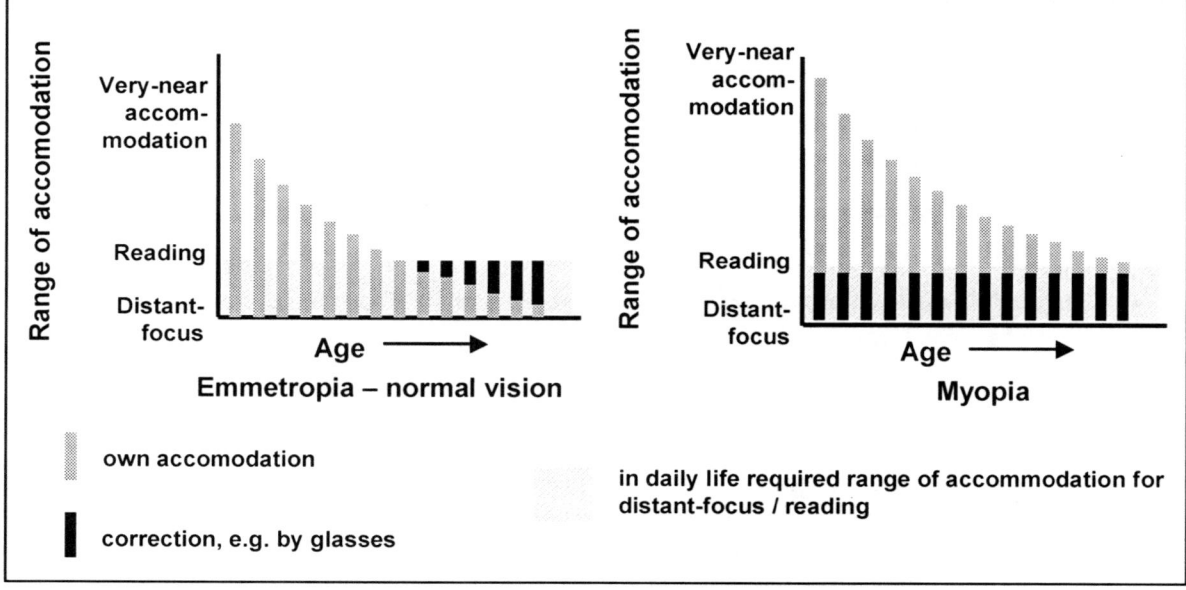

Figure 4 The change of the accommodation amplitude with age

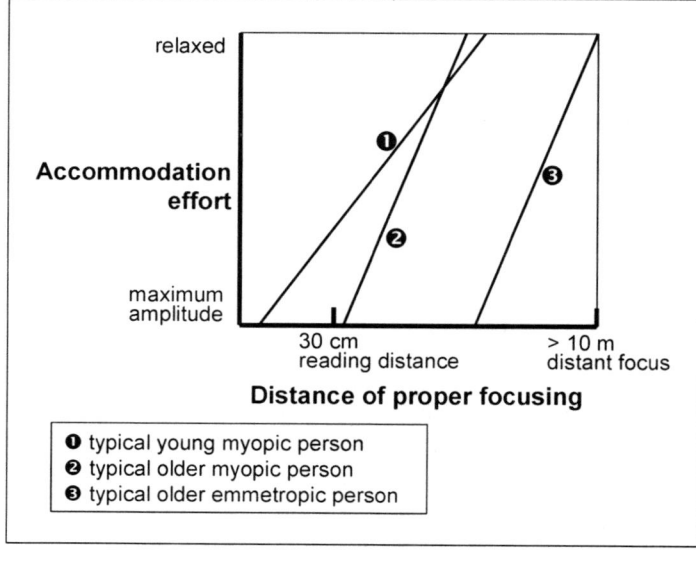

Figure 5 The accommodation effort with respect to age and distance

Figure 5 is a somehow different representation of the relation between the accommodation effort and the distance for which proper focusing can be achieved with increasing age. Even emmetropic persons need glasses to cover the range from reading distance to distant focus. Their glasses have to take care of the reading distance, the myopes's have to take care of the long distance.

It has been claimed that only very few non-myopic people over 60 are still able to accommodate, and it was concluded from research that a hotter climate accelerated the decrease in accommodative power[15].

Note:
Quite frequently older people report that their myopia is decreasing, attributing this to presbyopia. The reason, however, might be as well a beginning of diabetes, which changes the refractive power of the lens (see section 3.16.1).

1.10 Some more Age Related Geometrical Changes of the Eye

The anterior chamber decreases after the age of 20 because the lens is thickening. There appear to, be, however, variations depending on ethnicity. Whether this thickening is happening for men and women in the same way is disputed[15].

A study[44] with non-myopic children between age 6 and age 16 in Tibet showed:

- A decrease of the lens power by 2.59 D
- An increase of the anterior and the posterior radii of the lens
- An increase in vitreous chamber depth (by 0.69 mm).

It was concluded in this study by Garner et al.[44], "that the balance between the decrease in crystalline lens power and the increase in vitreous length is the major factor in maintaining the tendency to emmetropia in these children."

Note:
According to these results a disturbance in the described reduction of the lens power might already contribute to the appearing of myopia.

1.11 The Refraction

To determine if myopia exists, people have to see an optometrist or an ophthalmologist. It is generally recommended, especially for children,[6, 11] that any remaining accommodation (i.e. stress of the ciliary muscle) is eliminated as much as possible before doing the test. **Cycloplegic agents** can achieve this, i.e. by the application of eye drops, which relax the ciliary muscle. If this relaxing of the ciliary muscle is not done, pseudomyopia may still exist. In reality, however, hardly any practitioner appears to use these cycloplegic agents – maybe because it takes too much time until the agents work (about 30 minutes).

A comparison between non-cycloplegic and cycloplegic autorefraction showed that non-cycloplegic measurements generally result in too high minus diopters. The error is largest for hyperopes and smaller for myopes, but still -0.41(+/- 0.46D) for myopia of -2.00 D or more[45]. So, by not using the drops, they often can sell more glasses.

Notes:

- *According to other results and corresponding theories there is also a substantial accommodation hysteresis besides the one caused by the ciliary muscle and other ocular muscles, i.e. a hysteresis (i.e. a time lag for getting back to the original shape) of the ocular shape (see section 3.6.5) and even of the lens (see section 3.6.4). Cycloplegic agents **cannot eliminate all these hysteresis (pseudomyopia) effects**.*

- *The omission of cycloplegic agents can contribute to the progression of myopia because the prescribed glasses can be too strong, which causes a further progression of myopia (see section 3.2 and 3.3).*

- *Another potential source of errors is a chart for reading, which is badly illuminated: In this case, hidden **night myopia** may lead to an over-correction (see section 1.4.1).*

- *Psychological stress can have an immediate impact on refraction (section 3.13). Stress could occur in school, or during an eye examination. If glasses are prescribed as a result, they in turn can initiate myopia that didn't previously exist. The Bates method (section 3.2.2.1) focuses on this issue.*

- *As it is shown in the following sections, this **over-correction can induce a further increase of "real"** axial myopia.*

In 95% of the cases the results can be reproduced within 0.5 D - assuming there is no effect of pseudomyopia or hysteresis of accommodation at all. These hysteresis effects can make refraction difficult, and can finally contribute to a permanent **"lens-induced" progression** of myopia (see section 3.3).

In different countries, and by different authors different units are used to describe the amount of myopia and loss of visual acuity:

- **Diopter**, abbreviated **D**: The refractive power of a lens (to correct the myopia) can be expressed by the reciprocal value of the focal distance: -1 D corresponds with a focal distance of 1 m. People with myopia of -1.0 D can see still clearly at a distance of 1 m (at -2.0 D the distance is 0.5 m). The refractive power of the prescribed glasses is given in D with a minus in front.

- **Snellen chart**: This standard is more than 100 years old. 20/20 means that you can see at a distance of 20 feet what a "normal" person can see from a distance of 20 feet. 20/40 means that you can see at a distance of 20 feet what a "normal" person can see from a distance of 40 feet, and so on. Standard distance for myopia tests is 5 to 6 m. 20/40 is required in most States of the US to pass the Driver's License Test.

- **Decimal quotients:** In some countries the basic principle of the Snellen chart is used - the quotient of the distance where the patient can read to the distance where "normal" people can read. The result is given, however, in decimal units. A vision of 1.0 corresponds therefore to the visual acuity of a "normal" person. Some people, especially kids can have better resolutions up to a vision of about 2.0. Sometimes this decimal number is given in %, i.e. a visus of 1.0 corresponds to 100%.
- **Visual acuity or visual efficiency:** Sometimes another conversion from the Snellen chart numbers to percent is used. The table below contains the corresponding information.
- **Angle-resolution:** The visual acuity of the "normal" person (i.e. vision 20/20 or 1.0) corresponds with an angle-resolution of rays, which are incident on the eye, of 1 minute.

Besides plain spherical myopia, often **astigmatism** is diagnosed: This is the contribution of non-spherical irregularities of the eye, which can be compensated by added cylindrical lens-components. The power of these cylindrical lenses is given in D, too (same definition as above). The prescription will give additionally the circular direction of the astigmatism in degrees. Combined spherical and cylindrical glasses are called toric.

The "best spherical fit" for toric glasses (i.e. for eyes with astigmatism) can be roughly estimated as: Spherical D + ½ · astigmatism D

Visual acuity is determined by several parameters, of which the D figure or its equivalent is one. Other factors include astigmatism. A very rough cross-reference is shown in Table 1[46, 47]:

Diopter D	Snellen chart, 20/ ...	Decimal	Visual acuity / efficiency[48]
- 0.5	20/25 to 20/30	0.8 to 0.7	95% to 90%
- 1.0	20/30 to 20/50	0.7 to 0.4	90% to 75%
- 3.0	20/300	0.07	15%
- 4.0	20/400	0.05	10%

Table 1 Some different methods to measure visual acuity

If you want to **keep track on your myopia by yourself you can use Snellen Charts**, which can be downloaded from the Internet and printed[48], or which can be displayed and used directly on your computer monitor[49].

Very frequent visits to an optometrist for measurement of refraction bears the risk of a subsequent overcorrection, if the optometrist is not very well informed about myopia prevention and all the recent research results.

2 What Causes Myopia in General?

Chapter 3 will summarize the research. This chapter gives an overview of some of the main hypotheses concerning the development of myopia.

2.1 Is Myopia Inherited?

In the past, the official medical view considered myopia to be simply inherited.

No question, heredity plays a key role[50, 51] – everybody is determined by heredity and environment. In the same way, however, as there are talents of various levels, which can be compensated for to a great extent by personal energy, hard work, and methodology, all the possibilities should be tried to influence the "chemical factory" of the body by optimizing external parameters, e.g. by appropriate nutrition and adequate behavior.

Fact is,

- Myopia is **dramatically increasing** compared to the past[1, 6, 52, 53], and many children are becoming progressively myopic with **none of the parents or grandparents being myopic**, and even populations like Eskimos, where myopia was extremely rare before, are getting highly myopic.
- Myopia can be easily **created artificially** in experiments with animals[54].
- Myopia occurs in different frequencies in **different regions of a country**[55].
- Myopic parents have more often myopic children[56]: if both **parents are myopic**, the risk for the children to become myopic is sevenfold.

Two arguments about this controversy:

- Goldschmidt states[57], " Twin studies indicate a strong genetic influence and a weak environmental impact, while extreme myopia prevalences among selected population groups (university students) point to the opposite."
- Morgan states[58], "... evidence for low prevalences of myopia in Indians growing up in India, while Indians in Singapore have much higher prevalence rates."

The conclusion is that myopia itself is not inherited. Rather, biochemistry is, and it reacts differently to various environments.

As Lyhne et al.[59], who did research with twins expressed very well:

> "... results indicate a high heritability for ocular refraction and its determiners and thus suggest that environmental impact on refraction is not significant. However, the epidemiological association between educational length (near work) and myopia, the evidence on increasing myopia prevalence within a few generations, and the theory of gene-environment interaction imply that **some individuals might be genetically liable to develop myopia if exposed to certain environmental factors**".

A reader of this Myopia Manual expressed another likely possibility with respect to the inheriting of myopia: "The parents probably become myopic because they live in similar conditions as their offspring."[60]

Another point of view stated by Morgan[58]: "Thus, parents with longer than average eyes would tend to have children with longer than average eyes ... however, if average eye size is increasing due to environmental effects, a high proportion of children would become myopic."

In principle almost all the facts about myopia that will be presented in the next sections are either connected with the way of living of people, or with biochemical processes. Largely, however not completely, these biochemical processes are determined by heredity.

A few authors have reported a connection of few specific chromosomes with myopia[61], but contradiction with other results followed immediately[62, 63]. One expert states: Future genetic therapies of myopia are highly unlikely, because it appears that numerous genes are having an impact on myopia[56].

On the other hand, many papers show the fact that myopia often runs "in the family"[64, 65], and that myopia is very clearly more common in some populations than in others (see section 3.1).

By the way: Influences like nutrition during pregnancy have a high congenital impact on the child's health. And in other cases the "individual biochemical factory" is built very early in life and cannot be changed later. An example is the copper metabolism - which might have an impact on myopia[66, 67].

Basically any biochemical heritage can become effective via one of these two alternatives:

- Via a biochemical process which cannot be modified, and whose results cannot be modified either.

- Via a biochemical process which can be modified, or whose results can be modified. An example: People suffering from favism, an enzyme defect (a variant of G6PD deficiency) which leads to acute anemia after eating e.g. fava beans. Simple advice after somebody is diagnosed with this deficiency: Do not eat these beans. The literature gives further examples of "Nutritional Regulation of Gene Expression[68]".

It is my aim to offer assistance in the second case and to motivate people not to become fatalistic. Further, biochemistry is not in itself good or bad: An effect that has a disadvantage in one respect, can have an advantage in another respect (e.g. the G6PD deficiency mentioned above is said to offer protection against Malaria).

A simple analogy: If the engine of a car is prone to overheating through a design fault, the damage can be avoided in most cases by carefully watching the cooling water level, selecting top grade motor oil, and avoiding mechanical overload. Why not apply the same strategy to the human body, instead of hiding behind the word heredity?

Some facts, which can contribute to the answering of the question whether myopia is inherited can be found in section 3.1 ("Distribution of Myopia by Region, Age, Gender and Ethnicity").

2.2 Connective Tissue Disorders

In the case of connective tissue disorders, the structure of components of the myopic eye shows significant deficits. These structural deficits can have various origins:

- Clearly inherited (like in case of the Marfan syndrome).
- Appearing as a form of genetic variation, which happened after birth.
- An acquired disorder, e.g. caused by interactions of the immune system, or by inappropriate nutrition, or by other environmental or behavioral circumstances.

An example for the impact of the connective tissue on the highly myopic eye by Chang et al.[69]: "... that the fiber bundles of highly myopic eye were of thinner lamellar arrangement, with looser collagen matrix distribution and decreased collagen fiber diameter."

Section 3.3.3 describes some results with respect to the connective tissue.

2.3 Active Growth by Imaging Effects

After birth, the eye is too short for an optically correct focus. During growth, the eye expands by some feedback mechanisms to the proper length. This process is called **emmetropization**[70]. Animal experiments have investigated this process in detail, but there are still a lot of open questions about what goes wrong when some people become myopic, when others in the same environment don't. This active growth mechanism will be described in more detail in section 3.3.

2.4 Mechanical Effects

There is quite general agreement that myopia has some connection with accommodation. One explanations is the influence of the strain of the various muscles which are involved when doing near work – not just only the **ciliary muscle** for accommodation, but also various **extraocular muscles** which are controlling the position of the axis of the eye (see section 3.6).

2.5 General Overview of the Causes of Myopia

A very schematic overview of possible paths to myopia is shown in Figure 6. Each of these possibilities could be greatly expanded.

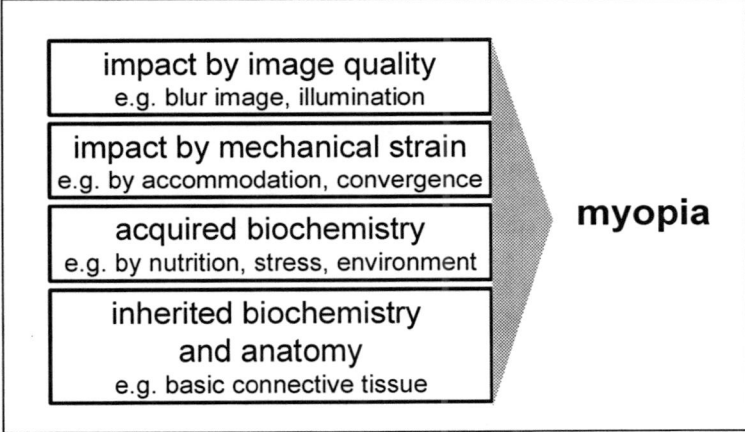

Figure 6 The potential paths to myopia

From the fact that under the same external conditions (i.e. near work, illumination etc.) not everybody gets myopic it can be concluded that the influence of the personal biochemistry / personal anatomy plays a deciding role.

3 Myopia – Observations and Experimental Results

This section contains:

- Environmental, behavioral or biochemical parameters found to be connected with myopia
- Therapies that have been proposed to prevent myopia or progression of myopia.

As there are sometimes interactions between these individual issues, a certain amount of repetition cannot be avoided.

Some observations and conclusions of the individual authors appear to be rather controversial. If we are to accept their observations as accurate, we must conclude that either

- There is a connecting logic in the background which has yet to be revealed, or
- There are various independent mechanisms, which have myopia as the common result.

3.1 Distribution of Myopia by Region, Age, Gender and Ethnicity

We can draw conclusions about the impact of different lifestyles, different environment, different nutrition, and different genetic heredity by comparing the variation in rates of myopia according to age in different regions. Some results are:

- An evaluation of statistical data for reported blindness due to malignant myopia in different states of the USA was done by compiling a chart with the rate of myopia per state, and distance to seacoast, annual hours of sunshine and the nutritional concentration of calcium, fluoride and selenium in each state. The results were:[55]
  - less **sunshine**,
  - less **calcium**,
  - less **fluoride**,
  - less **selenium** and
  - closer to a **seacoast**

  resulted in a higher probability of malignant myopia.
- Myopia rates are higher in urban than in rural areas[71, 72, 73].

  Note:
  Of course, farmers don't have much time to read.

- The frequency of myopia at children in various countries is[74]:
  - Germany - 10%,
  - Taiwan, South Korea - 70%,
  - Japan - 95%.

- Myopia recently worsened as a problem, as stated by Lin et al.[75]: "In Taiwan, myopia was not a problem some 50 years ago"; today about 15% of the population have over - 7.0 D.

- 50 to 60 % of the Japanese are said to be myopic, but only 2 % of the people in South America are myopic[76]. The author of this publication hints at a substantial difference with respect to spontaneity between these two populations.

- The incidence of myopia in Japan was increasing from 15% in 1920 to 36% in 1940 to between 50 and 60% in 1985[76].

- Sherpa and Tibetan children in Nepal have the same ancestry and genetic history, but the prevalence of myopia is 2.7% for Sherpa children and 21.7% for Tibetan children[77]. This difference was attributed to more rigorous schooling and higher advanced technology in Tibet.

  Note:
  Generally more rigorous schooling and higher advanced technology are going hand in hand with a change in nutrition and increased mental stress. For the impact of nutrition on myopia see section 3.16, for the impact of stress see section 3.13.1.

- Results of a study on Eskimos[78] are shown in Table 2.

Age	% Myopic
Over 50	0%
41 to 50	Less than 5%
31 to 40	23%
26 to 30	43%
21 to 25	88%

Table 2 Percentage of myopes among Eskimos

- Data about the degree of myopia in various populations[79] are shown in Table 3.

Population		Low myopia -1.00 to -5.00 D	High myopia -5.10 to -10.00 D	Extreme myopia more than -10.00 D
Asia, age 5 to 65[80]	Chinese	41%	14.7%	0.8%
	Malays	37.8%	8.5%	3.0%
	Indians	34.3%	7.7%	0.9%
USA, age 4 to 74[79]		43%	3.2%	0.2%
North America, Sioux Indians, age 3 to adult[81]		32.4%	4.1%	

Table 3 Percentage of myopes among various populations

- A study from 2001[82], giving the percentage of myopic males (at least -0.5 D) between age 16 and 25 in Singapore:

82.2 % Chinese

68.7% Indians

65.0% Malays

- Another statistic from USA (children, age 5-17 years)[83] is shown in Table 4.

Ethnicity	Myopes (shortsighted)	Hyperopes (farsighted)
Asians	18,5%	6,3%
Hispanics	13,2%	12,7%
Whites	4,4%	19,3%
African Americans	6,6%	6,4%

Table 4 Percentage of myopes among various populations in the USA

- Typical childhood progression rates were found to be between – 0.2 D and – 0.6 D in Europe and USA, and between – 0.5 D and – 0.8 D in Japan[84].
- In spite of similar myopia rates of Malays and Chinese, the age dependent progression profile appears to be rather different[85].

- Results from Singapore and Hong Kong show that myopia is 1.5 to 2.5 times more prevalent among adult Chinese than in corresponding European-derived populations, and that women have significantly higher myopia rates than men[86, 87].

  Moreover, as stated by Choo[88], "...severity of myopia rises by about 1.5 D per year in Singapore children, compared with 0.5 D per year in US children."

- The higher rate of female myopes is confirmed by results about Greek students: 46% female students, and 29.7% male students are myopic[89].

3.2 Accommodation and Near Work

In principle, results and experiences about accommodation (that is, changes in lens shape for near work) are related to artificially negative-lens-induced myopia, and myopia which was induced by forcing the eye to permanent near focus (see section 3.3).

3.2.1 Experiences and Results

3.2.1.1 General Experiences and Results

In general the influence of near work alone is not easy to isolate, as extensive near work means extensive in-door work (often at **low levels of illumination**, see section 3.7.2), which is mostly connected with a **potential lack of vitamin D** because of a lack of exposure to sunlight (see section 3.16.3). Moreover, children who are interested very much in reading often have a **more introverted personality** (see section 3.13.2) and are less interested in **physical activities** (see section 4.2.3.8 on the impact on the blood sugar level).

There are numerous indications that people, who are doing extensive near work, i.e., who accommodate extensively, are more often myopic. Some observations are:

- The appearance of myopia at people in USA and Greenland coincides with the **introduction of universal schooling**,[90] and the rate of myopia of school children in Berlin depended very strongly on the **level of the school** they visited: the more advanced the type of school, the higher the rate of myopia. Rates were between 55 and 35%[91].

- The progression of myopia of school kids is **slower during summer holidays**[92, 93, 94].

- Comparisons between myopia rates in 1882 and 1964 showed that the rate is very different for **individual professions**[52] (students in the 30% range, unskilled workers in the 2 to 3% range): While the total rate of myopia was increasing, the myopia rate for all the individual professions except unskilled work was decreasing. Explanation: The overall increase in myopia, according to these results, can be largely attributed to a changed ratio of job distributions from unskilled work towards professional and office work.

Highly elevated rates of myopia were found for craftspeople of various professions, who have to do extensive near work, e.g. for typesetters (in year 1930[95]), tailoring (in the years 1953[96] and 1961[97]). Up to 77% of the persons in these professions were found to be myopic.

- A test with monkeys (already in 1961)[98], whose **visual space was restricted** to an average of fifteen inches distance, showed that all of them developed some myopia.

- There are indications that extended accommodation can create a **chronic spasm of the ciliary muscle**, and experiments on monkeys showed that this stretching will begin after spasms for 2 to 4 months so spastic myopia and axial length myopia exist at the same time[99].

Note:
A permanent load can damage any muscle, not only the ocular muscles[100, 101].

- A study of university students showed a strong relationship between reading and other near work with myopia was found, however no relationship between myopia and working on **video display terminals** (VDT) or watching TV[102]. Watching TV at close distance however was promoting myopia[103, 104].

Note:
These results appear to be contradictory. As will be shown in section 3.3 the effect of VDTs and TVs can be expected to depend largely on the quality of the displayed images. Due to the limited image resolution of TVs and VDTs (LCD screens are better) a watching of these screens from near distance will create a blur image on the retina, with the potential consequences as described in section 3.3.

- For Chinese schoolchildren a correlation of myopia with the **reading** of books was found[105], in Finland a relation between myopia progression and time spent on **reading/close** work and on **reading distance** was found[106].

- It was measured (with partial coherence interferometry) that **the eye generally elongates during accommodation**, with this explanations by Drexler et al.[18]: "... by the accommodation-induced contraction of the ciliary muscle, which results in forward and inward pulling of the choroids, thus decreasing the circumference of the sclera, and leads to an elongation of the axial eye length." and by Shum et al.[19]: "... the elongation was more pronounced in emmetropes than in myopes."

Notes:
- *Is it possible that the difference is a structural weakness of the myopic eye, i.e. that the myopic eye shows some kind of "**memory effect**" or hysteresis after this stretching?*

- *Elongation means stretching of scleral tissue, and stretching of scleral fibroblasts is changing significantly the gene expression of these fibroblasts[107]. This means, **accommodation has a direct impact of the biochemistry** of the eye; this builds a link between mechanical and biochemical models of myopia, and a link between functional and structural models of myopia as well.*

- Rosenfield et al. stated[108] that "...results demonstrate that **myopes are less sensitive to the presence of blur**, and may at least partially explain why previous reports have demonstrated a larger **lag of accommodation**...". On the other hand, the compensatory eye growth in experimental myopia (see section 3.3) was **always in the right direction, even in the presence of very poor images**[109].

- Rosenfield et al. stated[110] that "... findings do **not support** the proposal that the development of myopia in young adults is accompanied by a **reduced accommodative response** during near work."

- Myopic children have less **tonic accommodation (i.e. dark focus accommodation)** than normal, i.e. emmetropic children[111, 112, 113]. After near work, however, the tonic accommodation of myopes increases more than for emmetropes. A large shift in tonic accommodation after near work was found to be typical for periods of acquisition and progression of myopia (some kind of accommodative hysteresis)[114].

- Very contrary to these results is the statement by Kushner[115]: "**Overcorrecting minus lens therapy** for intermittent **exotropia** [see section 3.4] **does not appear to cause myopia.**"

Note:
*A potential explanation is that the risk is **not so much originating from the excess accommodation** caused by the negative lens, but by the **increased esophoria** caused by the negative lenses (esophoria means that the axes of the two eyes are adjusted too much inwards when accommodating). Esophoria is frequently associated with myopia (see section 3.4.1 about phoria).*

- Near work, i.e. accommodation was shown **to increase the temperature** of the anterior segment of the eyeball, and to cause a **hyperproduction of intraocular fluid**[116].

Note:
This hyperproduction of intraocular fluid can increase the intraocular pressure; and an elevated ocular pressure was often found to correlate with myopia (see section 3.6.2). About the impact of the temperature on myopia see section 3.10).

- **Stress** in connection with near work was made responsible for the development of myopia: It was stated that stress induces distant-accommodation, which conflicts with the actual task near-accommodation. This conflict was claimed to cause either a spasm of the ciliary muscle, or phoria[117] (phoria means the exes of the eye are not adjusted appropriately; see section 3.4 about phoria and section 3.13 about mental issues).
- A helpful support of accommodation by **illumination** was found: see section 3.7.2.
- Obviously **near-work induced transient myopia (NITM) is increased by mental stress**: see section 3.13.1.

Summary as worded in one paper by Schaeffel et al.[50]: "The current theory is that lag of accommodation during reading shifts the image plane behind the retina and thereby stimulates retinal neurons to release growth promoting factors that enhance scleral growth. This is thought to be mechanistically equivalent to the effects of a negative lens in animal experiments."

Note:
The word "growth" appears to be somehow misleading, as – at least for higher grades of myopia - there is no growth of structurally intact tissue (which is normally meant by the word growth), but a stretching of degraded tissue (see section 3.3.3).

3.2.1.2 The Strength of Accommodation

Some results about the strength and amplitude of accommodation of myopes are:

- Abbot et al. stated[118]: "A **reduced accommodation** response to negative lens-induced accommodative demand was found in progressing myopes but not in stable myopes." In addition, eyes with myopia were found to have **lower amplitude of accommodation**. Fong stated[119] "Eyes with lower amplitudes of accommodation must use more of their accommodative reserve for near work. Myopia may be an adaptation that develops in eyes with reduced accommodative amplitudes", and **less accurate** accommodation[120]. And a reduced accommodation was speculated to create a blur signal, which might be responsible for development of myopia[63]. Consequently, under-accommodation may precede the development of myopia as clinical data suggest[121].

  In contrast to these results in other experiments it was found by McBrien et al.[122] that "...late onset **myopes having the largest amplitude of accommodation**, followed by early onset myopes, emmetropes, and hyperopes."

  Note:
  *In this respect it is interesting that wearers of glasses accommodate less than emmetropes or wearers of **contact lenses** due to optical reasons[123], but that hard contact lenses were often found to stop progression of myopia (not soft contact lenses).*

- Some positive effects of **pharmaceuticals like atropine** can be at least partly attributed to their attenuating effect on the accommodation (see section 3.17).
- **Chinese people have lower amplitudes of accommodation** than Caucasians[124], and **Chinese have a higher probability of becoming myopic.**

    Notes:
    *From an evolutionary point of view there might be a **linkage between both facts**:*

    - *Without any accommodation the only one way to focus is to adjust the length of the eye as happens in emmetropization (see section 3.3.5), and for dominating near work this means to become myopic.*

    - *Question: is there a rule like "the lower the accommodation before the onset of myopia, the higher the probability and the degree of the myopia that will develop later"?*

For information about the related issue **tonic accommodation** (resting state accommodation) see section 1.4.1.

3.2.1.3 Timing- and Hysteresis- Effects of Accommodation

Some results about the time it takes to accommodate and to recover are:

- Accommodation causes a substantial **hysteresis of the ocular shape:** With normal people, after accommodation, as Walker et al. stated[125], "... ocular shape had become more prolate [i.e. stretched]. This shape remained unchanged after 1 hour of sustained accommodation and then returned to baseline dimensions after 2 h of accommodation ... Ocular shape returned to baseline dimensions after 45 min of accommodative relaxation." (see section 3.6.4).

- Myopes showed reasonable **aftereffect of accommodation**[16], i.e. it took an average of 35 seconds for early-onset myopes and 63 seconds for late-onset myopes until the accommodation of the ciliary muscle was released. Non-myopes, however, showed no myopic aftereffect. It was speculated that this transient pseudomyopia is either the cause or a precursor of permanent myopia[126].

    Additionally, it was shown that during the progression of myopia there is a significant near work after-effect (sometimes called nearwork-induced transient myopia - **NITM**[16]), causing **transient myopia** that still existed 10 seconds and 30 seconds after the near task[127, 128].

    Correspondingly, there is a reduced facility, i.e. a **reduced maximum frequency of accommodation:** "Mean distance facility was significantly lower (9.7 cycles per minute (cpm)) in the myopic group compared with the mean distance facility in the emmetropic group (15.6 cycles per minute). There was no significant difference in the near facilities of the two groups (11.5 cpm in myopes versa 12.9 cpm in emmetropes)."[129]

More recent experiments confirmed the fact that myopic children are showing a significantly larger nearwork-induced transient myopia, but demonstrated additionally that this **nearwork-induced transient myopia was still evident after 3 minutes, which is significantly longer than what was previously reported for adults**[130].

- There is a **time lag of accommodation** for myopes [108, 131]. However, Rosenfield et al. stated[110] that "...stable myopes also exhibited the largest lag of accommodation."
- For children it is generally recommended *(Note: but very often not done)* to do the refraction after **applying a cycloplegic agent.** The residual accommodation, which exists if no cycloplegic agent is used results in **overcorrection of myopia**[45].

Notes:

- *Maybe the hysteresis of the **reshaping of the lens** before accommodation and after accommodation contributes to this effect as well (see section 1.3.3).*

- *This **aftereffect and hysteresis of accommodation can be responsible for a steady progression** of myopia in school kids: If the kid has to change in class permanently and fast between near work and reading from the distant blackboard, the mentioned delay can give the impression that the current glasses are too weak; new, stronger glasses, however, can easily induce additional myopia as described in section 3.3, and these cycles can repeat again and again. The long duration of the aftereffect (which was still evident after 3 minutes) strongly supports this model. **Bifocal glasses** might help in these cases, but care has to be taken when fitting these bifocals (see section 3.2.2).*

- *Maybe the anomalies of myopic accommodation can be explained by a lack of nitric oxide (NO) in the smooth ciliary muscle (see sections 3.12.4 and 4.2.3.4).*

- *Open **question**: What is responsible for the time delay and the aftereffect of the accommodation, a muscular problem, or a hysteresis problem of the flexibility of the lens? It appears to be rather likely that **a muscular problem is a key issue for myopia, i.e. not a consequence, but a reason**.*

3.2.1.4 Is there a Connection between Blur Sensitivity and Accommodation Deficits?

As the detected blur of an image can trigger the accommodation function there is the possibility that the reduced blur sensitivity of myopes is the reason for deviations of the accommodation performance.

The results are, however, contradictory:

- Rosenfield et al. stated[108]: "These results demonstrate that myopes are less sensitive to the presence of blur, and may at least partially explain why previous reports have demonstrated a larger lag of accommodation in this refractive group."
- Schmid et al. stated[132]: "There was no correlation between blur thresholds and refractive error magnitude, refractive error progression over the past year, or contrast sensitivity."

Note:
The reason for the contradictory results must be seen in differences in the setup of the experiments.

3.2.1.5 Accommodation and the Nervous System

The ciliary muscle, which performs the accommodation, is triggered by actions of the sympathetic and the parasympathetic nervous system. The parasympathetic system is responsible for the contraction of the ciliary muscle, and the sympathetic system is responsible for the relaxation.

There are two different hypotheses existing, both supported by numerous papers[16]:

- Myopia is caused by "a deficit in the sympathetic innervation."
- Myopia is caused by "a deficit in the dual [i.e. both sympathetic and parasympathetic] innervation."

The nitric oxide (NO) metabolism plays a role in the functioning of the sympathetic and the parasympathetic nervous system[133]. Results with respect to the connection between NO metabolism and myopia are discussed in section 3.12.6.

3.2.1.6 Summary of Results about Accommodation

Quite a number of people react with myopia when exposed to extensive near work and accommodation, and myopes have an accommodation problem. The open question is still[134], **whether myopia is caused by:**

- **Too much accommodation**, i.e. near work, potentially at a **too short working distance**.
- **Too weak accommodation** (under-accommodation), by which the focus is put at a distance behind the retina – at least temporarily, or **accommodation hysteresis**, i.e. a delayed relaxation of accommodation after near work.
- The impact of the accommodation-caused **temporary stretching of the sclera on the biochemistry of the sclera** (see section 3.6.1)

- **An unbalance of the vergence system** (vergence is the adjustment of the axes of the two eyes to each other according to the distance of the object, see section 3.4)

- **Too weak connective tissue** to cope with the extra stress on this connective tissue during accommodation.

- **An overreaction on the imaging effect, which** accompanies (potentially inadequate) accommodation (see section 3.3).

- **Abnormal physical or physiological properties** of components of the eye.

Apparently, however, near work creates myopia only in connection with other, so far in detail still unknown processes.

Moreover, the reason for myopia can be rather specific, i.e. **different for different people, and different for different grades of myopia.**

3.2.2 Proposed Therapies Based on the Accommodation Issue

3.2.2.1 Relaxing and Exercising

According to the "Bates – method" (Bates was an American ophthalmologist, first introducing his method in 1903) the prescription of glasses, with which a full correction is achieved, is accelerating the progression of myopia[135, 136]. This idea, which was claimed to be based on experience, was promoted at approximately the same time by the German ophthalmologist Wiser (around 1900)[137], and the American ophthalmologist Raphaelson [138] applied a similar approach.

Their basic ideas, still supported today by many publications and classes[139,140, 141, 142]:

- Make regular **relaxing exercises** of the eye: Exercise the ciliary muscle and all the other muscles which move the eyeball – make training to see distant objects in a relaxed way, as Attenborough stated[135] "... **re-learning the art and skill of seeing** ... good sight is the result of a relaxed state of mind and body ... poor sight is the result of tension...". Seeing is actually considered to be strongly connected with the personal mind.

    Notes:
    - This sounds a little bit esoteric, but what is happening in **the mind is having a strong impact on the body's biochemistry.** *Therefore, as the biochemistry has definitely an impact, the modification of the mind must have an impact as well.*

    - However, this is a two way process: biochemistry has an impact on the mind as well.

- Do "bathing in **light**" as an exercise, and make an exercise called **palming**, in which the palms of the hands cover the eyes to use transitions from full darkness to illumination.

- **Avoid full correction** of myopia, and avoid using your glasses as frequently as possible (see section 3.2.2.3). The proponents of this method claim to have very positive results.

  Note:
  The positive results rise the question, whether they can be explained by the mechanical theories mentioned in section 3.6.

Optometrist Bowan[143] recommends therefore the following easy exercise: "After 20 or 30 minutes of close work, look away from your work to something that has printing on it, like a clock, a poster, a sign outside the nearby window – whatever target you have that has a notable detail on it. While staring at the details, numbers or lettering, tighten your toes downward inside your shoes, then progress up your legs, through your torso, fists, arms and neck, tensing all your muscles intently for about five seconds and then quickly release them all at one time ... (The technical explanation for why this works is a basic fact of the brain that when you stimulate the voluntary nervous system as you did, the involuntary system is forcibly relaxed)".

The Bates method actually goes beyond the exercising of accommodation; it is also a method to fight the negative effect of stress on the eye (for more specific reports about the impact of stress on myopia see section 3.13).

The claim of some people that real axial myopia (not pseudomyopia) **can be really reversed** is very strongly rejected by the scientific world, and hardly any hard facts for this claim can be presented.

Notes:
- *Also with respect to the relatively new results presented in the next section it **makes sense to do some exercise** for accommodation and relaxing! There is a difference, however, between concentrated gymnastics of the eye and occasionally relaxing during near work. Additionally, the hysteresis of accommodation offers good reasons for these relaxing exercises (see section 3.2.1 about accommodation, section 3.6.5 about ocular shape and section 3.6.4 about the ocular lens).*

- *A clearly elongated eye cannot be made shorter by the proposed exercises, but there appears to be a good chance to avoid overcorrection and therefore a progression of myopia.*

- *Some followers of the Bates method seem to ignore scientific results instead of **synthesizing their personal experiences with research findings** (as is attempted in this book).*

- *In fact, it looks like the basics of these methods are **confirmed by recent scientific results**, but sometimes the somehow esoteric and rather emotional promotion of some followers is misleading.*

The partly related method **vision training**, also called **vision therapy, visual training, behavioral optometry, developmental optometry**, is described in section 3.8.

3.2.2.2 Biofeedback

The results of biofeedback exercising[144] are said by most authors to be **limited to improving "visual acuity"**, but **with little effect on refraction, i.e. the myopia**[56, 145, 146]. In the light of the results about image quality (see section 3.3) this improved visual acuity might be able to avoid the progression of myopia.

There is a (rather expensive) "Accommotrac® Vision Trainer" on the market[147], which uses the biofeedback principle.

Notes:

- *There is the claim of Accommotrac®: "Blood pressure and heart rate, for example, can be controlled; so can the ciliary body." Not only this statement will get little approval from cardiologists, but also myopia involves far more than the action of the ciliary muscle. Therefore, the use of this device is questionable.*

- *The fact that biofeedback appears to improve visual acuity, but not refraction reminds of computer software, with which the sharpness and the contrast of copies of an images can be improved, but – naturally – the "real" picture cannot be improved. How about if biofeedback works somehow similar? Evaluation of the retinal image is improved, but the retinal image itself stays as before (i.e. no change in the refraction).*

3.2.2.3 Undercorrection for Near Work, Plus-, Bifocal- and Progressive-Glasses

For information about **permanent** undercorrection see section 3.2.2.8.

The principle of this treatment is to avoid full correction, i.e. to **avoid full accommodation** for (extensive) near work – it was already mentioned in section 1.3.2 that the **eye elongates during accommodation, which corresponds with axial myopia**.

The results about **emmetropization** lead to the conclusion by Wildsoet[148] that "**full refractive correction of myopia will lead to accelerated progression**" Fitting lenses with zero power in front of myopic eyes, however, led to a recovery from myopia, whereas the application of corrective glasses, (like the fitting of glasses which is usually done!) prevented the recovery from myopia[149] (see also section 3.3.5 about emmetropization).

This principle of **undercorrection for near work** was found to result in a reduction of the progression of myopia, or even to result in a reduction of myopia[150, 151, 134, 152, 153, 154, 155]. In other studies and papers, however, the positive results could not always be confirmed[13], [134, 156, 157, 158], or showed a positive effect for the first year of the treatment only[159].

In detail Morgan stated[58]: "The COMET study reported that the progressive addition lenses were **more effective with children with lower myopia**, lower accommodative responses and closer reading distances, and **less effective with children with higher myopia**, better accommodative responses and longer reading distances."

Note:
*This matches with my suspicion that cases of **lower myopia are caused primarily by an "over-emmetropization" by intensive near work** (see section 3.3.5), but that cases of **higher myopia are caused primarily by defects of the connective tissue** (see section 3.21 for corresponding conclusions about the treatment). Clearly, both effects will be frequently or even mostly combined.*

The following methods for undercorrection are used:

- Usage of **glasses with less power** for extensive near work

- Usage of **bifocal glasses** (the top part of the glasses is adjusted for distant vision, the bottom part is adjusted for near work and has less power, i.e. some plus added

- Usage of **progressive glasses** (similar as bifocal glasses, but there is a step-less transition between the part for distant vision and the part for near vision)

- Usage of **plus glasses** for extensive near work, **together with contact lenses**, which are fitted for distant vision. Similarly, **non-myopic people** can use the **plus glasses for near work for prevention of myopia**.

    Plus glasses have a prismatic effect as well, which has an impact on the vergence mechanism[160], i.e. they are **reducing esophoria**[161] (vergence is the adjustment of the axes of the two eyes for proper focusing at the respective distance, esophoria is a fault in this adjustment, i.e. the axes are too much inwards; for details see section 3.4).

Common additions for near work are **between + 1.0 D and + 2.0 D**.

Consequently, for people who are wearing low power glasses the recommendation is to take them off for extensive near work. For kids who are **not myopic yet**, but might be at risk, there are recommendations to **use plus glasses** for extensive near work, as Weale stated[15]: "...several studies suggest that the degree and **prevalence and early onset of myopia can be reduced worldwide by the early provision of reading glasses**. They are to be viewed less as corrections than as bars to accommodative excess. The obstacles to the implementation of the requisite health policy are cultural rather than scientific or economic."

The **reported contradictory results** could be based on these reasons:

- The **detailed process** of the fitting of plus glasses or plus additions was different in the various studies. The use of cycloplegia (i.e. agents to relax the ciliary muscle) and autorefraction (i.e. automatic measurement of the refraction), e.g., can make a difference by avoiding overcorrection.

- The myopia of the involved persons was based on **different biochemical or mechanical/anatomic processes.**

    One study, e.g., reports about significantly larger effects of progressive lenses at lower accommodative responses at near, and with lower myopia[159].

    Note:
    This decreased effect of progressive lenses for higher myopia can be explained by the conclusion that higher myopia is less determined by optical effects, and is more determined by an overall weaker connective tissue. Correspondingly, in these cases a strong emphasis should be put on systemic improvements, e.g. by nutrition (see section 4).

Potentially **negative consequences of permanent (!) undercorrection** are discussed in section 3.2.2.8.

At a first look **bifocal (or progressive) glasses** appear to be an easy solution. Various studies, however, gave mixed results[162, 163]. Grosvenor et al. stated [164]: "...some showing myopia control with bifocals and some not ... there is evidence that bifocals slow myopia progression in children with nearpoint **esophoria**, but not in children with **exophoria** at near [esophoria and exophoria are faulty adjustments of the axes of the two eyes for short distance – at esophoria the axes are too much inwards, at exophoria they are too much outwards, see section 3.4 for details]." Another trial showed that bifocals slowed the progression of esophoric myopes in the **first 24 months only**, but later on myopia progressed at a similar rate as for children with single-vision glasses; the previously achieved difference in the degree of myopia was maintained, however.[165]

Note:
Maybe the "mixed results" mentioned above are caused mainly by the difficulties to fit the "right" bifocal or progressive glasses, take care of the very individual AC/C ratio (see sections 3.4.2 and 3.4.3) as well.

Special care has to be taken when **fitting bifocals** to achieve the undercorrection for near work[166]:

- The ratio of action between accommodation (A) and convergence (C), called the **AC/A ratio** can be upset in a negative way (see also section 3.4) – especially if just one power (e.g. +1.50 D) is added (see also section 3.4.2).

- When using progressive bifocals the kids may **look through the wrong part** of the glasses without knowing it, i.e. to look at short distance through the upper part, which is fully correcting for distant vision. This cannot happen with presbyopes for which bifocals are normally fitted, because they can see clear through the right part anyway.

- Special attention has to be paid to the setting of the **bifocal height**. According to their reading habits, the kids need bifocals set at the pupil, not level with the eyelashes as for adults.

> **Overall, the use of plus glasses** (for non-myopes) **or plus additions** (for myopes) **for extensive near work offers an easy first step to prevent further progression of shortsightedness, or to prevent shortsightedness at all.**
>
> And still more logical, you must keep a proper distance for reading – the more distant the paper the better! A larger distance has the same effect as a plus addition (not counting the vergence effects which will be discussed in section 3.4)!

Notes:

- *Maybe the claimed positive effect of plus glasses can be attributed primarily to the treatment of the esophoria (which is often associated with myopia, see section 3.4.1), and less to the reduction of load for the ciliary muscle by the accommodation.*

- ***Correspondingly, negative lenses and overcorrection with negative lenses increase esophoria***[115].

- *According to the generally and scientifically agreed fact of* ***emmetropization*** *(section 3.3.5),* ***accommodation*** *(section 3.2), accommodation induced* ***elevated IOP*** *(section 3.6.2) and artificially* ***negative lens induced myopia*** *(section 3.3) the positive effect of adding of plus power for near work is convincing.*

- *As there were no negative results published for the use of simply adding some plus power for extensive near work, the recommendation should be:* ***Try it!***

- *Astonishingly,* ***there is a lot of discussion about plus glasses and bifocals, but hardly anyone is talking about keeping a proper (i.e. not too near) reading distance!*** *Doing near work with a larger distance, however, is equivalent with plus glasses and a shorter distance (not mentioning the potentially disturbing vergence effect of a shorter distance, and the prismatic effect of plus glasses, see section 3.4).*

- *Nevertheless, it is* ***hardly likely that optical means like this undercorrection for near work alone are enough to fight pathological or progressive myopia.*** *It has to be supported by following the other recommendations, too (see section 4.8).*

For **older people** there is another, additional mechanism of plus glasses / plus additions: With the beginning of **presbyopia** the lens loses flexibility, it "freezes" its shape (see section 1.4.3). A lens, which is mostly in the accommodated shape, stays in this shape even when the ciliary muscle is relaxed, resulting in the symptoms of myopia. As a consequence plus glasses / plus additions for near work should be helpful for these people, too, because they keep the lens in a more "far-distance-shape". On the other hand, if all the accommodation efforts are taken off from the lens, it is loses its flexibility still earlier.

Moreover, a device called "**Myopter**", which is designed to eliminate the accommodative effort, is sold[167].

3.2.2.4 Intermittent, Short Term Wearing of Plus Glasses

I have shown evidence that plus lenses help through undercorrection during near work. There are also very strong indications that intermittent, short term use is also effective:

It is well known that chicks become myopic by wearing negative lenses (see section 3.3). However, Zhu et al. stated[168] that "Even when chicks wore negative lenses for the entire day **except for 8 minutes of wearing positive lenses**, the eyes compensated for the positive lenses, as though the negative lenses had not been worn. ... Brief periods of myopic **defocus imposed by positive lenses prevent myopia caused by daylong wearing of negative lenses. .... regular, brief interruptions of reading might have use as a prophylaxis against progression of myopia.**"

Note:
This reminds not only of the therapy by wearing plus additions (section 3.2.2.3), but also of the brief relaxing exercises, which were proposed by Bates (section 3.2.2.1).

In contrast to the positive results of the experiments on chicks, Morgan stated[58] that "similar experiments carried out on tree shrews and primates have not been successful." Nevertheless is was expressed in the same paper: "...the recently described properties of the STOP signal [which stops eye growth] evoked by positive lenses offer considerable potential."

3.2.2.5 Plus glasses – are they Effective via Reduced Accommodation or via Modified Vergence?

Wearing glasses (not contact lenses) has **not only an effect on accommodation, but generally also on vergence** (see section 3.4.5) – and vergence, **especially the esophoria** (see section 3.4.1) is closely associated with myopia.

From this point of view, there is a significant difference between an increased reading distance, an undercorrection, bifocals or progressive glasses, and plus glasses, e.g. combined with contact lenses if necessary.

Explicit wearing of plus glasses was claimed to be effective against myopia[138, 142] (not only for prevention, but also for improving an already existing myopia) **and offers the best means to reduce the potentially dangerous esophoria.**

Note:
The supporters of the plus-lens-therapy mainly argue on the basis of personal experience only without going into much detail of explanations, i.e. without mentioning its positive effect on vergence. There is, however, a scientific linkage between plus lenses, phoria/vergence, and myopia via the degraded-image-quality-model (see sections 3.3 and 3.4).

3 Myopia – Observations and Experimental Results

3.2.2.6 Comparison of the Various Optical Methods

In Table 5 various optical methods discussed in the sections above, are compared. However, some of the criteria mentioned here will be in subsequent sections. Of special **importance appears to be the column "Effect on vergence"**.

Optical method	Near accommodation	Effect on vergence (section 3.4)	Near vision	Distant vision	Usage / overall vision	Potential effect on myopia
Large reading distance	Reduced accommodation	Reduced near esophoria	Good	Good	Easy	**Highly positive** for everybody
Plus glasses		Reduced esophoria		Reduced / insufficient acuity	Myopes: for near work only	**Highly positive** primarily for prevention (section 3.2.2.4)
Glasses - full correction	Full accommodation	Increased esophoria		Good	Easy	**Negative** (section 3.2)
Glasses - permanent undercorrection	Reduced accommodation	Increased esophoria (but less than with full correction)		Insufficient acuity	Only for near work o.k.	**Negative** (section 3.2.2.3)
Glasses - undercorrection for near work				Good	Need two glasses	**Positive** (section 3.2.2.3)
Glasses - bifocal or progressive					Easy, if fitting is o.k.	
Hard contact lenses - full correction	Full accommodation	None		Good	Easy	**Positive** (section 3.19.1)
Hard contact lenses - permanent undercorrection	Reduced accommodation			Insufficient acuity	Only for near work o.k.	**Positive** (section 3.19.1), but also **negative** (section 3.3)
Hard contact lenses and plus glasses for near work		Reduced near esophoria		Good	Easy	**Highly positive** (sections 3.19.1, 3.2.2.4)

Table 5 Comparison of various optical methods

Notes:

- The column **"Potential effect on myopia"** reflects my **personal overall assessment**, based on the referenced sections about accommodation and about vergence/phoria.

- -As discussed in detail in section 3.4, **myopia is closely associated with esophoria and a high AC/A ratio**, which both result in a too-much-inwards-adjustment of the optical axes of the eyes at near focus.

- **Soft contact lenses** are not associated with a positive impact on myopia (see section 3.19.1) and were therefore not included in the table above.

3.2.2.7 Psychological Problems with Special Glasses for Near Work

The described principle of undercorrection, or bifocal- and plus-glasses is very often hard to accept by people:

With fully correcting glasses there is immediately good vision for all distances (at least for young people with full range of accommodation), which gives the feeling that **"everything is o.k. from now on"**, and if people don't worry about the future myopia is no longer an issue. And in general, **people don't want to recognize a problem until there is already some damage**.

Using undercorrection, bifocal- and plus-glasses people are **faced permanently with the issue of non-perfect vision**. This will be tolerated only, if people are concerned about the future, but many people are hardly willing to face problems in general, and still less to face problems which arise in the future.

Therefore, this therapy may meet with resistance.

In the best case, people who are at risk to become myopic will use plus glasses for extensive near work already before becoming myopic to **prevent myopia**. I guess, however that people will read my book (and everything else about myopia) only if the problem is already there (it's like with everything in life, **"damage makes you wise"** - a translation of the German proverb "Aus Schaden wird man klug").

On the other hand, people who are already myopic **may have the feeling that "now, being myopic anyway, it does not matter anyway."** This group, however, should be fully aware that high myopia is not just a lens-related optical problem, but that it can have **very serious consequences** for the general preservation of the eyesight, potentially leading to blindness (see section 1.7).

3.2.2.8 Permanent Undercorrection instead of Undercorrection for Near Work only

Many followers of the Bates' method propose a **permanent undercorrection**. A trial, however, showed that a permanent undercorrection of +0.75 D was **increasing the progression of myopia** at children instead of slowing it down[169].

The authors of this paper, however, state explicitly that their results apply for **permanent undercorrection only**, and that previous **positive results of progressive reading addition**[151] **are still valid**.

The result of this paper is in contrast to earlier and similarly designed analyses. In this study they examined four groups: full time wearers of glasses, myopes who switched from distance to full-time wear, distance wearers, and non-wearers. The result stated by Ong et al.[158]: "...that the 3-year refractive shifts are **not significantly different** among the four groups."

Notes:
- *On one hand this result matches the results given in section 3.3, where **optical blur**, which is a consequence of **permanent undercorrection**, is shown to cause for myopia as well.*
- *On the other hand this result is in contrast to the results given in section 3.3, where **plus lenses** caused the eyes of animals to shorten, i.e. to become **hyperopic**.*
- *Maybe the relation between the time which is spent for near work and which is spent for distant viewing could explain this conflict: It may depend simply, whether the eye can spend **enough time with successful focusing** (i.e. when it has a sharp image), or whether for a **very long time the eye detects a blur image only**.*
- *By the way, the development of my daughter's myopia is an indication that permanent undercorrection (which is promoted very emotionally by some people) is not necessarily the right therapy in every case.*

Permanent overcorrection is increasing myopia without any doubt (see section 3.3 as well).

Very careful determination of **the right refraction** is therefore an extremely important issue (see section 1.11).

3.2.2.9 Is the Accommodation System Getting too Lazy by the Plus Glasses?

There could be the argument that in the long term the lack of accommodative effort is making the accommodative system unable to work any more, i.e. to accommodate properly for near vision.

Notes:
Counter-arguments are:

- *Many people are doing hardly any near work during their daily life and they are still able to focus exactly for near if it is appropriate. Our ancient ancestors did not do nearwork of extremely long duration like for reading at all. On the other hand, they did fine handicrafts like embroidery, leather plaiting, flint chipping etc. – many dark winter days were spent like this.*

- *Even if plus glasses are used for extensive near work there are many occasions in daily life where short term accommodation for near is taking place without the usage of the plus glasses, which results in permanent training anyway.*

3.2.2.10 Refraction with a Cycloplegic Agent

For children it is generally recommended to have their visual acuity tested after **applying a cycloplegic agent, i.e. after a relaxation of the ciliary muscle**. The residual accommodation of the ciliary muscle, which exists if no cycloplegic agent is used results in **overcorrection of myopia**[45].

Herewith a cycle of a permanent increase in myopia can be initiated, if no cycloplegic agent is used.

Note:
According to personal experience cycloplegia is rarely done (this attitude might be very different in different countries).

3.2.2.11 Summary of the Accommodation Based Therapies

A schematic overview of the accommodation-based therapies is shown in Figure 7.

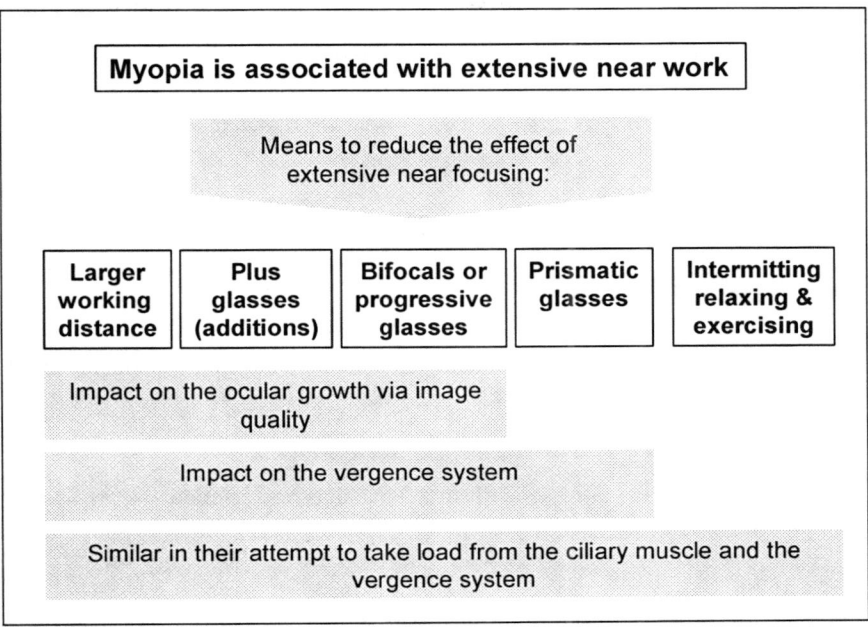

Figure 7 The accommodation based therapies

In spite of the fact that the promoters of this method argue mainly from personal experiences only, scientific explanations for its potential efficiency exist[149] (see also sections 3.2.1 and 3.4).

> *Note:*
> *Even if some of the claims of the promoters of the accommodation-based therapies appear to be exaggerated ("reversing of myopia is always possible"), there is no doubt that any reduction of accommodative stress (like large reading distance, plus lenses, bifocals, good illumination) is helpful and necessary to avoid the appearance of myopia and to stop the progression of myopia.*

In one paper, however, Schaeffel et al. stated[50]: "If variable genetic factors are major determinants of myopia in children, then modifying the visual experience (that is, doing near work with reading glasses), may not be very effective in inhibiting myopia development."

Note:
The logic of this statement appears to be questionable, as the following, controversial statement says: "... results indicate a high heritability for ocular refraction and its determiners and thus sug-

gest that environmental impact on refraction is not significant. However, the epidemiological association between educational length (near work) and myopia, the evidence of increasing myopia prevalence within a few generations, and the theory of gene-environment interaction imply that some individuals might be genetically liable to develop myopia if exposed to certain environmental factors."[69] *Extra glasses for reading are creating a modification of these environmental factors, and therefore may be effective in protecting against myopia.*

3.3 The Effects of Image Quality

3.3.1 Basic Results

Not too long ago (between 1977 and 1979) it was discovered that a lack of visual acuity on the retina leads to myopia in animals[56, 170].
This axial myopia can be artificially generated by[70, 98, 171, 172]:

- Covering the eyes of animals with **frosted glasses (form-deprivation myopia, FDM)**, or showing defocused pictures

    Note:
    Is there a connection between this effect and the residual tonic accommodation mentioned in section 1.4.1 (residual accommodation at low image contrast)? Permanent accommodation creates myopia (see point below), and with age this residual tonic accommodation was found to decrease. This corresponds to the fact that newly developed myopia also decreases with age.

- Applying **strong minus glasses**[173] **(lens-compensation myopia,** called LCM; added plus glasses cause lens-compensation hyperopia, called LCH)

    Note:
    This matches the results shown in section 3.2, where information about the correlation of permanent accommodation with myopia was given, and where it was warned of overcorrection. Additionally it was reported before that near accommodation results in an immediate elongation of the eye.

- Forcing the eye into **permanent near focus by restricting the distance of objects** that can be seen (this effect is illumination dependent).

- Keeping a developing **eye closed** by suturing an eyelid (not by keeping the animal in a dark environment).

- **Defects in the retina,** which are caused by toxication[174] or malformation lead to myopia, and nystagmus, an instable trembling of the eye, leads to high-grade myopia as well.

3 Myopia – Observations and Experimental Results

Some findings and facts for this artificial myopia are:

- At partly lens-covered eyes **only the respective part** of the sclera is changed.
- The **worse the acuity of the image** on the retina, the higher the myopia.
- The feedback mechanism between bad focus / elongated eye is **taking place already in the retina.**
- Applying **glasses works both ways**, i.e. applying plus glasses results in a shortening of the eye, resulting in hyperopia.
- Feldkaemper et al. stated[175]: "… **the eye becomes more sensitive to image degradation at low light,** the human eye may also be more prone to develop myopia if the light levels are low during extended periods of near work."
- A defocused image and especially a reduced **contrast** have not only an impact (extension) on the **vitreous body**, but also on the **length of the anterior chamber**[176]. In the early stage of myopia for children it was found, however that the vitreous chamber was already elongating, but the anterior chamber depth was still unchanged[177].

   Note:
   *This implies that the impact of image degradation affects not only the area of the eye which is close to the retina, i.e. the back of the eye, but also the rather distant front part of the eye. Conclusion: The **growth adjustment of the eye appears to be an almost systemic process**, which matches with some of the results given in section 3.3.3.*

- **Flickering light** can stimulate the release of dopamine and reduce the degree of the artificially induced myopia[178, 179], and increase choroidal blood flow[2].
- Eyes grow in length **only during the day**; at deprivation by translucent glasses they grow during night and day[29].
- Ohngemach et al. stated[180]: "**Intermittent periods of normal vision** inhibited deprivation myopia more if they occurred in the **evening than in the morning**" and **relatively short periods (1 to 4 hours) were very efficient** to reduce or to prevent form deprivation[181].

   Regular **interrupting the deprivation** can reduce the induced myopia, as Napper et al. stated[182]: "... several short periods of normal visual stimulation per day were more effective in preventing ... myopia ... than was one single period of the same total duration..."

   Note:
   *These results give a scientific **justification for the** experience driven recommendations of the Bates-method (see section 3.2.2.1).*

- After artificially introduced myopia the eye **recovers to emmetropia** after the cover is removed from the eye. If the myopia is corrected with glasses, no recovering to emmetropia took place[183, 184].

- Negative lenses, which cause myopic, elongated eyes, also cause a thinning of the choroid (the layer between the sclera and the retina). Vice versa, positive lenses, which are causing hyperopic, shortened eyes, also cause an also rapid increase in the thickness of the choroid[185, 186].

3.3.2 Biochemical Results

Some results about the impact of the imaging process on the biochemistry of the eye are:

- A drop in the level of the neurotransmitter **dopamine** (released by specific retina cells) in the vitreous body accompanies experimental myopia, and agonists for dopamine (i.e. agents that are supporting the action of dopamine) can at least slow down this deprivation myopia[171, 187]. Correspondingly, dopamine antagonists (i.e. agents which are blocking the action of dopamine) can enforce myopia[188].

- About **Amacrine cells** (types of neurons), Whikehart stated[189]: "...evidence indicates that amacrine cells (some of which use dopamine) serve as intermediate cells for the lateral transfer of signals across the retina", i.e. between the ganglion cells. Junqueira et al., however, stated[537]: "...their function is also obscure". Stone stated[190]: "... results ... suggest that dopaminergic amacrine cells may well be involved more generally in physiologic modifications of eye growth, not just in the form-deprivation myopia". This result, however, is disputed[191]. Colchicine, which destroys amacrine cells, promotes eye growth substantially[192].

- Devadas et al. stated[193] that the level of dopamine is (among others) controlled by "a retinal dark-light switch ... in the light-state it secretes **dopamine**, while in the dark state it secretes **melatonin** ...". Dopamine and melatonin are blocking each other[188].

- After induced form-deprivation myopia the **electrolyte balance in the vitreous was disturbed**: potassium and phosphate decreased, while chloride concentration increased. It was hypothesized that this change is caused by a reduction in the metabolic activity of the retina.[194].

- Mertz et al. stated[195]: "...visual conditions that cause increased rates of eye elongation (diffusers or negative lens wear) produce a sharp decrease in **all-trans-retinoic acid** synthesis [from retinol, i.e. vitamin A] to levels barely detectable ... visual conditions which result in decreased rates of ocular elongation (recovery from diffusers of positive lens wear) produce a four- to fivefold increase in the formation of all-trans-retinoic acid". Correspondingly, Morgan stated[58] "synthesis [of retinoid acid] is increased under conditions that suppress eye growth..."

Note:
It was shown that retinoic acid administered in the dark mimics the effect of light for some proteins expressed in the eye[196]; this offers a link to the results about the level of illumination, which will be presented in section 3.7.2.

- The peptide **glucagon**, and the gene ZENK play a role in experimental myopia of chicks[58].

This remodeling is typical for the adjustment process during growth, when the normally growing eye is optimized for best image resolution. Myopia occurs only when this feedback mechanism is disturbed.

3.3.3 Connective Tissue Related Results

The results of deprivation and defocus as described so far sound like a normal and healthy growth of the eye, controlled by optical effects. The connective tissue of the modified sclera, however, is neither normal nor healthy (this is valid for the sclera of highly myopic humans as well)[197].

The following list is a summary of some of the most significant research results. They demonstrate that there is a very strong correlation between higher grades of myopia and defects of the connective tissue.

- Scleral samples of artificially myopic tree shrew eyes (an animal frequently used for these experiments) were significantly **thinner and torn more easily.**[198] Similarly, highly myopic human eyes show scleral thinning at the posterior pole[197].

- The **structure of the fibers** of the sclera was found to be different compared to normal eyes[199].

- There is a **reduction of the amount of collagen and of the synthesis of proteoglycans**[200] [proteins, which are a main component of connective tissue besides collagen].

- Any agent that blocks the **cross linking of newly formed collagen dramatically increased myopia**[70].

- Norton et al. stated[201] "... deprived sclera contained **less proteoglycan**, or that the proteoglycans were less glycosylated or less sulfated." This led to his conclusion, "...that form deprivation **slows or reverses the normal process of extracellular matrix accumulation** in the sclera of this mammal."

- Rada et al. stated[202]: "The **turnover rate of ... scleral proteoglycans** is vision dependent and is accelerated in the posterior sclera of chick eyes during the development of experimental myopia. The loss of proteoglycans from the scleral matrix involves proteolytic cleavage ..."

- Jones et al. stated[203]: "... eye growth induced by retinal-image degradation involves increases in the **activities of multiple scleral proteinases** [enzymes with the capability to dissolve proteins] that could modify the biomechanical properties of scleral structural components and contribute to tissue remodeling and growth."

- Funata et al. stated[199]: "... a gradual increase in the **size of the collagen bundles and fibrils** from the inner to the outer layer of the sclera was observed in the control eyes, but was not evident in the myopic eyes."

- Kusakari et al. stated[204]: "**Collagen fibrillar diameters** of the fibrous sclera in the posterior segment of myopic eyes were smaller than in control..." and "...**collagen bundles** of the fibrous sclera [of myopic eyes] spread into the cartilaginous sclera, whereas in control eyes the distinction was clear."

- McBrien stated[183]: "... deprivation, which induced approximately 6 D of myopia, was accompanied by a three-fold **increase in the active form of gelatinase A** ... an enzyme involved in collagen degradation." Rada et al. stated[205]: "... visual deprivation is associated with an increased amount of the 72-kd progelatinase and a decreased amount of TIMP [tissue inhibitors of metalloproteinases] within the posterior sclera." This means, there is an **imbalance between tissue degrading agents and agents, which stop tissue degrading** towards tissue degrading.

- It was suggested by Siegwart et al.[206] that the sclera in deprived eyes "... offered **less resistance to vitreous-driven expansion** of the eyes."

- Form-deprivation resulted in the **building of hypertrophic cells** (chondrocytes), i.e. in the **enlargement of cells instead of the building of new additional cells**[207]. In other words, there is **no growth, but a stretching by a degradation of the quality of the tissue.**

    Note:
    *It appears plausible that these enlarged cells are showing a **reduced stability**, which would explain the stretching of the sclera in an extended myopic eyeball.*

- Gentle et al. stated[208]: "**Collagen type I expression was reduced** in the sclera of myopic eyes, however, collagen III and V expression was unchanged relative to control..." "...reduced scleral collagen accumulation in myopic eyes results from **decreased collagen synthesis and accelerated collagen degradation.**"

Summary:

Obviously, the remodeling, which is a normal process during emmetropization, has also rather **destructive and degrading features** This makes it easy to understand that if a feedback mechanism is out of tune, it will lead to myopia. Some people may develop malignant myopia through such a mechanism. In other words, the process leading to myopia is **not so much a passive one**, which is determined by simple mechanical stretching of a healthy sclera, **but an active one** with significant biochemical alterations[197], which includes that a biochemically degraded sclera is mechanically stretched.

It is still an open question whether the degradation of the sclera is completely biochemical. In this view, the reduced mechanical stability of the sclera is simply the effect of a changed biochemistry. The alternative is that **mechanical forces initiate biochemical modifications (a process called mechanotransduction**), which lead to the degradation[197].

A real and detailed understanding of the causation of deprivation myopia or lens-induced myopia, is still missing. There are some arguments that the experiments with animals are not fully valid for humans[209].

For general information about the connective tissue see section 4.2.1.

3.3.4 Remarks on the Image Quality Model

Some critical remarks against conclusions drawn from image quality experiments are:

- Most of the tests with experimental myopia were done with **chicks**; the chick, however, does not possess retinal blood supply[210], and also the sclera of chicks and mammals are very different[58]. For **monkeys**, at some species excessive accommodation is involved in experimental myopia, at other species it is not[210]. Moreover, Schaeffel et al. stated[50] that "there are also striking differences in the development of deprivation myopia in different populations of chickens."

- With all those experiments myopia can be initiated to a predictable degree. People, however, don't react obviously not uniformly, i.e. when exposed to the same environment, the same tasks and the same nutrition, some people become myopic and some will not. In other words, **for people there are ways to counterbalance the impact of myopia initiating events**, which seem not to exist for the tested animals. The target of myopia prevention should be, to promote and enforce these counterbalancing mechanisms.

- No explanation of the delay / lag of accommodation at myopes was given so far by the image quality model.

- For a potential impact of the vergence issue on the results of experimental myopia see section 3.4.

- These experiments can induce stress on the animals; stress, however, was found to be able to promote myopia as well (see section 3.13). Moreover, some of the experiments are increasing the temperature in the chick eye[211]; for the impact of the temperature on myopia see section 3.10. The stress model and the temperature model, however, cannot explain the different effects of positive and negative lenses (sign detection).

3.3.5 "Emmetropization" towards Myopia

The title of this section sounds very controversial, as **emmetropia is in contrast to myopia** (see section 1.3.1). This issue is, however, more complex (see Figure 8):

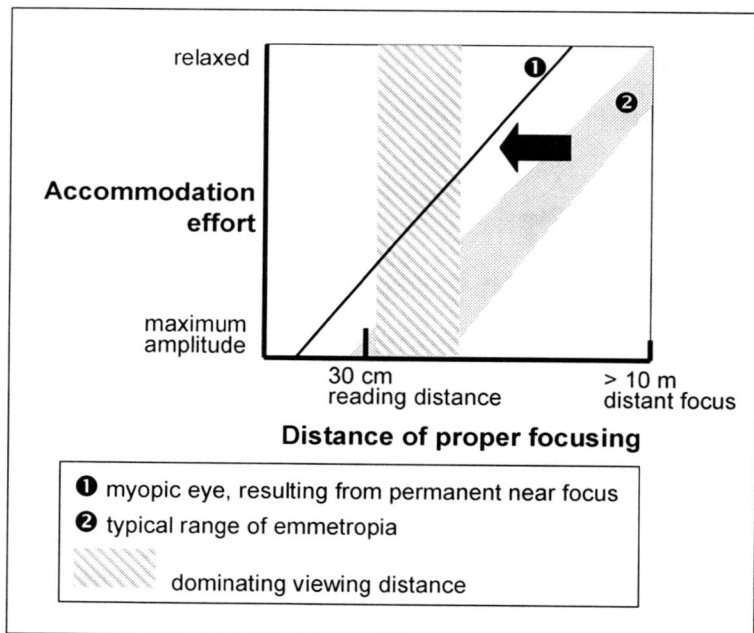

Figure 8 The shift of the accommodation effort caused by myopia

- Literally the word emmetropization means that the **eye is going to the state of emmetropia** (see section 1.3.1), i.e. to a state where proper focusing of distant objects can be achieved with a relaxed accommodation.

- Further the word emmetropization is used to describe the ability of the eye to adjust the eye-growth in length during development for optimal optical imaging. Wildsoet et al. stated[212]: "...when optical vergence **information is restricted to one plane, this plane becomes the endpoint of emmetropization.**" and "That eyes may emmetropize to distances other than real infinity is not a new observation ... laboratory-raised animals tend to be **more myopic ... when their environment is purposefully restricted**". In other words, emmetropization is used as well as the name of a mechanism, which **adjusts the eye length according to the preferred viewing distance.**

3 MYOPIA – OBSERVATIONS AND EXPERIMENTAL RESULTS

> In the **history** of human development both definitions matched, because mostly the dominating viewing distance was the far distance.
>
> Today, with often excessive near work, both definitions are controversial:
>
> If the eye adjusts to the dominating viewing distance it will often become not emmetropic, but myopic! Therefore, "emmetropization" in this case does not lead to emmetropia, but to myopia!

Experiments with animals showed that emmetropization can even lead to a **recovery from a previously induced myopia. Fitting lenses with zero power in front of myopic eyes led to a recovery from myopia, whereas the application of corrective glasses, (like the fitting glasses which is usually done!) prevented the recovery from myopia**[149].

There were **mathematical simulations of emmetropization and myopia** performed, taking into consideration interactions between **accommodation, vergence** and **optical blur**[213], and **level of illumination**[230] (see sections 3.4.7, 3.7.2). **Astigmatism** appears to play a part in emmetropization as well (see section 3.4.6).

The established effect of "emmetropization towards myopia" justifies the recommended use of **undercorrection - or of plus lenses as prophylaxis for non-myopes to prevent myopia** - and its progression as discussed in section 3.2.2.3 and as summarized in section 3.8. For the potentially negative effect of permanent undercorrection see section 3.2.2.8.

Notes:

- In a way, for a situation of permanent near work the development of myopia can be interpreted as permanent and efficient "emmetropization", i.e. not as a weakness, but as a very effective ability to adapt to a situation in the sense of evolutionary adaptation to the dominating distance of vision. So, shortsightedness develops as an adaptive response to a situation where short focus is called for. The biggest handicap is, however, the resulting potential damage to the back of the eye (see section 1.7).

- As emmetropization appears to work with a very different strength for various people, this process might be described by some kind of personal "emmetropization factor", which is different for each individual (apparently genetically determined) but which is also depending on personal habits like reading, illumination, accommodation response and last not least the individual biochemistry. Accordingly, myopia could be considered as an "over-emmetropization".

- As many people don't become myopic even when doing extensive near work, and without any plus glasses etc., the individual biochemical differences must be very essential, too. The main tool, which is available to us to influence this biochemistry, is nutrition. In sections 3.12.2, 3.16 and 4 these biochemical issues are discussed in more detail.

Besides the effect of "over-emmetropization" another potential reason for myopia was suspected: a **malfunction of the sign detection mechanism**[169], i.e. the problem would be not too much emmetropization, but **emmetropization in the wrong direction.**

Notes:

- *Even in this case, the resulting recommendation is undercorrection for near work (not permanent undercorrection!).*

- *Even if the published conclusion (that the problem is a malfunction of the sign detection mechanism) is true, this does not lead to a solution so far: The mechanism of the sign detection is not known yet*[56], *and therefore no tool to interfere here is available.*

3.3.6 Contrast and Spatial Frequency

It was found that contrast sensitivity is reduced for myopes with more than − 6.25 D. Contact lenses were able to improve clearly the contrast sensitivity in these cases.

Some authors attribute the loss of contrast sensitivity for severe myopia higher than − 12 D to retinal function disturbances[214] and not to mere optical imaging effects.

3.3.7 Monochromatic Aberrations

A spherical aberration is defined as a situation when a convex lens fails to focus parallel rays to a single point. This is due to deviations in the lens system. The spherical aberration of the eye is caused by the fact that the lens surface is not exactly spherical, but flattened at the periphery.

Obviously the mechanism of emmetropization works extremely exactly[56], as Artal et al. stated[215]: "In most of the younger subjects, total ocular aberrations are lower than corneal aberrations...", i.e. the **emmetropization works, not only for the complete eye, but also for local imaging areas within the eye.** For older persons these results were not valid, which could explain the fact that myopia is progressing fastest in young age, and comes often to a stop later.

It can be concluded from these results that **myopia is never completely caused by mechanical forces only** – optical imaging and biochemistry has to play an important part. On the other hand it was found by Wildsoet et al.[212] that "accommodation plays an important role in deciphering distance information in the visual environment during emmetropization".

Some details with respect to aberrations are:

- Aberration is called **positive** if the "minority rays" are focused in front of the rays, which are passing the spherical part of the lens, and is called **negative** if they are focused behind them.

3 Myopia – Observations and Experimental Results

- The **sign of spherical aberration was found to change by accommodation**, but there are results that it changes towards negativity[216] and there are results that it depends on the observer[217].

- **Rigid contact lenses**, which have a positive effect on the progression of myopia (see sections 3.19.1 and 5.2), reduce the amount of positive spherical aberration, which results in a better optical quality than the one achieved by soft contact lenses or spectacle lenses[218].

- Carney et al. stated[219]: "A tendency for the **cornea to flatten less rapidly in the periphery with increasing myopia** was shown."

- Nio et al. stated[220]: "Both **spherical and irregular aberrations increased the depth of focus**, but decreased the modulation transfer [i.e. the image quality and the image contrast] at high spatial frequencies [i.e. fine image patterns] at optimum focus."

- Spherical **aberration increases with increasing dilation of pupils**, and optical quality decreases as myopia increases[221].

Accommodation delivers signals to cause eye growth. This can be concluded from the facts that the local shaping of the eye is triggered even by local aberrations (could be called "**micro-emmetropization**"), and as the process of accommodation causes immediate spherical aberrations. There are conflicting results whether accommodation causes positive or negative aberration. The question is: **Does the sign and the magnitude of the accommodation-caused-aberration determine whether people become myopic?** This question matches with the suspicion which was expressed in one paper by Chung et al.[169]: "...strong evidence that myopia is caused by a malfunction of the sign detection mechanism in emmetropization..." However, Carkeet et al. stated[222] "...results do **not provide any evidence for aberration-driven form-deprivation as a major mechanism of myopia** development." Additionally Cheng et al. stated[223] "...spherical aberrations [at myopes] was not significantly different from emmetropic eyes."

If aberrations play a role in the development of myopia, there is be another strong argument in favor of bright illumination, because this results in a small aperture of the iris, and less aberrations.

Chromatic aberration is discussed in section 3.7.3.

3.3.8 Summary of the Effects of the Image Quality

Simplified the effects of the image quality can be summarized:

- Image quality can control the dimension, the shape and especially the quality of the sclera.

- The image quality has an impact on numerous biochemical processes.

- The reshaping of the sclera happens not via growth, i.e. cell multiplication, but via cell enlargement or stretching, and structural degradation.

The initiation and progression of myopia by the **image quality is compatible with a genetic influence on myopia**:

Genetics may be responsible for the metabolism, and the power of the feedback process that control eye growth[224]. This is in addition to genetically caused weak basic connective tissue, which can be a reason for myopia as well.

3.4 Phoria, Convergence and Astigmatism

When focusing on near object three things are happening automatically:
- **Accommodation**
- **Convergence**, i.e. the adjustment of the optical axes more inward compared to distance focusing
- **Narrowing of the pupils.**

3.4.1 Phoria

Phoria is a defect, in which this adjustment of the optical axes of both eyes to focus an object is not properly coordinated. This defect can be permanent, or it can be transient, e.g. under stress, nervousness, tiredness etc.

It can be that the axes of the two eyes are adjusted too much inwards when accommodating – **near esophoria** – or too much outwards – **exophoria**. Esophoria and exophoria are transient effects; if the maladjustment is permanent the corresponding effects are called **esotropia** and **exotropia**.

Some results are:
- It was reported that **higher myopia rates are occurring especially with esophoria at near**[121, 225] Chung et al. stated[226]: "The results support the hypothesis that **near esophoria is associated with high myopia**". The higher the esophoria was, the higher was the myopia progression rate. This matches plausibly with the correlation between elevated AC/A ratios (see section 3.4.2) and myopia. An explanation is the optical blur (i.e. not-perfect imaging) caused by esophoria.
- Brown et al. stated[163]: "In the progressive lens group, change toward **more exophoria at near was associated with less myopia progression.**"

- Esophoria at near was positively treated with added plus lenses, respective bifocals[161].
- Moreover it Brown et al. reported[163] that "... there was **only 46% as much myopia progression in the progressive lenses-esophoric group as in the progressive lenses-non-esophoric group.**" This means that progressive lenses (see section 3.2.2.3) were especially effective for myopes with esophoria.
- Additionally, a practitioner wrote that in his praxis pseudo-myopia, i.e. a **spasm of the accommodation was frequently accompanied by esophoria**[6].

    Note:
    Can it be that this elevated inwards convergence at near initiates an over-accommodation via the CA/C ratio (see section 3.4.3)?

- Mutti et al. stated[227]: "There is no association [between myopia and esophoria] when phoria is evaluated while children wear their current, habitual corrections. Yet many studies report a high prevalence of esophoria among children with myopia wearing a **new, rather than a habitual correction.**"

    Note:
    This could be explained by the AC/A ratio (see section 3.4.2). A new and increased correction implies a stronger accommodation at near, and a resulting increased convergence.

Whether a near esophoria is preceding myopia, i.e. causing myopia, or just accompanying myopia is not absolutely clear.

Note:
Additionally it might be possible that esophoria and myopia are not causing each other, but are caused together by another biochemical or biomechanical process.

3.4.2 The AC/A Ratio

A related parameter is the "**AC/A ratio**", i.e. the ratio of **automatic inwards convergence of the axes of the eyes with respect to the accommodative effort**. In other words: The nearer an object is, and the higher the accommodative effort is, the more the visual axes of the eyes will be adjusted inwards, triggered by the accommodative effort. The AC/A ration describes the degree of inwards adjustment in relation to the accommodative effort. In esophoria the AC/A ration is too high.

Often AC/A ratios, and results based on **measured AC/A ratios are hardly comparable**, because they are based on different definitions and different techniques for measuring[227, 131].

Some results are:

- Gwiazda et al. stated[131]: "Both types of **AC/A ratios are elevated in myopic children** ... Myopic children with esophoria underaccommodate at near. This suggests that a child who is esophoric must relax accommodation to reduce accommodative convergence and maintain binocular vision. The reduction in accommodation could produce blur during near work, which could induce myopia as in animal models". The problem of underaccommodation of myopes was already mentioned in section 3.2.

- Mutti et al. stated [227] that "... the response AC/A ratio was an important **risk factor for the onset of myopia** ... data suggest that the onset of myopia follows rather quickly, **within 1 year, if the AC/A ratio is high**.", i.e. it was not just accompanying myopia.

- A study by Chen et al.[228] with children in Hong Kong, however, could not confirm these results: "AC/A ratios appeared higher in progressing myopic children but the difference was **not statistically significant**."

Attention has to be paid to the AC/A ratio when fitting **bifocal glasses** to ease accommodation for near work (see section 3.2.2).

Notes:
- A high AC/A ratio corresponds in its effect to esophoria.

*- The AC/A ration might depend on the distance of the object in a non-linear way. Possible consequence: For reading a distance might be chosen, where **convergence is adequate, but where extra accommodative effort is necessary**, because the distance is actually too near. This excessive accommodation effort (see section 3.2 about the impact of accommodation) alone could contribute to myopia – as well via the image effect thesis (see section 3.3) as well via the mechanical thesis (see section 3.6).*

The schematic relationship between accommodation and convergence is shown in Figure 9.

3   MYOPIA – OBSERVATIONS AND EXPERIMENTAL RESULTS   59

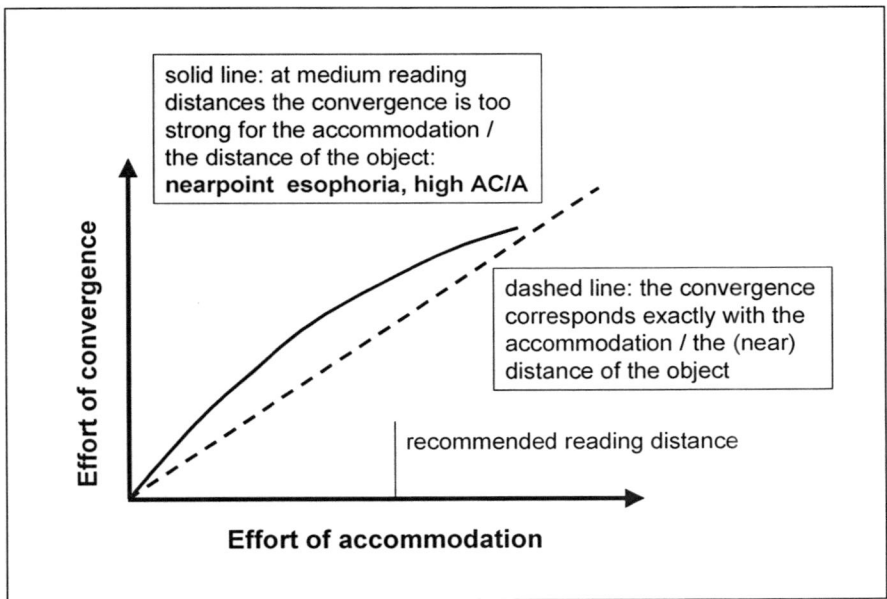

Figure 9 The relation between accommodation and convergence

Note:
It is not mentioned in the literature, but it appears to make sense:

*If the AC/A ratio is too high, and proper convergence is achieved only at a distance that is shorter than the distance recommended for reading, the use of **prismatic glasses, which compensate for the over-convergence at near distance** might be very useful. With glasses like this (**no undercorrection as mentioned in section 3.2.2.3**) a proper reading distance with normal accommodation could be achieved.*

3.4.3   The CA/C Ratio, and some more Types of Vergence

It is not only the case that accommodation initiates a certain amount of vergence (AC/A) as described in section 3.4.2. Vice versa **vergence triggers a certain amount of accommodation** ("convergence accommodation")[229]. This fact is described by the convergence accommodation/convergence (**CA/C**) ratio.

It was stated by Blackie et al.[230] that "...**a low CA/C ratio exacerbate the progression of near-work induced myopia**".

In section 1.4.1 the dark focus of accommodation, or tonic accommodation was mentioned. A corresponding effect for vergence exists: the **tonic vergence** or **dark vergence**, which is the adjustment of the axes of the two eyes in the dark or when closed. These two effects (i.e. tonic accommodation and tonic vergence) respond differently to an increase in illumination. There is a large individual bandwidth, as Jiang et al. stated[231]: " The critical luminance level at which the two responses were coupled for the 12 observers ranged from 0.01 to 0.45 cd/m2, with distinct individual differences."

Disparity vergence or **fusional vergence** is the effort to match the images of an object on the retinas of both eyes by the adjustment of the two visual axes.

At a more permanent fixation to near points (e.g. while reading) the disparity vergence and the accommodative vergence are gradually replaced by **vergence adaptation**.

It was said that the AC/A ration rises with age, and that CA/C is falling with age (considered range of age 16 to 48 years)[232].

Notes:
- *Obviously the mechanisms of vergence are highly complex, and are closely related to accommodation. A **strategy to handle progressive myopia should therefore pay high attention on a well-balanced vergence** (see also section 3.2.2.3).*

- *It appears that in the results of **experimental myopia** (see section 3.3) little attention was paid to the vergence issue; it looks like models that consider convergence, could explain some of these results from a different point of view[230].*

- ***Reading in bed**, especially lying on the side might be rather critical: Besides the effect that it leads mostly to a too near reading distance, the reading distance can be different for the two eyes, with unknown consequences of accommodation, vergence, AC/A and CA/A ratios.*

3.4.4 Hysteresis of Vergence

In section 3.2.1.3 hysteresis effects of accommodation were discussed. In fact, an analogue **hysteresis effect exists for the vergence**[233].

Note:
As a consequence, an impact on myopia could happen via this effect as well, either via the "reduced image quality model" (see section 3.3) or via the mechanical stress model (see sections 2.4 and 3.2).

3.4.5 Glasses, Contact Lenses and Vergence

Glasses have a **prismatic effect,** which is proportional to the degree of myopia and works towards nearpoint esophoria. This effect does not exist for contact lenses. For contact lenses, however, there is a higher degree of accommodation. As a consequence, Grosvenor et al. stated[234]: "If the AC/A ratio is moderate, the two effects tend to cancel each other out, but with a high AC/A ratio, the accommodative convergence effect may predominate, and with a low AC/A ratio, the lens centration effect [i.e. the not existing prismatic effect of contact lenses] may predominate."

The **claimed positive effects of plus lenses on myopia** (see section 3.2.2.3) can be at least partially based on this prismatic effect of the plus lenses, i.e. a **smaller exophoric** shift[160].

The data in Table 6 correspond well with the claim that **minus lenses tend to increase myopia,** whereas **positive lenses are said to decrease myopia** (see section 3.2.2.3), and the result that myopia is often associated with esophoria (see section 3.4.1).

Optical application	Shift towards esophoria, reduction of exophoria (associated with myopia, see section 3.4.1)	Shift towards exophoria, reduction of esophoria
Minus glasses	X[234]	---
Overcorrecting minus glasses	X[115]	---
Plus glasses	---	X[160, 161]
Plane (zero D) glasses	---	X[160]
Contact lenses	---	---
High AC/A ratio	X[235]	---

Table 6 The influence of optical devices on the convergence

3.4.6 Astigmatism

Another optical defect, **astigmatism,** was found before to have hardly an impact on myopia progression rates in two papers[236, 237]. More recently it was reported by Gwiazda et al.[238] that "... children with significant against-the rule astigmatism as infants are more myopic...", and the high prevalence of astigmatism and myopia at American Indians[239, 240] makes a correlation between astigmatism and myopia more likely.

3.4.7 Summary of the Vergence Related Effects

It appears plausible that an obvious disturbance of the **control circle: near focus – accommodation – convergence** can happen. These disturbances can lead to poorly focused, blurred images on the retina, which in turn can lead to myopia as shown above. A remedy, however, to prevent myopia or myopia progression by interfering with this convergence feedback circle, has not yet been established.

Together with the results of the influences on image quality, there are indications that there is a chain of processes for a development towards myopia[63, 131], which looks like Figure 10:

Environmental factors like near work, illumination, and mental stress
⬇
Optical blur by weak accommodation, strabismus (esophoria, AC/A and CA/C ratios, astigmatism) etc.
⬇
Retinal output signals (image-controlled model, see section 3.3),
or
excessive mechanical stress (mechanical model, see section 3.6)
⬇
Axial "growth" or stretching of the sclera, i.e. axial myopia

---

Figure 10 Paths to myopia

There exists a **quantitative mathematical model** in which the interactions between accommodation, vergence and optical blur were used to explain the development of emmetropization and myopia[213].

Notes:
- *This sequence looks rather straightforward. What appears to be **missing** frequently in the literature is the consideration of the fact that (especially highly) myopic eyes have **substantial structural and biochemical deficiencies and anomalies**, and that therefore the feedback mechanism as outlined above is not working in a moderate manner, but often excessively with some **pathologic** attributes. And why exactly is this chain of events **not having any impact on some people at all?***

- *Obviously, the knowledge of the interaction between the "opto-mechanical world" and the biochemical world is still missing. Nutrition (see section 3.16) might be one of the keys.*

- *Maybe there are **blood sugar** related effects on the AC/A ratio as well (see section 3.16.2).*

3.5 Saccades and Focusing

To focus an object, the eye is making **about 30 to 80 fast eye movements (oscillations) per second**, with an angle amplitude of about 10" to 30" (one " equals to 1/3600 of one degree)[241]. The purpose is to trigger permanently the sensitivity for contrast. Images are said to become grayish on the retina if the stable focusing is longer than 1 to 2 seconds. These saccades are said to play a role in the interaction accommodation / vergence, too[242].

Some people (not really the scientific world) are recommending special training glasses with a pattern of fine holes in a dark surface, called pinhole glasses, to encourage the eye to perform these saccades.

Note:
*In the scientific literature about myopia research there is **hardly any mention of saccades**, which is rather astonishing, as it appears to be essential for image acuity, and appears to be quite related to the experiments, where induced myopia in animals was successfully reduced by flickering light[171].*

The myopic eye has a specific problem correlated with saccadic eye movements, as David et al. stated[243]: " ...if account is taken of the increased force required to provide normal saccadic movement of myopic (larger) eyes, then the **shear force** [a force that occurs in the thin eye wall shell supporting the vitreous body] is up to **seven times greater** than that experienced for emmetropes."

Note:
This additional force for saccadic movements might create two problems:

- *If the extraocular muscles cannot sustain this additional power, a **degraded image** and/or focus might result again, contributing to a further **progression of myopia**.*

- *Due to this **increased force**, which is necessary for the myopic eye, a **progression of** myopia could be caused, according to the thesis presented in section 3.6.*

For myopes with **more than 6 D** a significantly **slower eye velocity in saccadic movements** was found, and if (soft) **contact lenses** were used instead of glasses, a significantly slower eye velocity was recorded as well. A potential explanation was the additional mechanical effort due to the increased mass.[244]

Moreover, **glucose metabolism** has an impact on the saccadic eye movements[245, 246], e.g. diabetic patients have **disturbed saccades** (asymmetry between the two eyes, longer latency). For the impact of the glucose metabolism on myopia see section 3.16.1.

3.6 Mechanical Stress, Strain and Pressure

3.6.1 Impact of Mechanics on Biochemistry

Theories, which are attributing myopia exclusively to image related effects, or biochemical effects, or mechanical effects are not necessarily in competition with each other: It is still an open question whether the process leading to a degradation of the sclera is completely biochemical, and the reduced mechanical stability of the sclera is simply the effect of a changed biochemistry, or whether mechanical forces are initiating biochemical modifications (a process called **mechanotransduction**), which lead to the degradation[197]. There can be also a combination of both effects.

This model was supported by the result that **scleral fibroblasts** (i.e. cells of the connective tissue), **which were mechanically stretched, showed significant changes in gene expression.** These changes were already observed after 30 minutes of stretching[107]. This time length is typical of near-work accommodation.

Note:
Accommodation generally results in a temporary elongation, i.e. stretching of the sclera of the eye (see sections 3.2.1.1 and 3.21.2). Conclusion: **Accommodation can result in gene expression of scleral fibroblasts!**

3.6.2 Intraocular Pressure (IOP)

Overall there is a general agreement in the literature that a **higher intraocular pressure is associated with myopia**[247, 248, 249, 250, 251].

For **children aged 9-11 years, however, no association between IOP and myopia** was found in one study[252], **whereas** another study by Lin et al. stated[253] that "...**IOP of patients less than 19 yrs is significantly higher** than patients more than 30 yrs..."

Note:
It is claimed that with new technology the measurement of the IOP is completely independent from the rigidity of the sclera, but maybe there are still limitations of the measurement process ("completely independent" is hard to believe from the point of physics).

Consequently for myopes there is an elevated probability of glaucoma[254]; a study showed typical probabilities for glaucoma of 1.5% for eyes without myopia, 4.2% for low myopia and 4.4% for moderate to high myopia[255].

3 Myopia – Observations and Experimental Results

When people with **progressive myopia** do near work, there is an uncompensated **hyperproduction of intraocular fluid** which causes elevated ocular hypertension because there is an insufficient outflow[116]. Correspondingly, for the time of recovery from experimental myopia an **increase in the fluid transfer** during emmetropization was found[256].

A **general increase** of IOP with **accommodative stress**[153] and with **accommodation and convergence** to close distance[257] was found.

Some authors, however, state that **a higher IOP follows the onset of myopia and does not cause myopia**[258, 259].

Note:
Is the structural change of the myopic eye's connective tissue also blocking the fluid to flow off, causing an elevated IOP?

Experiments have shown that growing eyes of chickens elongate during the day and shorten during the night, which correlates with the IOP (high at daytime, low at night). There were, however some phase differences between the rhythms in IOP and ocular elongation – with the IOP ahead of the elongation. It was therefore proposed by Nickla et al.[278] "**that the rhythm in IOP influences ocular elongation in ways other than by simply inflating the eye, for example, by influencing underlying rhythms in scleral extracellular matrix production.**"

Notes:
- *The observed phase difference between IOP and elongation could as well be explained by the effect of a **hysteresis of the mechanical properties** of the connective tissue.*

- *On the other hand, the pressure within the eye is uniform, but the control of the length of the eye due to emmetropization (section 3.3.5) can be **very local** as well, if this serves a better image quality. This is an argument against a completely IOP-driven myopia.*

One author claimed to have success in treating myopia with the IOP-lowering **beta-blocker** metipranolol[260], but other authors could not confirm this by using the different beta-blocker timolol[261].

From other experiments it was concluded that a higher IOP affects **neuronal functions** of the eye[262].

Note:
This would give a link with the fact that myopia is connected with dopamine metabolism and elevated IOP.

Several components of nutrition were found to be able to influence the IOP[250]:

- Rutin, a bioflavonoid was reported to lower IOP[263].
- A deficiency of chromium was reported to increase IOP[264].
- Elevated blood glucose was reported to increase IOP[265].
- Folic acid from food was reported to lower IOP[266].

All these dietary components were related to myopia besides their impact on IOP (see section 3.16).

Moreover, an elevated IOP appears to be highly related to emotional effects and stress[267], i.e. sensitive people are more at risk of an elevated IOP (see section 3.13 for the impact of stress on myopia, and section 3.13.2 for the relation between personality and myopia).

A study by Lee et al.[268] "identified a modest cross-sectional **positive association between current smoking and intraocular pressure.**"

3.6.3 The Muscles

Greene[269] has explored whether the elongation of the eyeball can be simply explained mechanically, by "the **stresses** experienced by the posterior sclera as a **result of accommodation, convergence, vitreous pressure, and the extraocular muscles.**"

Basis of the engineering-like analysis was that:

- Substantial forces are applied to the eyeball, e.g. the **extraocular muscles** can generate 150g (peak) and routinely produce 40g during large amplitude **saccades**[270] (see section 3.5 about saccades). In contrast, the force applied by the ciliary muscle was found to be only 0.6g.

  Congenital nystagmus, which is characterized by extreme saccadic movements, is mostly accompanied by myopia[271].

- A substantial increase of the **intraocular pressure** (IOP, see section 3.6.2) of up to additional 14mm Hg was found during accommodation and convergence at close distance[272].

The result of the analysis was that the **mechanical forces are strong enough** to explain the elongation of the eyeball seen in myopia. There are a variety of individual geometrical parameters (like geometrical arrangement of the muscles) and material-dependent parameters (like the quality of the connective tissue of the sclera), which can explain, why not everybody who is doing a lot of near work is becoming myopic (there is a lot of individuality for parameters like this[273]).

In other words: Myopia can be explained as the result of the joint effects of **muscular force and hydraulic pressure (IOP) on a weakened tissue structure.**

A specific theory about the interaction of the muscles was mentioned in section 1.3.3.

Notes:
- *The alternative theory of accommodation mentioned in section 1.3.3 is similar to this analysis - both are emphasizing the effect of the extraocular muscles.*
- *The long term, substantial load on ocular muscles can contribute to a **degradation of the connective tissue** of the sclera via an elevated **temperature** (see section 3.10). Near work was in fact found to increase the temperature of the eye (see section 3.2.1).*

3.6.4 The Lens

There exists another potential mechanical model, which might be used to explain myopia. Points to consider are:

- As reported in section 3.2.1 there is a **time delay for the return of a myope's lens shape** after accommodation (referred to as hysteresis).
- The experiment reported in section 1.3.3 showed that it can **take very long (several years!) until a lens goes back to its original shape**, if the accommodative stress was long lasting.

Together with the (optical) model of negative-lens-induced myopia (see section 3.3) a hysteresis of the shape of the lens might:

- Induce myopia by blurring the image when focusing a distant object, but when the lens is still at a residual accommodative state
- Induce myopia by an inappropriate negative lens, which is fitted according to this transient residual accommodative state.

This hysteresis of the shape of the lens might be caused by an effect of the **ciliary muscle**, or by an effect of the **elasticity of the lens.**

No information exists about what might cause different modes of elasticity of the lens for myopes and non-myopes; maybe the swelling of the lens in a hyperglycemic state contributes to this effect (see section 3.16.1).

3.6.5 The Ocular Shape

Some results about the ocular shape are:

- Schmid et al. stated[274]: "Eye shapes (a) **varied substantially among subjects** and (b) differed considerably from the corresponding shapes of spherical model eyes with identical axial eye lengths." This result is correlating with the individuality described in section 4.1.3.

- The ratio of the length to the transverse dimension in eyes shows that the higher the myopia the higher the ratio, i.e. the eye is **stretched primarily in length**[275].

- Partial coherence interferometry was used to measure the eye. The result showed that **the eye generally elongates during accommodation**, with this explanation by Drexler et al.[18]: "... by the accommodation-induced contraction of the ciliary muscle, which results in forward and inward pulling of the choroids, thus decreasing the circumference of the sclera, and leads to an elongation of the axial eye length ... the elongation was more pronounced in emmetropes than in myopes".

  Note:
  To understand this model, just think of a balloon, which is squeezed, and which expands as a consequence in the other direction.

- There is a substantial **hysteresis of the ocular shape**: Walker et al. stated[125] that with normal people, **after accommodation** "... ocular shape had become more prolate {i.e. stretched]. This shape remained unchanged after 1 hour of sustained accommodation and then returned to baseline dimensions after 2 hours of accommodation ... Ocular shape returned to baseline dimensions after 45 min of accommodative relaxation." See also section 1.3.3 about the impact of accommodation on the ocular shape.

  Note:
  *This hysteresis should be a major problem for the accuracy of refractive measurements for fitting glasses. One could even consider this elongation with accommodation as some kind of "slow accommodation". It appears rather plausible that with extensive near work, this **elongation becomes permanent, which corresponds to myopia**.*

- Mutti et al. stated[276]: "The eyes of myopic children were both elongated and distorted..." ... "Increased **ciliary-choroidal tension** is proposed as a potential cause of ocular distortion in myopic eyes."

  Notes:
  *- If an ocular body has a **weak support by the connective tissue**, the increased ciliary-choroidal tension and the **increased hydraulic force** during extended accommodation could explain the permanent axial extension: In the transverse direction the ocular shape*

is maintained by the ciliary muscle, but there is less or insufficient support in the axial direction (length) of the eye. The weak connective tissue might be correlated to the effects mentioned in section 3.3.3 and 3.16.12.

*- Can a specific **inborn ocular shape** cause an increased risk of developing myopia (e.g. via different resulting stress on the ciliary fibers)?*

- For Eskimos and for Chinese, both populations with an elevated rate of myopia, the anterior chamber angle declines more rapidly with age[277].

3.6.6 The Zonular Fibers

Note:
The following model has apparently not been discussed in the literature, but seems to be plausible:

*If the zonular fibers (which are attached to the lens, and whose pulling action on the lens regulates accommodation, see section 1.2) are lacking strength and elasticity, they have a problem in pulling the lens into a flat shape when the ciliary muscle relaxes. The result will be a **myopic refraction, leading to the prescription of glasses even if the eyeball is not elongated** yet, or to a blurred image with potentially corresponding negative effects (see section 3.3).*

*Furthermore, **reduced accommodation amplitude** can be expected.*

The basic reason for the weakness of the zonular fibers should be weak, degraded connective tissue. Weak, degraded connective tissue is closely related to myopia, especially to progressive myopia (see e.g. sections 2.2, 3.12.7).

3.7 Illumination / Light / Day- and Night-Rhythm

3.7.1 Day- and Night-Rhythm

Investigations have shown that growing eyes of chickens **elongate during the day and shorten during the night,** following the changes of the IOP with some delay.[278] There is, however, a rhythm in axial length and choroidal thickness even in constant darkness[279], apparently due to the circadian rhythm (i.e. night-/day-rhythm), which is triggering numerous biochemical processes.

The result of a study in 1999 was that **night-lights** increase substantially the probability of myopia for kids[280]: the probability was found to be increased more than three-fold for night-lights and more than five-fold for full light in the sleeping room.

Later other studies came to different results[281, 282], and the dispute between the researchers is still open[283], focusing on the question which study was properly, i.e. neutrally designed.

The issue cannot be judged here, but there are some related observations, which offer some potential explanations:

- Illumination has a high impact on **melatonin production** (Glickman et al. stated[284]: "Less than 1 Lux of monochromatic light elicited a significant suppression of nocturnal melatonin."), and melatonin and dopamine block each other[188]. While direct injections of melatonin were found to have no impact on myopia[285], other researchers like Kusakari[29] believe in an "intimate relation between the development of myopia and the day-night rhythm of melatonin in the pineal and the retina". And Ohngemach et al. stated[180] that "... results show that the **pineal gland** [which produces melatonin] has a surprisingly large influence on both the retinal dopamine receptor gene transcription and dopamine release". Additionally, eyes were found to grow in length only during the day[29], and myopia probably increases with shortened sleep[103]. The amacrine cells in the retina were found to play a key role in the control of the dopamine signaling, and these cells are influenced by melatonin metabolism[193].

  Furthermore, oxidative stress appears to be present in myopic eyes, combined with a lack of the antioxidant gluathione peroxidase – and melatonin (which is produced by the pineal gland) was found to stimulate production of gluathione peroxidase[286].

- A night-light is normally kept on, if there is a serious **sleeping disorder**. This disorder can be caused by a disturbed dopamine/melatonin balance, or by a lot of other biochemical or psychological disturbances. In this case, the night-light is not the reason for myopia, but a symptom of a disorder, which leads to myopia via other mechanisms. Just one example: Vitamin B6 metabolism was found to be related to insomnia[287], and vitamin B6 is a key substance for connective tissue integrity[288].

  This implies that switching off the night-light doesn't necessarily stop the development of myopia. The underlying reason for the sleeping disorder needs to be addressed.]

- A test with students had the result that a reduced **daily exposure to darkness** resulted in increased probability of myopia progression[309], while other influences like amount of near work were controlled.

  Note:
  This result could be caused by the illumination-triggered metabolism of melatonin (see section 3.7.1).

For general information about the day- and night-rhythm see section 4.2.3.7.

3.7.2 Level of Illumination

Some results about the impact of the level of illumination are:

- A once promoted theory was that excessive **heating up of the background of the eye** (or the whole body) is responsible for myopia[6]. The eye was said to be overheated because of too much incident light through over-large pupils. It was said that this large opening of the pupils is common to all myopes (claimed to be based on many references), and is additionally caused by stress. At near accommodation the width of the pupil of myopes was said to be even larger than of other people.

  Newer publications, however, report that the opening of the pupils of myopes is not wider[289], and that low levels of light can help myopia to progress[175, 290]. Generally the pupil is narrowing when accommodation is occurring[291]; maybe this was helpful during evolution of mankind to use better depth of focus for near objects (each photographer knows that depth of focus is a problem for near objects, which can be solved by a smaller aperture of the iris of the camera).

- A test with monkeys (already in 1961)[98], whose visual space was restricted to an average of fifteen inches, showed that all of them developed some myopia, but that **groups with high and low level of illumination showed less myopia** than the one with medium level illumination. The high level matches about the number of 300 Lux for reading which was mentioned above, the medium level matches a level "provided in a ten by ten foot room with an eight foot ceiling and a 100 or 150 Watt bulb at the ceiling" as Young stated[98] – which is considered to be common for reading. The illumination level of the low level group made reading impossible.

  Note:
  These results are similar to the one found about thirty years later when the deprivation issue and the effects of an inappropriate minus lens were discovered as initiators of myopia.

- Light was found to increase (among others) **dopamine levels**[171, 292]. This fact matches with the statements in section 3.3.1.

- A result by Feldkaemper et al.[175] from the experiments about myopia caused by low image quality is: "... the eye becomes more sensitive to image degradation at low light, the human eye may also be more prone to develop myopia if the light levels are low during extended periods of near work".

- It was also described[6] that a higher level of **illumination increases significantly the capability for accommodation**, and that presbyopes (i.e. older people with reduced accommodation) can read more easily in high illumination – clearly independent from the increased depth of focus, which is caused by a narrower opening of the pupil.

- A **mathematical model** by which the appearance of emmetropization (i.e. eye growth to achieve emmetropia) and myopia was quantitatively explained by the interaction between accommodation, vergence and optical blur[213] was extended to include the effect of the level of illumination. Result: **bad light increases the development and progression of myopia, especially of late onset myopia**[230].

- **Depth of focus** has an impact on image acuity as Atchison et al. stated[293]: "For uncorrected myopes of 3.0 D or less, visual acuity was nearly as good with a 1-mm pupil as for corrected myopes". Therefore, a steady opening of the pupil above average might trigger a feedback circle in case of already existing imaging deficiencies, i.e. promote myopia.

- For dilated pupils (which are accompanying low levels of illumination) **increased spherical aberration** and decreased optical quality was measured[294] (see section 3.3.7 about aberration, and section 3.3.5 about aberration and emmetropization).

  Notes:
  *Corresponding with this fact, the **individual relation of the pupil size per level of illumination** may have an impact in both directions – too large and too small might be both negative:*

  *- A **below** average pupil size results in a low level of illumination on the retina, with the mentioned negative effects.*
  *- An **above** average pupil size results in a degraded depth of focus, with the mentioned negative effects.*

- To some extent the illumination level has an impact on the important issue of the **vergence** (see section 3.4.3):

  It was stated by Owens et al.[295]: "... convergence is a more important distance cue than accommodation under low illumination..." and by Kersten et al.[296]: "Accommodation to a dim target corresponded closely to the convergence accommodation".

  Note:
  *It can be concluded that under **low light** a convergence problem like esophoria can have a negative impact on accommodation, e.g. **create over-accommodation**.*

- Vannas et al. stated[297]: "...there was a trend towards a higher prevalence of myopia among conscripts living above the Arctic Circle, consistent with the hypothesis that **ambient lighting might influence refractive development**. Other novel associations with myopia were the **decreased use of sunglasses and brown iris color**."

  Notes:
  Several explanations for these results of "a higher prevalence of myopia among conscripts living above the Arctic Circle" could be offered: The lack of complete darkness during sum-

mer (see section 3.7.1), the lack of sufficient light during winter, and a lack of vitamin D caused by the lack of light during winter (see section 3.16.3).

The association between myopia and a decreased use of sunglasses could be explained, e.g., by temperature effects (see section 3.10).

Summary: Good illumination is highly recommended for near work – as Feldkaemper et al. stated[175]: "Because the experiments show that the eye becomes more sensitive to image degradation at low light, the human eye may also be more prone to **develop myopia if the light levels are low during extended periods of near work.**" Apparently, our grandmothers were right, when they warned, "kids, don't read in bad light!" (See also the recommendations in section 3.8).

Additionally it has to be noted that in the past the majority of people **worked outdoors**, where in general a by far higher level of illumination exists.

3.7.3   Color of Illumination

As light of longer wavelength (red) is dispersed less than light of shorter wavelength (blue), the exact image of a multicolor (e.g. white) object exists in different planes, e.g. the exact image on the retina exists for one wavelength (color) only. For the **other wavelength the image on the retina is not perfectly focused** (chromatic aberration; this effect is often used by the optometrist to check for overcorrection). Corresponding with this fact is that persons who wore blue filters showed initially some degree of myopia[298].

It was concluded that the eye does **not use this chromatic effect to detect the sign of a defocus** (too near / too far)[56], i.e. that chromatic aberration is not essential for emmetropization. This is in contrast to a statement by Schmid et al.[299]: "...data hint that **chromatic aberration may have some role as a cue to defocus in emmetropization.**"

An experiment by Kroger et al.[300] about the accommodative response during near work showed, however that "The refractive state was largely independent of the color temperature of the illumination light (white paper) and the color of commercially available papers (white illumination). Selective **elimination of long wavelengths, however, significantly reduced the accommodation stimulus by about 0.5 diopters.**" These authors "suggest that the visual system primarily uses long wavelengths, if available, during reading tasks."

Other authors came to the same conclusion – i.e. a recommendation to eliminate infrared light, which is close to visible light – via a completely different model. They concluded from experiments that the **hyperthermia, which is caused by the infrared light**, increases the activity of enzymes, which causes a **loss of the spatial structure of hyaluronic acid and collagen biomolecules.**[301]

Moreover, there are reports about positive results of **treating patients with more general visual disorders** by the effect of an illumination with specific colors[302].

The mechanical stability of corneas was improved by treatment with vitamin B2 (riboflavin) **and UV irradiation**, which introduced additional cross-links (see section 5.2.12).

3.7.4 Flickering Light

Flickering light can stimulate the release of dopamine and reduce the degree of artificially induced myopia, and increase choroidal blood flow (see section 3.3.1). The retinal blood vessel dilation is increased[303], but this retinal vessel dilation by flickering light is reduced if the level of nitric oxide (NO) is reduced[304] (see section 3.11 about myopia and blood circulation, and section 3.12.6 about myopia and NO).

There is also an interaction between this vessel dilation by flickering light and a hyperglycemia (see section 3.16.1 about myopia and hyperglycemia).

3.8 Vision Training

Vision training[305, 306, 307, 394] (also called **vision therapy, visual training, behavioral optometry, developmental optometry**) is a concept to improve the eyesight by specific **training of all the components and functions of the eye**, i.e. the lens, the ciliary muscles, the extraocular muscles, and the brain, which is involved in the coordination of seeing.

Vision training is related to the Bates-Method (see section 3.2.2), but goes far beyond, incorporating additional issues like Convergence (see section 3.4), saccades and focusing (see section 3.5), mechanics (see section 3.6), illumination (see section 3.7) and mental issues (see section 3.13).

Vision training uses many devices like lenses, prisms and computer software, but there are also exercises for which no specific tools are necessary.

It is emphasized that the exercises have to be specifically tailored to the specific problem of the individual patient, which means they need to be based on a professional eye examination. The person who is directing the vision training is normally a professional optometrist.

Note:
The success of this method should depend highly on the skill and experience of the supervising optometrist. Care should be taken to find an optometrist who has in fact a strong professional overall-background in eye care and is not just a self-made follower of the vision-training concept.

3.9 Recommendations from Optical and Mechanical Results

Some results of the research about **image quality, accommodation** and related issues are summarized in a few recommendations[308]:

- **Interrupt your near work every 30 minutes by focusing on distant objects and maybe by wearing plus glasses, and relax your eyes especially in the evening**[180].

- **For near work, keep the book or computer screen reasonably distant, or better, use undercorrecting or bifocal glasses** (not for driving a car! And general under correction can result in a blurred picture on the retina, which will result in deprivation myopia, too[120]; about bifocals see section 3.2.2). **Plus glasses** for extensive near work should be of advantage for people who are not myopic yet, but are at risk, and for people who wear contact lenses.
  Note: Reading in bed leads mostly to a too short reading distance.

- **Read printing with large letters.**

- **Do not read at bad light, 300 Lux is the minimum** (see also section 3.7.2).

- **Some exercising of the accommodation by alternating focusing near and far objects can be helpful** (but don't expect miracles from classes which are offered about this issue).

- **Do not keep a light switched on in the kid's room at night** (there is a controversy in the literature about this issue, but better be on the safe side, see also section 3.7.1) – and take care to have **enough sleep** at the proper time and in darkness[309].

A more **complete summary of recommendations**, not restricted to image quality is shown in **section 4.8**.

Note:
Science confirms now some old and basis ideas of Bates and Wiser mentioned above. It does not confirm, however, the exaggerated promises of some of the followers, i.e. to reverse myopia.

3.10 Temperature

It was mentioned in section 3.7.2 that an **elevated temperature** of the eye, caused by illumination, has been **suggested as a cause for myopia**. The suspected mechanism was the fact that accelerated biochemical reactions degrade the connective tissue of the sclera[310]. Numerous reports in the literature show that e.g. the activity of collagenase, an enzyme that degrades collagen, can be increased substantially by inflammations and related elevated temperatures. Additionally it was reported that the strength of connective tissue is generally rather temperature dependent.

There is little question that an elevated temperature is damaging the structure of the sclera, resulting in myopia[301, 311, 312].

The temperature of the eye can be elevated by various circumstances:

- **Excessive illumination** was claimed to increase the temperature of the retina (see theory outlined in section 3.7.2).

- It was shown that **light with long wavelength** could be expected to be harmful for myopia by raising the temperature (this increases the activity of enzymes, which causes a loss of the spatial structure of hyaluronic acid and collagen biomolecules, see section 3.7.3).

- **Near work** was shown to increase the temperature of the eyeball[116].

  Note:
  The substantial forces applied during accommodation and vergence (see section 3.6) could explain this temperature rise.

- **Stress**, like during examinations, was found to elevate body temperature: the higher the scores in the examination, the higher the temperature difference between examination and no-examination[313].

- **Feverish sicknesses**[314], or generally an activated immune system, are increasing overall body temperature.

Note:
Maybe there is an interaction with blood circulation (see section 3.11) – poor blood circulation may reduce the transfer of the heat generated during the hard work of accommodation.

Summary:

An elevated temperature is a candidate for causing myopia. This alone, however, gives little help to prevent it, as it is a consequence of other processes.

The fact that an **elevated temperature significantly decreases the stability of connective tissue** (i.e. of the sclera) is important in connection with the thesis that during near work substantial **mechanical forces are applied** to the eyeball – forces which act in the direction of axial myopia (see section 3.6). This mechanism also has significance in connection with **increased activities of the immune system**, which elevates the temperature, too, and which was found to be relevant for myopia (see section 3.12).

3.11 Blood Circulation

It was found by Ravalico et al.[315] that "with regard to increasing axial length and refractive error a progressive **reduction in ocular pulse amplitude and pulsatile ocular blood flow** was noted". Lam et al. stated[316]: "The pulsatile ocular blood flow was negatively correlated with axial length" (i.e. the longer the eye the lower the pulsatile ocular blood flow), and Reiner et al. stated[317] that "myopic eye growth produced from vision degradation leads to dramatic reductions in choroidal blood flow". Very specific Dimitov et al. stated[318] that "Central retinal and posterior ciliary blood velocity decreases with the increase of the degree of myopia." There was a significantly increased **resistance** index for the blood flow in the posterior ciliary artery[319]. This **decreased blood** flow was seen in both human and animal studies.

Some authors were concluding that this **reduced blood flow is a consequence, but not a reason for myopia.**

On the other hand an increased blood circulation explained the success of a specific surgical treatment[320], and development of experimental (form–deprivation) myopia was suppressed by **flickering light**, which increased choroidal blood flow (and dopamine release)[2].

Overall, it was concluded that **increased choroidal blood flow is protecting the eye from lengthening**[321].

Additionally in **eyes that are recovering** from artificial (form deprivation) myopia a temporally **increased choroidal blood flow** was observed together with an increase in choroidal thickness[322].

A severely **reduced blood circulation** in the retina (retinal ischemia) can **severely damage retinal neurons**[361].

Notes:
- *Nitric oxide was found to increase blood circulation (see section 4.2.3.4), and is related to myopia (see section 3.12.4).*

- *Even if a reduced blood circulation is not causing the onset of myopia, the decreased blood flow as a consequence of myopia can contribute to a further **progression** of myopia.*

- *The exact mechanism of reduced blood circulation in the myopic eye appears to be still open. Maybe the structural degradation of connective tissue in high myopia is responsible for this effect in a similar way, as people with problems of the connective tissue frequently appear to have a **low blood pressure** (no reports are known, however, about a correlation between low overall blood pressure and myopia).*

- *Maybe there is an interaction between blood circulation and temperature (see section 3.10) – a lack in blood circulation may reduce the transfer of the heat, which is generated during the hard work of accommodation.*

3.12 Some Specific Biochemical Issues

3.12.1 The Immune System

Some results about the significant interaction between the immune system and myopia (especially more severe myopia) are:

- **Antibodies to collagen** were found in the serum of myopic people. However, a control group, and surprisingly the most severe group of myopes, had no such antibodies The authors draw these conclusions[323]:

    - The immune response to collagen can serve as a definite indicator of pathologic changes in the sclera.

    - An accumulation of collagen antibodies in the serum can be considered a normal reaction to changes in collagen structure

    - The lack of collagen antibodies may be considered a prognostic factor of an unfavorable course of myopia.

- **Circulating immune complexes** (CIC) in the serum and the anterior eye chamber were measured. Patients with complicated myopia had a highly elevated CIC level, indicating autoimmune processes being responsible for biochemical changes in the eye tissue[324].

- Examination of patients with myopia has revealed disturbances of the immune system by a **decreased absolute amount of T-lymphocytes** and an **increased content of immunoglobulins** in blood serum. The shown sensitization of the body to eye tissue antigens hints at the participation of autoimmune processes in the pathogenesis of myopia. The authors conclude that an inhibition of the thymus function leads to degenerative changes in the sclera and destruction of collagenic fibers[325].

- A study found that asthma and other allergies, as well as myopia, were more frequent for extremely mathematically and/or verbally excellent students (see section 3.13.2)

- As mentioned in among the rate of asthma and other allergies, and myopia was substantially higher[326], which is showing a connection between myopia and **autoimmune reactions**.

- Several authors found a correlation of myopia with a variety of **infectious diseases** in childhood[327].

- It was described that children of mothers who suffered from **infections** during pregnancy were four times more likely than normal to become myopic before the age of 8 years[328].

- Fledelius et al. stated[329]: "The elevated myopia figure of 43% among juvenile **chronic arthritis** (JCA) patients suggests an association between myopia and JCA: In lack of more precise indicators and in accordance with older literature, an explanation might be a weakening effect of chronic inflammation on scleral connective tissue".

- Already in 1854 the autopsy of myopes led to the conclusion that myopia is connected with a process **of inflammation**[330].

- Markwardt et al. stated[331]: "... histamine caused **contraction of the human ciliary muscle** cells in a concentration-dependent fashion." Accommodation is (generally assumed to be) performed by contraction of the ciliary muscle (for information about the histamine release by the immune system see section 4.2.2).

- A disturbed **calcium metabolism** was found for myopes[153]. The relation between calcium and the immune system is discussed in section 4.3.1.1.

- In section 3.1 it was reported that myopia is less frequent in rural areas. A potential explanation is given by the result that children in early contact with agricultural animals have less asthma and **allergies**[332].

- For eyes with pathologic myopia an **elevated rate of apoptosis** (i.e. programmed cell death) **in photoreceptor cells of the retina** was observed[333]. Grodzicky et al. stated[334] that apoptosis "is a physiological process of cell death that normally occurs when cells are damaged or no longer needed." Apoptosis is **often strongly related to the immune system**, and can lead to autoimmunity.

    Note:
    Selenium deficiency can lead to decreased numbers of amacrine cells and of photoreceptor cells (see section 3.16.12.1).

- A personal observation: Many people with high grade myopia are hardly ever sick, but have problems with harmless insect bites, or are suffering from asthma, all of which are all indications of an overactive immune system.

    Note:
    Infections both raise temperature and activate the immune system. Both of these may induce myopia, for example immune system overactivity can produce higher levels of collagenase, a collagen (i.e. connective tissue) degrading enzyme (see section 4.2.2). Moreover, infections are very likely the initiators of later autoimmune diseases[335].

For general information about the immune system see section 4.2.2.

3.12.2 Oxidative Damage and Antioxidant Defense in General

Numerous research papers showed a correlation between higher grades of myopia and an elevated activity of oxidative processes:

- Generally myopia, especially progressive myopia was correlated with damages by **oxidative processes**[336, 424].

- Florence stated[337]: "The eye is an organ with intense AOS (activated oxygen species) activity, and it requires high levels of antioxidants to protect its unsaturated fatty acids".

- The higher the myopia of patients with retinal detachment was, the higher was the **lipid peroxidation**, which is a free radical caused process[336]. Malondialdehyde, a breakdown product of lipid peroxidation, was found in increased levels in diabetes and higher myopia[338].

- Among patients undergoing retinal detachment surgery the group of patients with more than 10 Diopter show a **significantly higher TBARS concentration**[339] in the subretinal fluid than any of the other groups studied. The TBARS (thiobarbituric acid reactive substances) concentration is an indicator for the concentration of damaging reactive oxygen-containing molecules.

- For children and adolescents with progressive myopia and retinal complications a **reduced ratio between the antioxidant activity and the radical formation** in the lacrimal fluid was found.[340]

- For eyes with pathologic myopia an **elevated rate of apoptosis in photoreceptor cells of the retina** was observed[333]. Grodzicky stated[334] that apoptosis, or programmed cell death "is a physiological process of cell death that normally occurs when cells are damaged or no longer needed." This process of apoptosis of retinal cells is often related to the proteases called **caspases**[341], and Nunes et al. stated[342] that "**antioxidant deficiency [in this publication a deficiency in vitamin E and selenium] significantly increased caspases-like activity**" in chick skeletal muscle cells.

- Generally it was stated by Behndig et al.[343]: "If inflammatory reactions occur, **ocular tissues are at risk for damage** induced by superoxide radicals and peroxynitrite, the reaction product with nitric oxide."

For general information about oxidative damage and antioxidant defense see section 4.2.3.2.

3.12.3 Enzymes Glutathione, Glutathione Peroxidase, Superoxide Dismutase, G6PD

The body produces several enzymes for the protection of cells and tissue against other enzymes or against oxidants. An **imbalance can cause an increased rate of cell and tissue turnover**, resulting in damage and degradation.

A decreased level of these antioxidants can be a reason for a vulnerability of the connective tissue; an increased level can be a reaction of the body to counteract against an oxidative attack. Some results are:

- Depending on the degree of the myopia of patients with retinal detachment an increased **lipid peroxidation** was found. Simulation of this process with animals resulted in a **decrease of the (protecting) glutathione peroxidase activity**[344]. Glutathione peroxidase contains selenium, whose impact on myopia has been mentioned before (section 3.16.12.1).

  For information about the glutathione cycle see section 4.3.1.6.

- Myopes with a **lack of copper-zinc superoxide dismutase** are at a substantially higher **risk of vitreous degeneration**[94].

- The activity of superoxide dismutase (**SOD**), which was increased (together with **NO**) by supplemental zinc (section 3.16.5), **prevented axial elongation** in myopia in animals[327]. Matching this result, the Chinese myopia medication "**Nacre**" is increasing the SOD activity in the eye[357].

- There was a higher activity of glucose-6–phosphate dehydrogenase (**G6PD**) at myopes with progressive myopia than in myopes with stable myopia[345] (see section 4.2.3.12 about G6PD).

  Note:
  From this result it cannot be concluded that a higher level of G6PD causes myopia! Most likely, when myopia occurs, the defense system against oxidative damage is activated, herewith triggering the production of G6PD. So far there are no reports available about the correlation between inborn G6PD deficiency and myopia. It appears to be plausible that inborn G6PD deficiency might accompany myopia.

For general information about G6PD see section 4.2.3.12.

3.12.4 The Blood-Retinal Barrier

Definition of the blood-retinal barrier: "Specialized nonfenestrated tightly-joined endothelial cells that form a transport barrier for certain substances between the retinal capillaries and the retinal tissue."[346]

Rizzolo stated[347]: "The retinal pigment epithelium (RPE) is a monolayer that separates the outer surface of the neural retina from the choriocapillaris. Because the choriocapillaris is fenestrated, it is the RPE that forms the outer blood-retinal barrier and regulates the environment of the outer retina."

Experiments with animals showed an abnormally **increased permeability of the blood-retinal barrier in experimental myopia**. The question, however, is as Kitaya et al. stated[348], whether "impaired blood-retinal barrier function might be a secondary effect of myopia development rather than the cause of myopia."

Notes:
- *Additionally, it is possible that the impaired blood-retinal barrier as well as the myopia are caused not by each other, but are caused together by a special biochemical process.*
- *If an impaired blood-retinal barrier was responsible for myopia, selenium supplementation might be efficient against myopia via its retina-protecting effect (see section 3.16.12.1).*

Glucose level appears to be related to myopia as well (see section 3.16.1), and glucose has a significant impact on the blood-retinal barrier[349].

The blood-aqueous barrier appears to be intact in young high myopes with healthy posterior vitreous body and retina[350].

3.12.5 The Vitreous Body

The vitreous body consists mainly of a mixture of fluid and gel, where the gel acts, besides other functions, as a shock absorber against sudden stress and strain, which includes the forces caused by the saccades (see section 3.5). Gel is composed of collagen. When collagen structure changes, the relation between gel and fluid will be affected, in turn possibly destabilizing the retinal surface, which can cause retinal detachment[189].

Liquid is about 20% of the vitreous body at age 18 and progresses to more than 50% in old age[351].

Morita et al. stated[352]: "The results ... suggest that **liquefaction of the vitreous begins at a relatively young age in patients with high myopia** and progresses with age and axial elongation, thus resulting in a frequent occurrence of posterior vitreous detachment."

It was concluded that liquefaction is caused by the functional disorder of the **blood-retinal barrier in myopia**[39] (see section 3.12.4 about the blood-retinal barrier).

Some recommendations for maintaining the health of the vitreous body were given[38]:

- Avoid and/or protect against bright sunlight or sunlamps
- Avoid excessive supplementation of vitamin C
- Avoid excessive, unbalancing supplementation of zinc or copper
- Avoid excessive intake of foods rich in phosphorous

3.12.6 Nitric Oxide (NO)

Nitric oxide has multiple effects on the eye[353].

On the one hand **NO reduces myopia**:

- There are indications that NO can serve to **relax ciliary muscles**[354, 355] and therefore Tokoro stated[356] that "... chemicals related to NO may be useful drugs to treat myopia."
- Zinc was found to **prevent experimental myopia**, accompanied by an **increase of NO and NO synthase** (NOS) and superoxide dismutase (SOD)[327]. The same was claimed for the Chinese medicine "**Nacre**"[357] (see section 3.17).
- Chiou stated[353]: "It is possible that high **myopia can be prevented/treated with inhibitors of iNOS activity** and/or iNOS induction."

On the other hand **NO increases myopia**:

- Experimental myopia was induced by the use of translucent goggles (form deprivation) or negative lenses. Injection with a Nitrous Oxide blocking agent prevented myopia[358, 359, 360].
- The retinal degenerative lesion, which is found in high myopia, can be attributed to an overproduction of NO[353].

  Note:
  A damage of the retina, caused by the degradation of NO which produces toxic peroxinitrate, can be avoided by extracellular zinc, magnesium, and most likely by the vitamins B6 and B12.[361]

Additional effects are:

- Chiou stated[353]: "The **retinal degenerative lesion is caused by iNOS** induction and overproduction of NO which leads to apoptosis of retina."

- Experimental myopia caused a reduction in iNOS, which is the most powerful one of the NO generators[362].

- NO has a significant effect on the **intraocular pressure IOP**, as well an increase as well as a decrease was reported[363, 364, 365]. For the impact of the IOP on myopia see section 3.6.2.

- NO can **reduce retinal dopamine**[366, 367]. For the impact of dopamine on myopia see section 3.3.1. For the biochemical process of **light adaptation** there is an interaction of **dopamine and NO**[368].

- Tamm et al. stated[369]: "The presence of intrinsic NOS-positive nerve cells concentrated in the inner parts of the ciliary muscle might indicate a physiological **role of nitric oxide for disaccommodation or fluctuations during accommodation.**" For the impact of accommodation on myopia see section 3.2.

- Ando et al. stated[370]: " These data indicate that NO is an important stimulator of **choroidal neovascularization** and that reduction of NO by pharmacological or genetic means is a good treatment strategy."

An **explanation**:

Chiou stated[353]: "**Both underproduction and overproduction of NO could lead to various eye diseases.** ... Providing NOS substrates or NO donors to lower the intraocular pressure, increase ocular blood flow, relax ciliary muscle etc. On the other hand, immunological NOS (iNOS) is inducible only in pathological conditions by endotoxins, inflammation and certain cytokines...retinal degenerative lesion is caused by the iNOS induction and overproduction of NO..."

A simplified **summary**:

It appears that NO is good, but the excessive amounts of NO produced by iNOS are bad.

For general information about NO see section 4.2.3.4.

3.12.7 More Biochemical and Biomechanical Effects

Various biochemical and biomechanical effects, which were found in connection with experimental myopia (i.e. with animals), have been described in section 3.3.3. Some more of these effects, which were found at myopic people, are:

- Increased **excretion of acid mucopolysaccharides** was found in the urine of patients with advanced myopia[371, 327]. Mucopolysaccharides are basic components of collagen and the connective tissue, which was found to be defective in the sclera of highly myopic patients. This indicates disturbances in their immune system.

- People with a **reduced content of collagen** and a delayed decrease of soluble fractions of collagen with age in the posterior scleral regions of the eye were found to be at risk for myopia related problems[372]

  Matching these results is the experience that myopes have a **decreased corneal thickness**, as well as **decreased endothelial density**[373].

- Myopic eyes have a tendency to show a reduced content of collagen in the posterior scleral region and **diminished tensile strength of the fibers**[372].

- **Fibroblasts** (which are constituents of collagen, and which are the only cell type in the sclera) **decrease** with increasing myopia, but increase during recovery from myopia[88].

- Myopes have a high probability of **posterior vitreous detachment** (PVD), i.e. a liquefaction of the hyaluronic acid matrix of the vitreous and a collapse of the interfused network of collagenous fibrils, and finally detachment of the vitreous from the retina[38]. This indicates that myopia is very often accompanied or caused by structural deficits of the connective tissue, which are caused by biochemical effects.

- Some deviations from the normal **status of the hormones** testosterone, 17-ketosteroid, 17-beta-estradiol and cortisol were found[374], however no straightforward conclusions could be drawn.

  Note:
  *Estrogen increases **endothelial nitric oxide**[688] (see section 3.12.4 about the impact of NO on myopia, and section 4.2.3.4 about NO metabolism), and extended **estrogen treatment** increases the activity of lysyl oxidase, an enzyme which is essential for the cross linking of collagen the structure of the collagen of the sclera is degraded in myopia)[375].*

- For people with extreme myopia the concentration of the amino acid **glutamate** was 10-fold increased[457].

  Note:
  Glutamate is important for the NO metabolism (see section 3.12.4 about the impact of NO on myopia, and section 4.2.3.4 about NO metabolism).

3.13 Mental Issues

3.13.1 Stress

Several authors have discussed **stress as a significant reason for myopia**[6, 376]. Stress cannot induce myopia directly, but it can change parameters that influence the functionality of the eye. Here are some of the observations and statements about myopia in connection with stress:

- The **opening of the pupil** is increased (called mydriasis): this can affect the depth of focus.

- Workers closely checking merchandise for faults (requiring **high and sustained concentration**) became myopic, while colleagues doing other near work were unaffected[52].

- Under stress, there is a reflex to adjust the eye to distant vision, i.e. relax the ciliary muscle and set the axes of the eye correspondingly parallel. Consequently, there is a **conflict between stress and near work**[117], where the ciliary muscle has to be activated, and the optical axes have to be adjusted to vergence. Result can be a degraded image, which may lead to myopia.

- Stress was shown to elevate the **body temperature**[292], and herewith damage connective tissue (see section 3.10 on the impact of the temperature on myopia).

- There are conflicting results about the level of **cortisol** in myopes: Results of an increased cortisol level[377, 378] and results of insignificant differences were found[379]. A solution for this contradiction was offered by stating that in general the cortisol level is increasing under **transient** stress. After **long-term exposure to stress**, however, there will be a decrease of the cortisol output[380]. Cortisol has a high impact on connective tissue by mediating reactions of the immune system, e.g. by decreasing inflammations, and by creating structurally defective connective tissue[381] (see sections 4.2.2 and 4.2.3.3).

    Overall, the impact of stress on cortisol level creates a definite risk for becoming myopic.

    It was stated that the Bates-method (section 3.2.2) had achieved its results at least partly be reducing stress, i.e. by creating more relaxed vision[135, 136].

    Note:
    It is unknown, whether the experiments where degraded vision led to myopia created substantial stress for the respective animals.

- Stress can increase the **intraocular pressure** (IOP)[382], and there is a substantial impact of IOP on myopia (see section 3.6.2).

- Stress can cause the **vitamin C** level to drop rapidly[383], and vitamin C is important for connective tissue integrity.

- Stress has a high impact on **calcium** metabolism. The impact of calcium metabolism on myopia is discussed in section 3.16.3.

- Stress can have an impact on **blood sugar level and insulin production**, which in turn can have an impact on myopia (see section 3.16.1).

- Stress can increase the excretion of **chromium**[384]. The impact of chromium metabolism on myopia is discussed in section 3.16.6.

- During the **summertime and school holidays**, there is less progression of myopia[91, 92, 94]. Several explanations are possible: Less stress, less near work, more physical activities, or more exposure to the sun (vitamin D?).

- **Psychosomatic**, i.e. stress and anxiety induced feelings were reported to be able to influence myopia[385].

- The analysis of ocular examinations after the **extraordinary stress of an earthquake** showed that 30% of people were diagnosed with pseudo myopia, and 8% with various forms of strabismus or phoria. These people had not complained about their vision before[386].

    Note:
    *From this observation it can be concluded that frequent mental stress can easily lead to a permanent prescription of inappropriately strong glasses, **resulting in a permanent progression of myopia**.*

- It was reported that the first prescription of glasses was frequently the time of **serious personal stress**[139].

- The **Bates method** (see section 3.2.2.1) emphasizes relaxation of the eye as well as exercises of accommodation.

- The higher level of **stress in some Asian countries** like Taiwan, Singapore and Hong Kong (triggered by ambitious schooling) has been at least partly blamed for the substantially higher prevalence of myopia in these countries.[387]

- Wolffsohn et al. stated[388]: "The data show that for EOMs [early onset myopes] the **level of cognitive activity operating during the near and far tasks determines the persistence of NITM** [near-work induced transient myopia]; persistence being maximal when active cognition at near is followed by passive cognition at far." The tasks were either passively watching or active arithmetic calculations.

Note:
Stress can substantially contribute to the rapid increase of myopia in populations like the Eskimos: For these populations the traditional lifestyle brought a lot of mental stability, now replaced by modern lifestyle and modern media.

For general information about stress see section 4.2.2.8.

3.13.2 Personality and Mentality

Compared with other variables personality and mentality are harder to cover in scientific research. Some statements that were made are:

- In section 3.2.1 I already reported a correlation between a better education, which is generally connected with more reading, and myopia. For general statements like "myopes are more intelligent" this has to be considered.

    Indeed, statistical surveys have shown that myopic children **perform better** in school, independent of the social status of the parents[327, 389, 326, 390, 391].

    Correspondingly, according to results from Singapore, educational levels, personal income, professional occupations, and better housing are associated with higher rates of myopia[86].

- In section 3.10 it was already reported that the higher the scores in an **examination** were, the higher was the difference in body temperature between examination and no-examination, and that an elevated temperature can damage the connective tissue of the sclera. Possible explanation: Students, who take examinations more seriously, achieve better results, but consequently they are more at risk of myopia.

- Besides the correlation with intellectual performance, there was an elevated rate of **introversion** for myopes found among students[392].

- 50 to 60 % of the Japanese are said to be myopic, but only 2 % of the people in South America are[76]. The same author hints at a substantial difference with respect to **spontaneity** between these two populations.

    Note:
    There are many other variables, like the pressure to excel at school.

- It was claimed that visual problems are frequently caused by the desire of a person, to avoid the confrontation with a specific aspect of her/his life or personality – i.e. **the person doesn't want to see it**[76].

- In section 3.2.2.1 it was mentioned, how the **Bates-method tries to influence also the mind of the myopic person**, and not just mechanically the eyes only.

- A hypothetical explanation for the potential reasons for the correlation between intellectual performance and myopia was given by Miller[393]: "... A single genetically controlled mechanism affects both brain size and eye size."

  Note:
  The correlation between brain size and intelligence is highly questionable. Smaller brain of women used to be a justification for unequal rights

- A potential link might be the **immune system**: Myopia, and asthma and other allergies, were substantially higher among extremely mathematically and/or verbally excellent students[326].

- Moreover, there is a close interaction between **vision and learning** in general, i.e. a person's way to face the complex situation of learning has an impact on the person's vision[394] – and vice versa.

3.14 Physical Exercises

No direct correlations between myopia and physical exercises are available. Two results, however, are giving strong indications:

- In **urban areas** myopia rates are higher than in rural areas (see section 3.1). Generally people in the city have less physical activity than people in the countryside.

  (Sure, there are many other differences. For example, immune system would be healthier in the country, more Vitamin D, less reading...)

- All forms of physical exercises reduces the **intraocular pressure (IOP)**[395]. For the impact of the IOP on myopia see section 3.6.2.

For general information about physical exercises see section 4.2.3.10.

3.15 Myopic Changes in Pregnancy

There is a tendency that during pregnancy a shift towards myopia or an increase of myopia takes place. This shift, however, is generally reversed after giving birth[396].

Note:
Consequently, fitting of new glasses during pregnancy should be handled with extra care to avoid an overcorrection at the time after the pregnancy.

3.16 Impact of Nutritional Components

This section contains published information about two issues:

- nutritionally affected biochemical parameters where myopes show a difference
- experiences where nutrition was found to have an impact on myopia.

The results summarized in this section are based mainly on statistics. To be fair it should be noted that interpretation of the statistics can be very difficult: does a parameter, found to occur together with myopia really have an impact on the mechanism of myopia? It might occur due to an unrelated **association** only. (Remember? It can be said, e.g. that most of the children who run across the street and get hit by an automobile were wearing tennis shoes, so therefore, tennis shoes must have caused the accidents. Obviously, the tennis shoes were only a common association, not a related factor.) As, however, people whose eyesight is threatened by myopia cannot wait for final scientific results the advice can only be to follow any recommendation, as long as following this recommendation does not imply a new risk.

Generally, nutrition can have a positive impact on myopia either

- by improving the stability of the connective tissue, especially of the sclera, and/or by
- suppressing an exaggerated feedback which is triggered by image quality effects as outlined in section 3.3.

3.16.1 Carbohydrates, Blood Sugar Level, Insulin Metabolism

Some research papers showed an interaction between myopia and glucose metabolism:

- **Hyperglycemia**, when the blood sugar rises, as in diabetes or after meals, causes hydropic **swelling of the crystalline lens, and myopia**. The reason of this thickening of the lens is a decrease in the tension of the zonule fibers. Vice versa there can be farsightedness as the blood sugar falls[397, 26]. The refractive error in cases of diabetes can change 1 or 2 D within a few hours[398].

    For diabetic patients, refractive changes can go up to – 4.00 D, and changes can take several weeks. The degree of myopia after medication for diabetes was started is not somehow proportional to the residual hyperglycemia, but there is a transient hyperopic change when control of the hyperglycemia is becoming effective[399].

- **Hypoglycemia** causes frequently **reduced contrast sensitivity**[400], which can have an impact on myopia as well (see section 3.3).

- Glucose metabolism has an impact on the **saccadic movements** of the eye, which are essential for focusing[245] (see section 3.5).

- Overall, **diabetics** appear to have a higher rate of myopia[401].

- **Accommodation** is reduced in diabetic schoolchildren[402].

- Malondialdehyde, a breakdown product of **lipid peroxidation**, was found in increased levels in diabetes and in people with high myopia[338].

- Dielemans et al. stated[265]: "Newly diagnosed **diabetes** mellitus and high levels of blood glucose are associated with **elevated IOP** and high tension glaucoma."

- Du et al. stated[403]: "Diabetes-like glucose concentration **increases superoxide production in retinal cells**, and the superoxide contributes to impaired viability and increased cell death under those circumstances."

Note:
Oxidative processes (see section 3.12.2) as well as retinal metabolism (see section 3.3) have been credited with causing myopia.

- Lane stated[153]: "Young myopes statistically consume **more than triple the ratio of refined carbohydrates** to total carbohydrates, as compared to hyperopes, and this difference is most highly significant..." Moreover, the consumption of sucrose per head has risen e.g. in England from 6.6 kg in 1815 to 54.5 kg in 1979[404].

Note:
Maybe the effect lies not only in the high consumption of refined carbohydrates, but also to a great extent in the overall sub-optimal nutrition, e.g. a lack of folic acid and numerous other nutrients.

- A change in nutrition toward a focus on food **rich in refined carbohydrates and sugar** was blamed for the dramatic increase in myopia: diets high in refined carbohydrates are **increasing blood sugar (hyperglycemia), insulin levels (hyperinsulinemia), and insulin resistance**, which in turn causes the growth of the eyeball[405, 406].

The **explanations**, which were given by Cordain et al.[405]:

- Elevation of insulin increases the levels of the insulin growth factor-1 (IGF-1), "a potent **stimulator of growth in all tissues**".

- "Reduced levels of the insulin like growth factor binding protein-1 (IGFBP-1) may reduce the effectiveness of the body's natural retinoids in activating genes that would normally **limit scleral cell proliferation**" (for the role of retinoic acid on myopia see section 3.3.1).

For example it is explained[407] that in pacific islands where people kept to the original diet of fish, yam and coconut no increase in myopia was observed, in spite of long schooling hours of the children. In contrast, a myopia rate of over 18% was reported for Hong Kong fishermen, who had never attended school[408]. The rate was even higher for those with schooling.

As **another evidence for this insulin-argument** it is noted by Cordain et al.[405] that "population studies have demonstrated that **people of Asian and Chinese descent tend to be more insulin resistant** (which, however, often increases to some degree the production of insulin) than people of European descent" – and the prevalence of myopia is especially high in Asia.

- Glucose level has an impact on the functioning of the **blood-retinal barrier**, which is related to myopia (see section 3.12.4).

- In experiments with mice **hyperglycemia combined with a lack of insulin** leaded to a significantly **increased number of mast cells in the sclera**[409].

  Note:
  An increased number of mast cells should result in an enhanced activity of the immune system, which can reduce the stability of the sclera. For information about myopia and the immune system see section 3.12.1.

- **Flickering light** can protect against artificial myopia (see section 3.7.4), most likely by retinal vessel dilation. High blood glucose significantly reduces this flicker induced retinal vessel dilation[303].

A number of **nutritional components are important** for the avoiding of **hyperglycemia. They were found to be related with myopia as well**: Manganese, Chromium, vitamin D and flavonoids (see section 3.16 and section 4.3).

Moreover, hyperglycemia influences **biochemical issues, which were found to be related with myopia as well**: NO level, cytokine production, oxidative stress, and microcirculation (see section 4.3).

This might support the thesis that hyperglycemia can play a role in the development of myopia.

Moreover, it was found that a disturbed blood sugar metabolism has an impact on the pulsatile ocular blood flow[410]. The blood flow appears to be connected with myopia (see section 3.11).

Notes:
- *Hyperglycemia (i.e. elevated blood sugar level) can be caused not only by nutrition (and inheritance), but also by **stress** and a **lacks of exercise**, etc. It is not restricted to people with type I diabetes (who are permanently depending on insulin), and older people with type II diabetes, but can*

occur temporarily independent of age, i.e. also in children, where the development and progression of myopia is most critical (see also section 4.2.3.8).

- *Additionally, it was emphasized that it is very important to keep a diet that **avoids steep increases in blood sugar level**, i.e. to have a "low-glycaemic index-low-fat-high-protein" diet[411, 412]. - Very frequently these steep increases in blood sugar (hyperglycemia) later cause significantly lowered levels of blood sugar (hypoglycemia).*

- *The findings summarized above **do not mean** that many myopes are diabetic, or that diabetes is a frequent reason for myopia. They mean, however that **carbohydrate and insulin metabolism might very well have an impact on the development of myopia**.*

- *In contrast to the report about low rates of myopia in the pacific islands, a very substantial increase in myopia was observed for **Eskimos** (see section 3.1), and obviously, their dietary habits had been changed significantly.*

- *Maybe another issue of the changed nutrition is the changed **sodium/potassium ratio** (see section 4.2.3.9).*

For general information about carbohydrates, blood sugar etc. see section 4.2.3.8.

3.16.2 Is there a Connection between the Blood Sugar Level and Negative-Lens-Induced Myopia?

In section 3.16.1 it was described that an elevated blood sugar level can induce at least transient myopia. In section 3.3 it was described that inappropriate, additional negative lenses can cause permanent axial myopia.

Note:
*Personal suspicion: If an eye becomes temporarily myopic due to elevated blood sugar level, and if therefore negative lenses are prescribed, these lenses are inappropriate during phases with normal blood sugar level. They might **cause in this interval lens induced myopia**, resulting in an elongated eyeball, i.e. axial myopia.*

*If these cycles are sufficiently long, and are repeated, a **permanent progression** to myopia might follow.*

Additionally, the hyperglycemic swelling of the lens might change the **mechanical properties of the lens**, contributing to an accommodative **hysteresis** (see section 1.3.3) and the **aftereffect of accommodation / the accommodative lag** (see section 3.2).

3.16.3 Calcium and Vitamin D

Calcium, magnesium and vitamin D have strong interactions. Because of this, they are described together.

- An evaluation of **statistical data for reported blindness due to malignant myopia in different states** of the USA was done by compiling a chart with the rate of myopia per state, and distance to seacoast, annual hours of sunshine and the nutritional concentration of calcium, fluoride and selenium in each state. One result was an inverse correlation between malignant myopia and calcium content in the water as well as annual hours of sunshine[55]. Annual hours of sunshine can serve as a measure of vitamin D supply.

- Starting in the 1930s Knapp, an American ophthalmologist was the first author to describe the impact of calcium and vitamin D according to his **experiences in his ophthalmologic praxis**[413]:

    - "In the course of being **fed vitamin D deficient, low calcium diets**, the eyes of dogs and rats revealed clinical myopia."

    - "Further research was conducted on humans, not patients with the usual slow progressive short sight, but painstakingly selected, highly progressive myopes from many thousands of patients. They were fed **supplements of vitamin D and calcium**. Over 50% of this rapidly progressive group, whose myopia would reasonably be expected to progress rapidly, instead showed a decrease in their myopia, or remained stationary. One third of the series registered a reduction in myopia."

- A publication of an ophthalmologist was getting high attention, because he claimed that by intake of animal protein progression of myopia in kids was reduced to only one third as before[414]. Later analysis revealed, however that what he accounted as the benefit of protein was the benefit of the **calcium in the calcium caseinate** he used[153].

    Note:
    Another possible explanation of this result is the fact that casein increases cNOS activity (see section 3.12.4 about the effect of NO on myopia, and section 4.2.3.4 about nutrition and NO).

- Experimentally induced myopia in animals was severely increased if a **calcium deficient diet** was used. Surprisingly, this was not the case with a vitamin D deficient diet. Overall, however, Hodos concludes[311], "... variables that effect eye growth include nutritional deficiencies of calcium and vitamin D."

- The highest **concentration of calcium in the hair** was measured in cases of increasing myopia, and calcium concentration was highest for myopes and lowest for emmetropes[153]. The literature about hair analysis states that elevated calcium levels are indicating not an

- oversupply with calcium but an accelerated calcium turnover in the body, caused e.g. by chronic stress, allergies or chronic infections[415].

- **Preterm children** are frequently myopic. Children with very low birth weight received supplementation with calcium and phosphorus – in the unsupplemented group 61% became myopic, in the group with supplements only 11% became myopic[416].

- During the **summertime**, the time of school holidays, the progression rate of myopia is significantly **lower**[92, 93, 94]. Part of the explanation may be a higher exposure to the sun, which means more supply of **vitamin D**, and more physical activities.

- The positive effect of a medication containing "Nacre" (see section 3.17) was attributed to an **increased content of calcium** in various tissues of the eye[357].

- The great increase in myopia found for Eskimos[78] may be related to nutritional changes, e.g. a reduction in fat-soluble vitamins (i.e. vitamins A and D) by a factor of 10[417]. Other possible factors are the reduced time spent outdoors and the increased amount of near work connected with schooling.

- There is a relation of **myopia and caries** of the teeth[327]. There is no doubt that caries is (among other reasons) related to calcium metabolism.

For general information about calcium see section 4.3.1.1, about vitamin D see section 4.3.2.6.

3.16.4 Magnesium

Due to an inherited disorder in the magnesium metabolism **hypomagnesemia** (i.e. a lack of magnesium), combined with hypercalciuria (i.e. increases excretion of calcium in the urine) can occur. Often this defect is accompanied by myopia and nystagmus[418, 419, 420].

It was concluded that the **Marfan syndrome** is related to metabolic magnesium deficiency[421] and to **excessive hyaluronic acid synthetase**[422]. People with Marfan syndrome are showing, among others, an extreme flexibility and mobility of their joints.

For general information about magnesium see section 4.3.1.4.

3.16.5 Copper and Zinc

Some results about the correlation between copper and zinc metabolism and myopia are:

- Vinetskaia et al. stated[423]: "Progressive myopia was found associated with **reduced copper content [in the tears]** and **changed ratio zinc to iron**, this indicating certain metabolic disorders in the connective tissue system, in the scleral membrane first of all, and in the antioxidant defense system."

- Qiang et al. stated[104]: "... there was a close relationship between juvenile myopia and ... **zinc/copper ratio** in hair ..."

- For myopes above – 6.0 D a **statistically significantly decreased concentration of copper** in the serum was measured[424]

  Note:
  *A reduced content of copper in the serum can be observed only for an **already substantial lack of copper**[765].*

- Avetisov et al. stated[425]: "Copper measurements in scleral tissue of 14 cadaveric emmetropic eyes and in 10 eyes with myopia of various degrees have shown a **significant reduction of copper** levels in the equatorial and posterior segments of myopic sclera and abnormal distribution of copper in the tissue, this indicating disordered metabolism of this trace element."

- Patients with progressive myopia received **injections with a copper-pyridoxine** (pyridoxine is vitamin B6) compound near to the sclera to stimulate the formation of collagen and improve the cross-linking of connective tissue fibers. After 3 year the refraction was stable for 64% of the patients[426].

- Patients with **low levels of diet-responsive copper-zinc superoxide dismutase** (CuZnSOD, an antioxidant enzyme) had a very substantially increased risk to develop structural defects in the vitreous body (*vitreous floaters*, which are common for myopes) than patients with a high level of CuZnSOD[38, 94].

- **Eye drops containing zinc were inhibiting experimentally induced myopia** in animals. It was concluded that this positive effect is due to a measured increased activity of superoxide dismutase (**SOD**), which prevents excessive processes of oxidation, and of nitric oxide (**NO**) and nitric oxide synthase (**NOS**)[427].

- **An Indian mixture containing "zinc, ascorbic acid and micronutrients"** was taken in capsules, and was reported to improve the myopia in certain cases[428].

- The Chinese myopia medication "**Nacre**" (see section 3.17) is containing zinc, copper and numerous trace elements, which results in **increased SOD, NOS and NO activity**[357].

  Note:
  Due to the numerous ingredients the principles of its efficiency are hard to judge.

- A **Zinc compound** (the Indian medicine "Yashad Bhasma") was evaluated. A two months use produced improvements in myopia. The results were, however, statistically not significant[429].

For general information about copper see section 4.3.1.3, about zinc see section 4.3.1.8., for general information about NO and NOS see section 4.2.3.4.

3.16.6 Chromium

Some results about the correlation between chromium metabolism and myopia are:

- Hair analysis was showing substantially **decreased chromium levels** for myopes, and especially for progressing myopia[153]. This was explained by a higher intake of refined carbohydrates, e.g. sugar. Sugar is said to deplete body stores of chromium. Matching with this is a result showing that myopes consumed only 39% as much fiber as hyperopes (i.e. farsighted people), which is interpreted as an increased consumption of refined food by myopes. Tissue chromium concentration was found to be negatively correlated with intraocular pressure (IOP) also (see section 3.6.2 on the impact of the IOP on myopia).

  The explanation given by Lane[153] is that "... the importance of chromium in visual function is probably due to its role as the potentiator of **insulin** at the insulin-receptor sites in blood vessels supplying the ciliary muscle."

  For the directly myopia related results of the impact of carbohydrates and insulin metabolism see section 3.16.1, for general information about the blood sugar level see section 4.2.3.8.

- The ratio of **chromium to vanadium in erythrocytes is depressed** for myopes.[430]

- The structure of the **retinal pigment epithelium** showed more damage for Chromium deficient rats[431].

- Chromium deficiency showed abnormal reactions of the **immune system** in the retina of rats[432].

- In myopic eyes of chicks a significant **decrease of chromium in the aqueous humor** was found[357].

For general information about chromium see section 4.3.1.2.

3.16.7 Manganese

Persons with **high hair manganese concentrations** were found to show increasing hyper**opia or decreasing myopia**[153].

A deficiency in manganese results in a **loss of photoreceptor cells and capillary anomalies** in the retina[433].

Note:
A connection with the antioxidant Mn SOD appears to be likely (see section 4.3.1.5).

For general information about manganese see section 4.3.1.5.

3.16.8 Potassium

The concentration of potassium in the hair of myopes was found to be **very significantly lower** than in emmetropes or hypertropes[153] (highest concentration at hypertropes).

For general information about potassium see section 4.2.3.9.

3.16.9 Iodine / the Thyroid Gland

A few results about the correlation between the metabolism of the thyroid gland and myopia are:

- The experience was reported that consequences of high myopia, like changes in the vitreous body or in the retina can be **positively influenced by iodine**[434]
- Increased rates of myopia were found for people with **enlarged thyroid glands** and people showing hyperthyroidism[435, 436]. It is well known that thyroid problems are often related to iodine metabolism.

Another essential constituent of thyroid hormones is **selenium** – Kohrle stated[437]: "The human thyroid gland has the highest selenium content per gram of tissue among all organs."

3.16.10 Vitamin A

In section 3.3.1 it was stated that retinoic acid is significantly involved in experimentally induced myopia (less all-trans-retinoic acid synthesis when myopia is built up). Whether vitamin A, the precursor of all-trans-retinoic acid, has any impact on this mechanism is unknown.

Besides this vitamin A (and zinc) are essential for night vision.

For general information about vitamin A see section 4.3.2.1.

3.16.11 B-Vitamins

Some results about the interaction between B-vitamins and myopia are:

- As reported in section 3.16.3 myopia is often accompanied by a disturbed calcium metabolism, measured by elevated calcium levels in the hair. Vitamin B6 (pyridoxine) is said to be able to **correct this disturbed calcium metabolism**[438].

- Vitamin B6 and B3 (pantothenic acid) are said to be helpful in regulation of **intraocular pressure** (IOP)[104].

- There was a correlation found between deficiency of vitamin B1 and of vitamin B2 and **nystagmus** and **disturbed eye tracking**[439]. Nystagmus is an uncontrolled, often rhythmical movement of the eyeball, and often accompanies myopia.

    According to the title of a Japanese publication juvenile myopia was treated with massive doses of vitamin B1[440].

- Peroxide oxidation of lipids is intensified in progressive, complicated myopia. Also, antioxidant defense parameters in the tear fluid are decreased, resulting in structural and pathological changes in the retina. Success was achieved by applying **locally an antioxidant medication containing vitamin B6** (and emoxypin, a structurally analogue of vitamin B6) via a film, which was placed behind the lower eyelid every evening for 15 days[441, 340].

- A lack of vitamin B6 is connected with an increase in the level of **homocysteine**, which can contribute to myopia. Homocysteine is discussed in section 3.16.13.

For general information about B vitamins see section 4.3.2.2.

3.16.12 Some More Antioxidants

3.16.12.1 Selenium

Some results about the correlation between selenium metabolism and myopia are:

- An evaluation of statistical data for **reported blindness due to malignant myopia in different states** of the USA was done by compiling a chart with the rate of myopia per state, and distance to seacoast, annual hours of sunshine and the nutritional concentration of calcium, fluoride and **selenium** in each state. As a result among others an inverse correlation between malignant myopia and selenium was found[55].

- Rats fed a diet higher in selenium (200 µg/kg diet) had **fewer cellular degenerating capillaries in the retina and a higher central choroid than those fed a diet of 100** µg/kg. Both levels of selenium, however, resulted in a normal activity of erythrocyte glutathione peroxidase, which is considered to be a marker for selenium sufficiency[442].

    Notes:
    - *Retinal defects are closely related to higher grades of myopia (see sections 1.7 and 3.12.4).*
    - *A reduced thickness of the choroid accompanies experimental myopia (see section 3.3.1).*
    - *Statements of sufficient selenium in the diet may be wrong.*

- The concentration of **selenium in the retina** of animals with excellent vision is up to 100 times as high as in the retina of animals with weak vision[443].

- Selenium deficient diets reduced the **amacrine cells and the photoreceptor cells in the retina** of rats and mice[432,444]. Amacrine cells were found to be important in deprivation experiments, where they were found to be involved in the dopamine signaling (see sections 3.3.2 and 3.7.1).

For general information about selenium see section 4.3.1.6.

3.16.12.2 Flavonoids and Related Compounds, and vitamin E

This family contains over 4000 different compounds. Some results of their effect are:

- It was claimed that **cyaninoside chloride** is effective to treat progressive myopia by protecting collagen against enzymatic attack by collagenase, showing antioxidant activity[445,446].

- The **magnesium chelate of flavones** named Flacitran was found in long-term treatments to have a positive effect on complications of malignant myopia. This was explained by its ability to hinder the buildup of degrading enzymes collagenase, elastase, hyaluronidase, and of histamines[447]. Collagen, elastase and hyaluronic acid are components of the connective tissues, and the ending "ase" indicates the degrading property. Histamines are mediators of inflammations.

- A medication containing **anthocyanosides** (e.g. bilberries) **plus vitamin E** had positive influence on progressive myopia and its consequences[448]. Similarly, diabetic retinopathies (which are caused by damages in capillary vessels) were successfully treated with anthocyanosides[449]. And there are numerous commercial claims that anthocyanosides from bilberries are helpful to treat myopia.

- A medication containing **troxerutin plus vitamin** E had a positive influence on the progression of myopia[450]. The effect was claimed to be based on the antioxidant anti-hyaluronidase properties of vitamin E, and the anti-hyaluronidase and anti-histamine properties of troxerutin.

- Bhutto et al. stated[451]: "...findings indicate that the **decrease in retinal capillaries** in vitamin E–deficient rats is secondary to retinal degeneration."

- Vitamin E can inhibit the **hyperglycemia induced elevated production of superoxide** in the retina[403].

- A **rutin compound** improved the **retinal microcirculation**[452]. For the relevance of microcirculation to myopia see section 3.11.

For general information about flavonoids see section 4.3.3.1, about vitamin E see section 4.3.2.7.

3.16.13 Folic Acid and Homocysteine

3.16.13.1 Observations

Some results about the interaction between homocysteine- and folic acid-metabolism and myopia are:

- A strong correlation of **food-folate intake with a reversal of myopia**, and with some reduction of the intraocular pressure (IOP) was found. Supplementation with the pharmaceutical form appears to be less effective than intake of food-folate[266].

    Note:
    The positive effect could be explained not only by the positive effect of folate, but also with food ingredients which are can frequently be found in food which is rich in folate, e.g. flavonoid.

- Numerous publications report high and very high myopia (among other symptoms) for people suffering from **homocystinuria**, an inherited defect that leads to abnormal high levels of the amino acid homocysteine in the serum[453, 454, 455, 456].

- The concentration of the amino acid **methionine** was 10-fold increased for people with extreme myopia[457] (for the role of methionine within the homocysteine metabolism see section 4.2.3.6).

- Mulvihill et al. stated[458]: "Young persons with marked and progressive myopia ... should be screened for homocystinuria."

For general information about folic acid see section 4.3.2.3, about homocysteine see section 4.2.3.6.

3.16.13.2 An Explanation

A very short explanation of the biochemistry that links the referenced observations[459, 460, 461] (for more details see section 4.2.3.6):

- **Homocysteine** is built from the other amino acid methionine by the metabolism as an intermediate product: Normally homocysteine is quickly recycled to methionine or finally transformed to cysteine. For these transformations especially folic acid, vitamin B6 and vitamin B12 are needed. A missing transformation can have genetic reasons, or a lack of appropriate quantities of folic acid, vitamin B6 and vitamin B12.

  Elevated levels of homocysteine, which is a powerful oxidant, can be the source of various serious health problems, including degraded cross-linking of collagen[288].

- A high intake of **proteins**, especially of meat, contains a high quantity of methionine and increases therefore the demand especially of folic acid and of vitamin B6.

Note:
A resulting lack of the amino acid cysteine can also degrade the generation of glutathione peroxidase (see section 4.2.3.2 about the impact of glutathione peroxidase, and section 4.2.3.6 about the homocysteine related cycle).

3.16.14 Other Components of the Diet

Some results about the impact of a few other nutrients on myopia are:

- Lane stated[438]: "Young myopes who are not increasing in myopia have a significantly lowered distribution of **flesh protein** intake compared to the distribution for young persons whose eyes are getting relatively more myopic..."

Note:
The more indirect reason might be that a diet more rich in meat would require higher amounts in other components of the diet (like vitamin B6 to keep homocysteine levels down, see section 3.16.13). Similar indirect nutritional effects appear to be very common.

3 Myopia – Observations and Experimental Results

3.16.15 Overall Nutritional Status and Myopia

So far nutritional components were mentioned, whose specific lack was found to be correlated with myopia. On the other hand, myopia exists primarily in developed countries, where under-nutrition is no problem at all.

Some **statistics**:

- Josephson stated[462]: "... noted that the percent of schoolchildren with **myopia rose and fell with the severity of the depression**, and linked that to nutrition: In 1925, it was reported that 25% of the schoolchildren attending a group of clinics in New York were afflicted with near-sightedness. With the advent of the depression, the figure rose steadily from over 40% in 1932 and to 72% in 1935. Reflecting re-employment and improved nutrition in 1036, the percentage incidence of near-sightedness dropped to about 51%. In 1937, the figure dropped to 42%."

- Edwards et al. stated[463]: "Children who developed myopia had a generally lower intake of many of the food components than children who did not become myopic. The differences were **statistically significant for energy intake, protein, fat, vitamins B1, B2, and C, phosphorus, iron and cholesterol**. Despite these differences, children who became myopic were neither shorter nor lighter..."

    Note:
    When children become myopic the nutrition-based conclusion does not have to be that they are getting less of specific nutrients. More likely, their individual demand for specific nutrients is higher (see the introduction of section 4)

Some **explanations**:

- The lack of specific nutritional components shows its effect on myopia only when it is **connected with extended near work**, i.e. in countries with a high rate of literacy. This high rate of literacy is often correlated with a lot of **indoor-time**, i.e. a potential lack of vitamin D (sunlight) and of physical activities.

- In developed countries the content of the individual components of the nutrition has been **changed** by far more than in countries where under-nourishing is still a problem, but where the traditional food is still the same as long ago.

    Moreover, the critical issue might be not the absolute content of a specific nutrient, but the **balance** between various nutrients (see section 3.16).

- Spanheimer et al. stated[464]: "Malnutrition is associated with **defects in connective tissue metabolism**..."

3.17 Pharmaceuticals

Overall, attempts to treat myopia by pharmaceutical agents (not considering the nutrients discussed in section 3.16) haven't led to generally accepted, positive results. Some results are:

- The main pharmaceutical agent tried for myopia, is **atropine**. Atropine is used commonly as a cycloplegic agent **to relax the ciliary muscle** completely before determining the refraction, especially for children. The summary of some reviewed publications is that atropine shows positive results in the first phase[465], but as Grosvenor et al. stated[466] it "does not stop the progression of myopia, but **only delays it**", i.e. a positive impact during application was counterbalanced by an increased progression after stopping the application. A result from experiments with chicks, published by Schwahn et al.[467], is: "Atropine suppressed myopia only at doses at which severe nonspecific side effects were observed in the retina."

  During application, attention has to be paid to avoid phototropic effects caused by an excess of light hitting the retina (as the pupil is staying wide open), and to provide binocular glasses for near work. There are other cycloplegic agents, which were examined (like tropicamide), with no convincing success, however[468].

  Tests with experimental myopia at animals showed that injections of atropine, which can help to increase dopamine levels in the eye, were successful only at high doses, which were accompanied by serious side effects in the retina[467]. In this experiment Atropine increased the **release of dopamine** (for the impact of dopamine on myopia see section 3.3.2).

  The effect of atropine on myopia cannot only be explained by its impact on the ciliary muscle (i.e. the blocking of accommodation) and the dopamine metabolism, but also by its reduction of the release of histamine[469], an agent of the **immune system**, which also helps to attack connective tissue (see section 4.2.2).

  There are concerns about **serious long time risks** caused by the permanent pupillary dilation[88].

- Related antimuscarinic agents like **pirenzipine** are being evaluated[470]. Some first and positive results were reported[471, 472]. Pirenzipine is said to be **more selective**, i.e. not having the side effects as severe as atropine on the iris (mydriasis), on the accommodation and the ciliary muscle[473, 474].

- **Adrenergic agents** (like timolol or metipranolol) are intended to decrease the intraocular pressure (IOP) as a potential reason for myopia. One author claimed to have success in treating myopia with the IOP-lowering **beta-blocker** Metipranolol[260], but other authors

- could not confirm this by using the other beta-blocker timolol[261]. Further research in this area is going on[475].

- The **Chinese medicine "nacre"** was used for tests with experimental myopia of animals. Nacre eye drops are made of the shell of pearls and consist of numerous trace minerals and amino acids. It was claimed that experimental eye elongation was reduced compared to control groups, and SOD activity and NOS activity, as well as NO content were increased. Moreover, the content of various minerals (calcium, zinc, chromium) in eye tissues was changed by this medication [357].

  Note:
  Due to the numerous ingredients the principles of its efficiency are hard to judge.

- For the treatment of choroidal neovascularization, which can accompany pathologic myopia (**CNV**, see section 1.7) there is a rather new therapy with the agent **verteporfin (trade name Visudyne)**. Activation of verteporfin by light (**photodynamic therapy**), in the presence of oxygen, creates short-lived reactive oxygen radicals, which results in local endothelium damage, resulting in occlusion of vessels.

- Chiou stated[353]: "It is possible that high **myopia can be prevented/treated with inhibitors of iNOS activity** and/or iNOS induction." Currently, however, there appears to be no practical treatment with these agents yet.

- Trier et al. steted[476]: "Methylxanthine, a metabolite of caffeine, **increases collagen concentration and the diameter of collagen fibrils in the posterior sclera**, and may be useful for treatment or prevention of conditions ... such as **axial myopia** ..."

  Note:
  Are coffee and tea therefore good against myopia?

For the future there are expectations of handling myopia more effectively by influencing the biochemistry of the retina, e.g. by increasing the dopamine level, than by influencing the strain on the ciliary muscle as was tried before[477, 478].

3.18 Congenital Myopia, and Inherited Diseases which are related to Myopia

There are two possible explanations for myopia at birth (**congenital myopia**):

- Without any pathologic biochemical malfunctioning **the eye can be simply too long already at birth** – according to the observed phenomena of large variations in size and shape of all kind of organs[273]. If the deviation from the normal length is too large, emmetropization can hardly fix it.

Open question: Will myopia progress in this case?

Amblyopia is a reduced visual acuity without visible pathologic defects. In most cases one eye only is affected. The affected eye is often highly myopic, which is named anisometropic amblyopia. To prevent the handicapped eye from being switched off the therapy consists generally of a part time occlusion of the well functioning eye (penalization). This switching off of one eye is often achieved also by the use of atropine eye drops. Unequal contact lenses need to be used if the handicapped eye has myopia of more than about 4 diopters, as glasses result in images of too different size on the retina.

Note:
It appears to be quite open, whether the myopia of the handicapped eye is caused by the amblyopia (according to optical effects described in section 3.3), or whether the congenital one-sided high myopia causes amblyopia.

- **Severe biochemical malfunctioning is already present** – malfunctioning which often shows symptoms other than high myopia. Most of these diseases are affecting the connective tissue. A number of these defects have been described (overall there are more than 150 genetic defects which are related to myopia[58]):

  - **Stickler's syndrome**, accompanied by bone, heart, ear and eye problems (besides myopia affecting vitreous body, retina, focusing, glaucoma), but usually patients do not have all the problems. Houchin stated[479] that Stickler's syndrome "is believed to be the most common syndrome in the United States and Europe, but one of the rarest to be diagnosed". Children with Stickler syndrome have a depressed nasal bridge, short nose and joint hypermobility[480].

    Note:
    These features remind of the features of many Asians, and Asians have substantially elevated rates of myopia.

  - **Marfan's syndrome**, accompanied by extreme mobility of the joints, dislocations of the lens of the eye, and heart problems (see section 4.3.1.4).

  - **Mitral valve prolapse (MVP)**, a heart problem (see also section 4.2.3.13), which is considered to be a generalized connective tissue problem. It is accompanied by an elevated rate of myopia (can be caused by Marfan's syndrome, but does not have to be caused by it)[481].

  - **Barlow syndrome** / mitral valve prolapse syndrome (a mild form of the Marfan's syndrome?), accompanied by heart problems, **and** extreme mobility of the joints.

  - **Ehlers-Danlos syndrome**, accompanied by accompanied by extreme mobility of the joints, osteoporosis, and ruptures of blood vessels.

- **Kearns-Sayre syndrome**, accompanied by paralyzed muscles of the eye, and heart problems.

- **Seckel syndrome**, accompanied by reduced growth and pigmentary retinopathy.

- **Cohen syndrome**, accompanied by psychomotor retardation and hyperextensibility of the joints.

- **Nystagmus**, i.e. uncontrolled, often rhythmical movements of the eyeball. Nystagmus can be congenital or develop at a later time.

As can be seen above, a **hypermobility of the joints**, which is based on a connective tissue problem frequently accompanies inherited myopia.

The result of a study about students in Turkey was that myopia is slightly more common among students with hypermobility[482].

Note:
The degree of myopia of the students with hypermobility was not investigated in this study – it would be plausible if the degree of myopia of the students with hypermobility is higher than that of the other students.

Until more research results will be published, **the best that can be done** in all these cases appears to be to follow overall recommendations which are given e.g. in this book. The malfunctioning biochemistry is unlikely to be exactly corrected, but hopefully some counterbalancing mechanisms can be activated. In this way, some degree of help may be found to correct the negative biochemistry. **At least it is worth trying!**

The syndromes mentioned above are describing **some very distinct diseases**. Far more often there are **just some deviations** from the "normal" status or from "normal" biochemical functioning, which has as one of its consequences the appearance of myopia. **Often this specific biochemical process is inherited, but it can be as well caused during pregnancy or by the circumstances of the birth. Or some behavior or habit or nutrition at a later age simply does not match with one of these biochemical processes.**

Therefore, pathological myopia can be considered as always congenital, in a certain way.

Note:
The reason for cases of congenital myopia does not always have to be a degraded connective tissue, which affects the sclera; it can be as well a metabolic defect which causes an exaggerated feedback process which is triggered by an image-quality-effect as outlined in section 3.3.

3.19 Other Means to Slow Down or Stop Progression of Myopia

3.19.1 Contact Lenses

Numerous experiences and experiments of ophthalmologists have shown that wearing **RGP (rigid gas permeable) contact lenses** instead of glasses can **slow down the progression of myopia** substantially[483, 484, 485]. A new study, however, **denied this**[486].

This positive effect has not been found for **soft contact lenses**[487]. In contrast, it was found that a switch from glasses **to soft contact lenses increased the progression of myopia** substantially, also adding a greater change in near-point phoria and a steepening of the corneal curvature[488].

Note:
A steepening of the corneal curvature increases refraction. Flat fitted hard contact lenses are flattening the corneal curvature; this effect is used in orthokeratology (see section 3.20.1.1).

The **positive effect of hard / rigid contact lenses** might be attributed to several different mechanisms:

- **Image quality and contrast** are better with hard contact lenses than with soft lenses[218]. Poor image quality and poor contrast are correlated with the appearance and progression of myopia (see section 3.3).

    Note:
    Is this the reason for **the missing positive effect of soft contact** *lenses on the progression of myopia?*

- A flat fitted lens can **flatten the cornea** (see section 3.20.1.1). However, this does not seem to help the slowing of myopia progression[489, 490, 357].

- Wearing **glasses results in less accommodation** compared with a normal eye, or compared with wearing contact lenses[123].

- It was said[139] that already Bates (see section 3.2.2) hinted at a connection between chronic visual problems and a lack of blinking. Wearing hard contact lenses **promotes blinking** by the slight irritation.

- Maybe the minor, but permanent irritation of the hard contact lens causes an **increases blood circulation**. Increased blood circulation was made responsible for the positive effect on myopia (see section 3.11), but in the literature this effect of hard contact lenses was not claimed to cause the positive effect myopia.

Note:
Maybe the fact that newer designs and materials of hard contact lenses are less irritating, can explain the result of a study[486], which found no positive result of hard contact lenses on the progression of myopia.

- Hard contact lenses can correct **astigmatism** up to a rather high degree. Whether astigmatism causes myopia appears to be not yet finally decided (see section 3.4).

- The transition to contact lenses has some impact on the **AC/A ratio** due to the higher accommodation, and due to an eliminated prismatic effect of the glasses[234] (see sections 3.4.2 and 3.4.4). These effects, however, are identical for hard and soft contact lenses.

- Rigid contact lenses reduce the amount of positive **spherical aberration** (see section 3.3.6)

Overall, the mechanism for a reduced progression by wearing RGP contact lenses is unclear so far, but apparently, it works well.

Note:
Contact Lenses and plus glasses for extensive near work *appear to be a useful combination.*

Contact lenses are necessary when there is a **substantial difference in the refraction of both eyes**, because with glasses the difference of both images on the retina is too large to result in one combined image (see also section 3.18 about amblyopia).

For more information about contact lenses see section 5.2.

3.19.2 Reinforcement of the Sclera

Some positive results for a reinforcement of the sclera were reported. The purpose of this treatment is, to place some support behind the sclera, and was done, e.g., by:

- An **injection** with a polymer composition, containing copper-pyridoxine (i.e. containing copper and vitamin B6) was placed near to the sclera to promote collagen formation[426].

- In a **surgical operation** the **synthetic material** mersilene was implanted, and a connective tissue capsule was built around it, with new collagen fibers growing through its cellular structure[491].

- In a **surgical operation** a **strip of the sclera from a donor eye** is placed around the eyeball to prevent further stretching[33].

It appears that these techniques are mainly applied in Eastern Europe, especially at the Helmholz Institute in Moscow. There are, however, negative reports from other countries[492]. According to the **high risk** of a treatment like this, it is normally restricted to very high grades of myopia.

3.19.3 Acupuncture

Some moderate decrease of up to –1.0 D by acupuncture was reported[493], and some success was reported for acupressure, too[494]. In trials with laser puncture it was concluded that the positive effect is based on improvements of the accommodation / convergence system[495].

Note:
Acupuncture depends to an extraordinary degree on the personal skill of the practitioner (and many people seem to work in this field with not necessarily this high qualification).

This reminds one of homeopathy: On one hand it seems to be esoteric, on the other hand there are numerous examples that homeopathy works in specific medical cases[496].

3.19.4 Electrostimualtion

One experiment reported that transconjunctival electrostimulation had positive effects on the accommodation, and slowed the progress of progressive myopia.[497]

3.20 Means to Correct Myopia

The methods described here are those that change the refractive properties of the eye itself, in contrast to external devices like glasses, and traditional contact lenses.

Surgical techniques should be used only when the degree of myopia has stabilized.

3.20.1 Manipulation of the Cornea

3.20.1.1 Orthokeratology

(General sources[498, 499])

If the base radius of the contact lens (see section 5.2.5) is substantially larger than the radius of the cornea of the eye, the lens is said to be fitted flat, and will cause the cornea to change towards the flatter shape of the contact lens. As a flatter cornea has less refractive power it can compensate for a low-grade myopia. Decreases of typically 1.0 to 2.0 D can be reached, which might be enough for many people to do without glasses or contacts lenses. As the flattened cornea will go back to its original shape over time, the procedure has to be occasionally repeated.

A report warned that overnight wearing of orthokeratology contact lenses may be harmful in children[500].

In more detail, an epithelial thinning in the center and a thickening at the edge is causing the refractive changes[501].

3.20.1.2 Radial Keratotomy RK

(General sources[502, 503])

Radial cuts are made in the cornea to change the radius of the surface. The method is used to treat myopia in the range of − 2.0 to − 6.0 D. Potential problems: Due to a limited acuity of the new refraction, glasses or contact lenses might still be required. Glare at night can occur.

3.20.1.3 Photorefractive Keratectomy (PRK)

(General sources[504, 357])

Removing corneal material by a laser reshapes the surface of the cornea. The method is used to treat myopia in the range of − 1.0 to − 6.0 D. Best results are achieved for myopia of up to − 3.5 D. Potential problems: Under- or over-correction can occur, but predictability is normally very good. Corneal haze can occur, and pain after the surgery is common.

3.20.1.4 Laser In Situ Keratomileusis (LASIK),
Laser Epithelial Keratomileusis (LASEK)

(General sources[477, 357, 505, 74])

The difference from PRK is that before operating the laser a surface segment of the cornea is flipped aside after cutting it off from the side. After the reshaping procedure with the laser, this surface segment is flipped back, allowing a very fast healing and providing an undamaged surface. While in **LASIK** the surgeon cuts a flap in the (deeper) stroma of the cornea, in **LASEK** the cut is done in the outer layers of the cornea, i.e. the epithelium.

The method is used to treat myopia in the range of − 1.0 to − 12.0 D (or even up to − 15 D). Predictability is normally very good (the lower the myopia, the better the predictability), and the lower the myopia, the better the stability of the new refraction[506]. Haze can still occur. Machet[507] stated: "Just as the good can be very good, the bad can be very bad".

For some hints before deciding on a surgery like this see section 5.3.

3.20.1.5 Intrastromal Corneal Ring

(General source[508])

A plastic ring is placed under the surface of the cornea, making the curvature of the cornea more flat. The ring is inserted in two semicircles in two surgically prepared channels in the surface of the cornea. The thicker the ring is, the higher is the achieved correction of the refraction. The method is used to treat myopia in the range of – 1.0 to – 4.0 D (or even up to – 6.0 D). The procedure is reversible by taking the ring out, or changing it. Results are not always predictable[479].

3.20.1.6 Artificial Cornea

(General source[509])

An implanted biocompatible polymer might be used one day to modify the refractive properties of the cornea. Xie et al. stated[509] that artificial corneas "…have the potential to become an alternative to spectacles and contact lenses for the correction of refractive error."

There are three different types of implants discussed: an implant that sits on the surface (i.e. replaces a segment of the epithelium, synthetic onlay), an implant that sits inside the cornea (i.e. in the stroma, synthetic inlay), and an implant, which replaces a full segment of the cornea (i.e. replaces a segment of the epithelium, the stroma and the endothelium).

3.20.2 Manipulation of the Lens System inside the Eye

(General source[510])

There are four alternatives changing the refraction of the lens system inside the eye:

- Removal of the biological lens
- Exchange the biological lens
- Addition an additional lens into the anterior chamber (i.e. in front of the iris)
- Addition an additional lens into the posterior chamber (i.e. between iris and own lens).

There is quite a substantial risk of severe complications for these operations e.g. like retinal detachment, or decrease in lens transmittance[511]:

"If today the only means available for correcting myopia consisted of [surgery] and tomorrow somebody invented glasses or contacts, he'd win the Nobel Prize hands down."[512]

Exchange of the biological lens: This surgery is similar to the common surgery for patients with a cataract and is done at refractions over – 10 D.

For older people successful posterior chamber implantation of multifocal intraocular lenses was reported[513].

For patients with a cataract there are new reports about artificial lenses, which are able to accommodate in quite the same way as the original lens[514]. The future will show, whether this will be an alternative for myopic patients, too.

Adding an additional lens: The additional lens can be inserted either into the anterior chamber (i.e. in front of the iris), or into the posterior chamber (i.e. between iris and own lens). This technique is applied for refractions over – 8 D up to over – 25 D.

First results of these techniques were quite promising[515], [516] (the last one by the American FDA with 523 eyes) but further trials are necessary.

An analysis of the actual and the theoretical risks for implantable contact lenses (ICL) for moderate to high myopia showed that the risk for visual loss by these lenses is even lower than for LASIK or PRK[517].

Note:
On the one hand these operations are rather similar to standard and low-risk operations in ophthalmology, on the other hand every operation is carrying some risk of infection, and additionally there is the serious general risk of long-term effects. These long-term effects are not so important for older cataract patients, but are especially important for young patients.

There are new developments in the design of the lenses: for bifocal applications diffractive lenses were found to be superior compared with refractive lenses[518]. Diffractive lenses are built by tiny microstructures on the surface of the lens; refractive lenses are like conventional lenses[519].

3.21   Summary: What Causes Myopia?

Three main mechanisms appear to lead to myopia:
- **Optically initiated effects**, including some effects caused by accommodation. These involve some so far unspecified biochemical processes. The normal balanced eye growth of childhood (emmetropization) doesn't occur.
- **Mechanical effects**, including effects caused by accommodation, which enforce an elongation of the eyeball – in connection with an unfortunate geometry and weak connective tissue.

- **Systemic connective tissue degrading processes**, which are sometimes rather pathologic, and which often appear to have a genetic reason.

All the other mechanisms, given above as potential causes of myopia, are possibly using various sub-mechanisms of one of these processes, and may take place simultaneously.

Near work and accommodation apparently play a key role in the development of myopia. However, not everyone is affected by these factors. Therefore other processes must be very important as well. These processes are obviously playing a big role in progressive and in pathologic myopia.

Maybe all the pathways mentioned above are biochemically or logically **combined, e.g.:**

- **Optical effects** might in fact result in **connective tissue degrading** effects to remodel the shape of the eye.
- **Mechanical effects** might induce transient **optical blur**, cause over correction, and cause myopia by these **optical effects**.
- **Mechanical effects** might cause **connective tissue degrading effects** (e.g. via temperature).

Consequently, preventing myopia or stopping the progression of myopia might be achieved one day by interrupting the (sometimes rather long) sequence of biochemical process-event-steps, which finally lead to modified or degraded connective tissue structures in the eye.

This can only be done in one of the following ways:

- Modify **personal behavior and/or environment**.
- Modify **nutrition**.
- Make a **massive pharmaceutical intervention**.

The advice resulting from personal behavior were referenced already in section 3.8 and section 3.19.1. **A total summary of recommendations is given in section 4.8.**

Section 4 will cover some of these potential biochemical process-event-steps, which might be influenced by nutrition (and which were already mentioned in section 3.16). No pharmacological correction for myopia is available so far.

Finally, it should be remembered (see section 3.13.2) that there are reasons that via biochemistry myopia is linked to the personality of the myopic person, which cannot be handpicked, either. **And if you are happy with your personality, you might consider myopia as a price to pay for it.**

3.21.1 School and Myopia

The simple, non-pathologic, non-progressive form of myopia is sometimes called school myopia. According to the results presented above schooling may, however, have some basic influences on myopia, which might play a role for progressive myopia, too.

- Being a student implies a lot of **near work** and accommodation, and additionally a **frequent change** between near work and viewing the writing on the distant blackboard. This environment, together with the **hysteresis of accommodation, of the ocular shape and even of the ocular lens** (see section 3.6) can result in children being unable to read the blackboard properly, and they will get glasses. This **cycle may repeat and repeat**, resulting in a progression of myopia.

- Depending on the personality of the child, and of the performance requirements set by the school, the child may be **stressed by educational requirements**; for the impact of stress on myopia see section 3.13.

- Frequently school is connected with a long period of immobilization, and a **lack of physical activity**; for the potential impact of physical activity on myopia see section 4.2.3.10.

3.21.2 Is Myopia Caused by Mechanical or by Biochemical Processes?

It looks like that there can hardly be a compromise between the proponents of a completely mechanical explanation ("accommodation-forces are responsible") of myopia and the proponents of a completely biochemical explanation ("image quality is responsible", "genetics are responsible", "nutrition is responsible").

There is, however, a linkage between the two kinds of explanation: mechanical forces initiate biochemical changes, a process called **mechanotransduction**, which was already discussed for explaining the development of myopia[197].

This model was supported by the result that **scleral fibroblasts, which were mechanically stretched, showed significant changes in gene expression**[107].

Note:
Together with the fact that accommodation generally results in a temporary elongation of the eye (see section 3.2.1.1) this impact of mechanical strain on gene expression and herewith on biochemical processes could alone explain a development of myopia.

3.21.3 Prevention of Progression of Myopia or Prevention of Myopia

The progression of myopia is fought with the same tools that prevent it in the first place.

Generally it is very difficult, however, to convince people (especially children) to take action **before** a problem appears. It is the more necessary to take this prophylactic action if there is a problem of myopia already in the family.

> The good news is, however that apparently there are means to fight against myopia and the progression of myopia – **you just have to face the problem and make the effort!**

3.21.4 Working against Myopia or against the Consequences of Myopia?

The proposed means can work to stop the progression of myopia, e.g. by stabilizing the degraded connective tissue, but they can also be helpful in preventing the serious consequences of higher grades of myopia (which were mentioned in section 1.7).

This prevention of consequences is in fact the most important issue, considering the tragedy of a potential blindness!

3.21.5 Inflammation towards Progressive and Pathologic Myopia

It appears to be very plausible that lower degrees of myopia are largely caused by optical effects, which lead via emmetropization to a moderate elongation of the eyeball. As Celorio et al. expressed[520]: "...[results] support the belief that **progressive myopia is a condition distinct from the more common mild degrees of myopia.**"

High, progressive or even pathologic myopia, however, can be said to have – additionally – the basis in **exaggerated reactions of the immune system, i.e. in processes of inflammation.**

Therefore people, who are affected by this type of serious myopia, should pay special attention to these key words when reading the following section 4.

3.21.6 Functional- versus Structural- Deficits

Structural defects can be responsible for more severe myopia, i.e. the process of viewing and focusing is working normally, but the structure of the tissue is degraded. Alternatively, myopia can be due to **functional defects**, i.e. the structure of the tissue is normal, but the process of viewing and focusing is not working normally.

To be more specific, there can be these cases:

- **Structural deficits alone** (e.g. Marfan syndrome)
- **Functional deficits alone** – they can be **optical** (e.g. heavy esophoria at near) or **biochemical** (e.g. an exaggerated feedback loop of image related effects, see section 3.3)
- **Structural deficits cause additional functional deficits** (e.g. degraded connective tissue results in decreased stability of the sclera and decreased performance of the ciliary smooth muscle)
- **Functional deficits cause additional structural deficits** (e.g. form deprivation experiments cause degraded connective tissue)
- **A third reason** causes both structural and functional deficits (e.g. **mental stress** with all its implications: degraded connective tissue, accommodative spasms etc.)

Note:
It appears to be logical that

- for functional deficits optical means are most appropriate (at least until there are means to control the feedback loop of image related effects)

- for structural deficits systemic means, i.e. via nutrients are most appropriate. Structural deficits are probably the major reason for progressive myopia and pathological myopia.

The mental issue can have a very strong impact on myopia (see section 3.13), and **mental conditions can influence functional processes as well as processes which may lead to structural problems.**

3.21.7 Are the Published Results really Contradictory? Maybe not!

Maybe the published results about the reasons for myopia and its progression are not as contradictory as they seem. Maybe the following personal view (which might have been expressed by other people before as well) explains many (not all) of the published results:

- During accommodation the eye is **squeezed by the ciliary muscle in transverse direction, and as a consequence elongates via the hydraulic intraocular pressure IOP** (see sections 1.3.3, 3.6.5 and 3.6.2).
- Poor **image quality leads to a local degradation of the connective tissue**, which allows remodeling of the ocular shape (see section 3.3.3). Possibly this remodeling is caused via

tissue-turnover-regulating processes, and mechanisms that involve processes of the immune system.

- **Both effects**, an increased pressure in the direction of elongation, and a biochemically-weakened structure work **in the same direction: myopia. Moreover mechanical stress can initiate biochemical alterations via a process called mechanotransduction.**

- Other observed influences, e.g., the impact of **mental stress, illumination, and weaker inborn connective tissue** support the mentioned basic effects of pressure and local tissue degradation. Obviously myopia is correlated with lower amplitude / lag of accommodation (section 3.2) and with a somewhat degraded connective tissue. **A softer relaxed ciliary muscle, and softer zonule fibers result in less tension for pulling the lens into the flat distant-focus shape.**

An important key word about all these potential mechanisms is **emmetropization**, i.e. the ability of the eye to adjust the eye-growth in length during development for optimal optical imaging – with a corresponding myopic adjustment if near focus is a major environmental requirement. Combined with the tissue degrading effects found at experimental myopia it could be concluded that **near work might control eye growth through tissue degrading effects**. Consequently, a **strategy to prevent (progression of) myopia should improve near work conditions, and/or tissue degrading biochemical conditions** (i.e. to reduce what is called in section 3.3.5 the "emmetropization factor").

As a consequence, the most important tools to prevent progression of myopia would be:

- **Reduction of accommodative and other stress** e.g. via reading with appropriate distance only or appropriate undercorrection for reading
- **Optimize image quality**, e.g. via good illumination
- **Strengthening of the connective tissue**, e.g. via optimized nutrition which helps to prevent degradation, which might be caused by local effects (e.g. via poor image quality) or by systemic processes (see section 4).

According to this model, the development of myopia can be simplified as shown in Figure 11 **and** Figure 12.

3 Myopia – Observations and Experimental Results

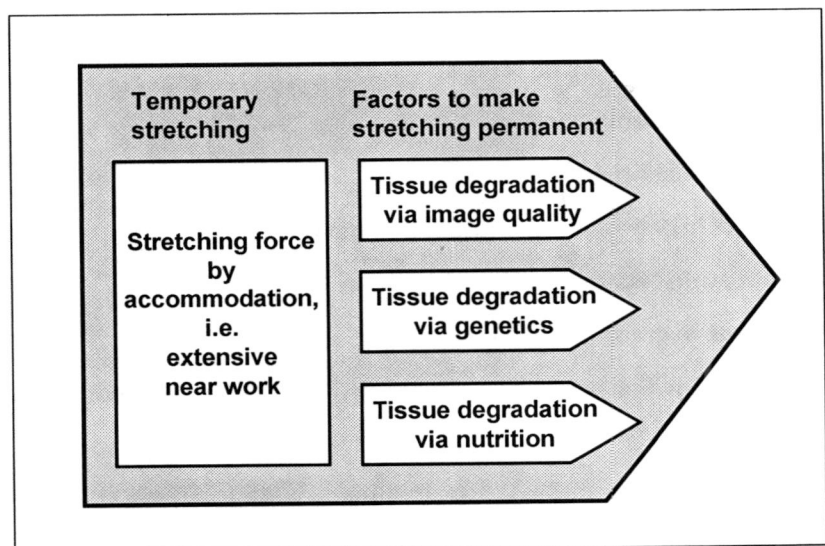

Figure 11 The process of myopia development - very simplified

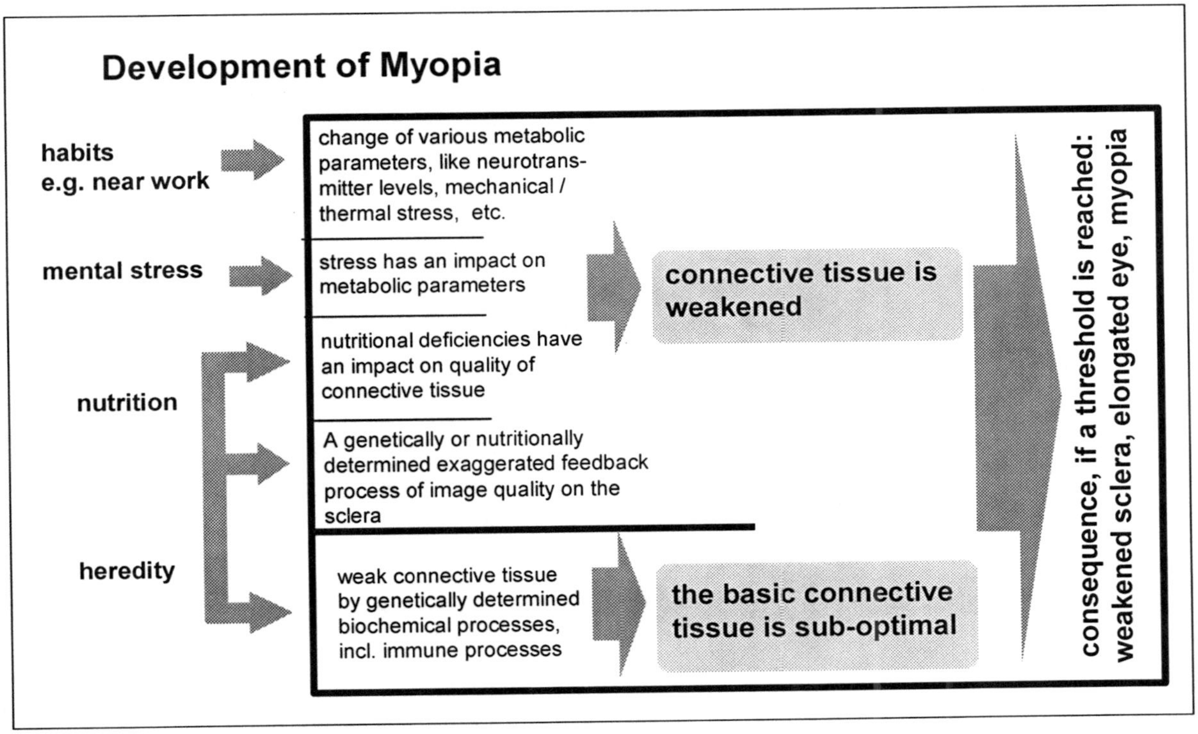

Figure 12 The process of myopia development – more detailed

As a summary for section 3 the main problem for **serious progressive and pathologic myopia** (not for the low grade school myopia) can be seen in

- an overreacting immune system
- an overreacting image-feedback system
- an abundance of highly reactive oxidizing radicals
- an insufficient antioxidant system
- connective tissue degrading processes
- a lack of nutrients, which are needed for the synthesis of connective tissue.

Some biochemical details will be discussed in section 4. They might offer some means to fight against pathologic myopia and its consequences.

The difference between not very problematic, stable myopia and progressive myopia can be explained as shown in Figure 13.

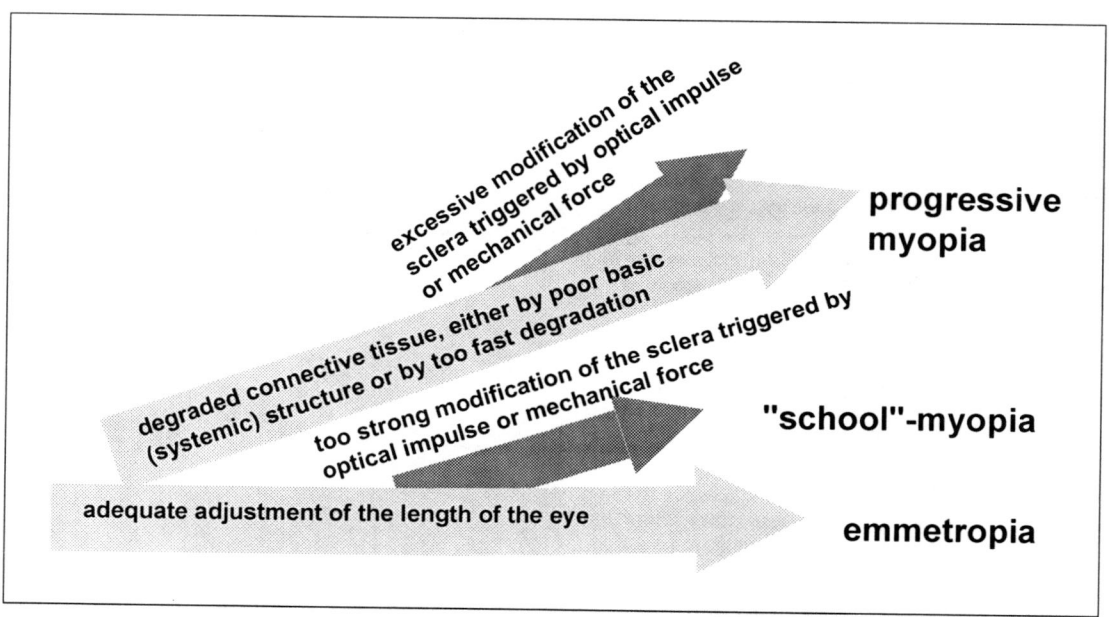

Figure 13 The different paths to "school"-myopia and progressive myopia

And the means for prevention and prevention of progression can be roughly described as shown in Figure 14.

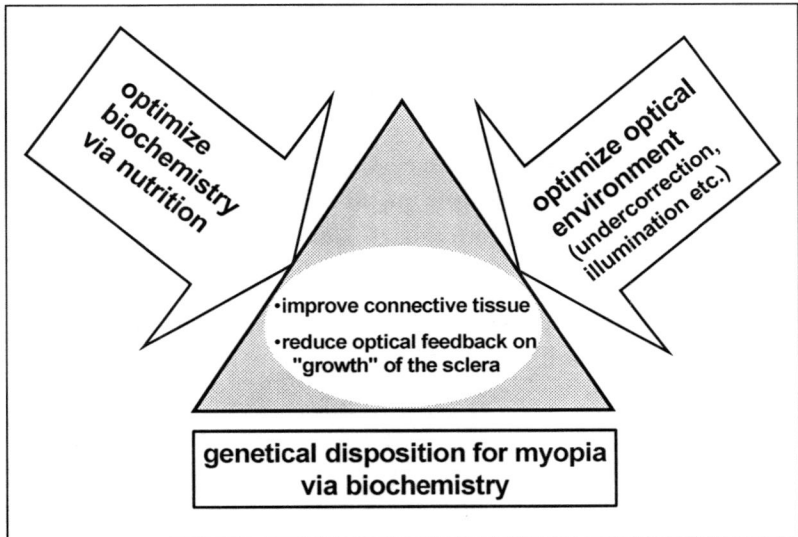

Figure 14
The means for the prevention of the progression of myopia

Optimizing the optical environment is important for **everybody**. In addition, optimizing biochemistry via nutrition is extremely important when fighting **progressive, more pathological** myopia.

4 A Synthesis – or how some Pieces might Fit together

So far, this book contained merely a compilation of summaries of significant publications about causes and treatment of myopia.

I will present some conclusions in this chapter by linking this information to published results in related biochemical areas.

The main target group of readers for this section is people with higher grades of myopia, i.e. with a probable systemic problem of the connective tissue. For this group it is most necessary to take some action to avoid the potentially very serious consequences (see section 1.7) of high myopia.

The point is that every event that leads to myopia is based on a long chain of biochemical processes. Research has already revealed some of these processes, but many causal connections are still unclear. In general, the situation looks as shown in Figure 15.

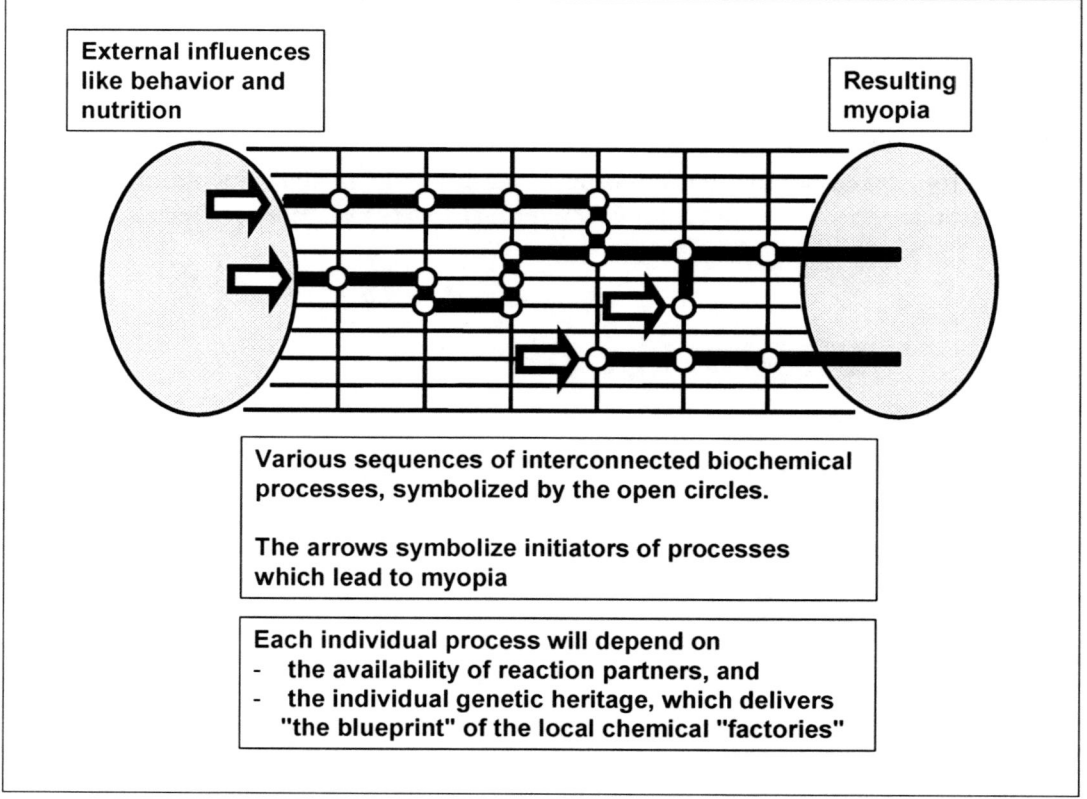

Figure 15 The biochemical paths to myopia – very schematic

4 A Synthesis – or how some Pieces might Fit together

Some facts are:

- **Several initiating events** might lead to myopia.

- Some of the initiating events are **external,** and can be influenced directly via external means (e.g. by behavior, environment and/or nutrition). Examples: See section 3.16.

- Some of the initiating events are **internal**, i.e. genetically controlled biochemical processes can cause them. Sometimes these processes can be still influenced by external means, e.g. by nutrition[521]. It was found that in many cases of inherited enzyme defects high doses of the vitamin component of the corresponding coenzyme can at least partially restore enzymatic activity[522, 523].

- There is **no general remedy** that can fix all problems.

- In contrast to experiments with animals, which apparently always lead to myopia, **people do not react uniformly,** i.e. when exposed to the same environment and the same nutrition, some people become myopic and some will not. In other words, for people there are apparently ways to counterbalance the impact of events that lead to myopia for other people.

- Numerous internal and systemic diseases have specific effects on the eye[524].

The target should be, therefore, to do the best possible to prevent myopia or prevent progression of myopia by **optimizing every process that can be externally influenced.** The mentioned counterbalancing mechanisms should be promoted and enforced, as they prevent some people from becoming myopic, even when people living under the same circumstances become myopic. Sometimes a less than optimal working biochemical process can be compensated to some degree by optimizing other processes by external influence, as mentioned above - like giving a badly designed engine the best motor oil available.

For some processes, it appears (as will be shown in the next sections) that there are linkages between processes that trigger myopia. They may not be isolated, as one would think from reading the scientific literature.

As already mentioned, there are clear guidelines for proper "optical" behavior (see Section 3.8), and therefore nutrition is the main alternative tool for corrective action.

4.1 Some General Remarks about Nutrition and Environment

4.1.1 Biochemistry versus Mechanical Effects versus Optical Effects?

The fact that this section 4 deals primarily with nutrition and biochemistry does not mean that mechanical aspects and optical aspects are considered to be of minor importance.

These mechanical and optical aspects are not questioned in any way. However, my recommendation is to find biochemical mechanisms that have a **positive influence on these mechanical and optical processes and properties.** Conclusions and recommendations which are directly following from the optical or mechanical observations are fully valid – see section 3.8.

4.1.2 Nutrition and the Environment have Changed Dramatically

The health status of numerous populations has significantly changed due to "modern" nutrition. Extensive research since the 1920s has shown this. This fact could be demonstrated best by analyzing populations whose nutritional habits have been changed within a very short time. Most obvious was the change in the development of the teeth - not only showing plain caries, but primarily serious complete disarrangements of the teeth, as described in the classic book "Nutrition and Physical Degeneration" by W.A. Price[525]. This is caused by substantial changes in nutrition, i.e. considerably increased intake of empty calories/carbohydrates, changes in the content of nutrition by depletion of the soil, increased intake of processed food, and consequently decreased intake of micronutrients like trace minerals, vitamins and amino acids[526].

For example the very large increase of myopes among Eskimos can be explained not only by an increase in near work (school), but also by very significant changes in nutrition. Price writes[417]: "The foods of the native Eskimos contained 5.4 times as much calcium as the displacing foods of the white man, five times as much phosphorous, 1.5 times as much iron, 7.9 times as much magnesium, 1.8 times as much copper, 49.0 times as much iodine, and at least ten times that number of fat-soluble vitamins."

In contrast, populations in Pacific islands, which kept their traditional diet, had no increase in myopia in spite of transition to extensive schooling[405]

The **general effect of changed nutrition was demonstrated** by comparing the arterial stiffness of Chinese recently immigrated to Australia with long-term Chinese residents in Australia. Dart et al. stated[527]: "...with recent migrants eating significantly more rice meals." Result: "Increasing duration of Australian residence appears to be accompanied by an increase in proximal arterial stiffness."

4 A SYNTHESIS – OR HOW SOME PIECES MIGHT FIT TOGETHER

Apparently the nutrition in early life is especially important. Bergner stated[528]: "Diet during pregnancy and childhood can determine the status of health in adult life..." Especially for parents of young kids there is the temptation, to please the children with empty snacks and give in to them if they don't like their proper meal.

Our genes are optimized for **best adaptation to the food available to our Paleolithic ancestors**, who were hunters and gatherers about 200 000 years ago to about 12 000 years ago. A comparison of their food and the food of today is shown in Table 7[529]:

	Paleolithic intake	U.S. Recommended Dietary Allowance	Current U.S. intake	Average ratio paleolithic intake/ Current U.S. intake
Vitamins, mg/day				
A (retinol equivalents)	17.2	4.80 – 6.00	7.02 – 8.48	2.22
B1	3.91	1.1 – 1.5	1.08 – 1.75	2.76
B2	6.49	1.3 – 1.7	1.34 – 2.08	3.80
C	604	60	77 - 109	6.49
Folic acid	0.357	0.180 – 0.200	0.149 – 0.205	2.02
E	32.8	8 - 10	7 - 10	3.86
Minerals, mg/day				
Calcium	1956	800 - 1200	750	2.61
Sodium	768	500 - 2400	4000	0.19
Potassium	10500	3500	2500	4.20
Iron	87.4	10 - 15	10 - 11	8.32
Zinc	43.4	12 - 15	10 - 15	3.47
Fiber, g/day	104	20 - 30	10 - 20	6.93
Energy, kJ/day	12558	9209 - 12139	7326 - 10465	1.41
Phytochemicals, i.e. flavonoids etc	Eaton et al. stated[529]: "...it is plausible to suspect that their [paleolithic] concentrations may be relatively high, like those of micronutrients."			

Table 7 Comparison of paleolithic nutrition with the nutrition of today

Note:
*To be fair it has to be mentioned that the evolutional adaptation and selection which took place in paleolithic times had most likely **different targets than we have today**: Physical strength and a strong immune system had a higher priority than today, whereas compared with today a different kind of psychological robustness was required. Maybe, however these previously very high requirements for the **immune system** and our adaptation to these requirements are a problem today (see sections 3.12 and 4.2.2).*

Evolution could not keep pace with the speed of nutritional, behavioral and environmental changes: According to Darwin's famous results, evolution was optimizing individual populations with respect to the local demand. The period for adjustments like this has to cover many generations. In contrast to these long-term processes nutrition (and overall life style) have been changed very much within a very short time. In line with this view myopia, even high-grade myopia, could be considered not just as a defect, but also as an optimization of the organism according to other priorities.

In fact, there are many changes overall which have happened to mankind within a very short time. The effects of these changes are shown in Table 8:

Changes	The reasons	The effects
Nutrition	- Changed **eating habits** (e.g. more empty carbohydrates and meat) - **Depletion of the soil** by intensive agriculture - Industrial **processing of food** removes nutrients - **Migration** of people results in confrontation with different eating habits	Disturbed **nutritional balance**, **lack** of individual nutrients, see section 3.16
Work and behavior	- More **near work** (school, office work, less "blue collar work")	- Disturbed **focusing** mechanisms, see sections 3.2, 3.3
	- More **mental stress** at work (examinations, qualifications)	- Disturbed **biochemical processes**, see section 3.13
Environment	- Less **physical activities** (mainly sitting at work, easy transportation) - Different exposition to **sunshine** (indoor work, living in the city)	- Impact on various **metabolic functions** (e.g. less vitamin D built-up, less vitamin B6 storage, modified folic acid protection), see section 3.1
	- Artificial **illumination and television**	- Modified **day- /night-rhythm**, see section 3.7.1
	- **Cleaner environment** (at home and in public), and extensive application of **vaccinations**	- Impact on the **immune system**, see section 4.2.2

Table 8 Modern lifestyle and its impact

Sure, not necessarily all the findings referenced in the following sections can be transferred completely to the biochemistry of the eye, and not all the results found in experiments with animals are valid for humans. These experiences are giving, however, enough reasons to try to make use of them, especially if their application can hardly do any harm.

Generally, an optimized nutritional supply can work via any one of the following mechanisms:

- **Improve the disturbed biochemical process** that leads to myopia, by modifying it.
- Improve the **result of the disturbed biochemical process** that leads to myopia, by supplying it with a modified balance of participating nutritional components.
- Help to **minimize the negative consequences** of the disturbed biochemical process, which leads to myopia.

4.1.3 There is a very Large Biochemical Individuality

There is no standardized "normal" biochemical functioning or anatomy of the body. Very large variations of the respective parameters exist, and consequently the specific demand for specific components of nutrition is very different for different people[273, 530, 531]. Often a high-dose vitamin therapy can help with genetic disorders and diseases[522]. Just two examples: Due to inherited metabolic anomalies some people require 5-50 times the normal dose of vitamin B6[523], and the need for the amino acid lysine was shown to have a seven-fold variation in a sample of 55 people[532].

Price stated[525]: "In line with the concept of "biochemical individuality", as expressed by Dr. Roger Williams, which postulates the inheritance of acquired partial enzyme blocks, many patients need vitamin and mineral supplements for optimal health, and even for normal metabolism."

Another proof of biochemical individuality is the statement by Connor[533]: "**Most drugs work in fewer than one in two patients mainly because the recipients carry genes that interfere in some way with the medicine.**"

This biochemical individuality can exist on a personal basis, or can involve very large populations – e.g. the prevalence of myopia in Asia. It can be considered as well as just a different description of individual genetic biochemistry.

A typical case of biochemical individuality is the specific nutritional need of people with G6PD deficiency (see section 4.2.3.12).

4.1.4 There are Biochemical Alterations before Clinical Symptoms Arise

Many people consider the supply with nutritional components to be sufficient as long as there are no clinical symptoms, and that in industrial countries there is hardly any nutritional deficit. In contrast to this "traditional" opinion it has been stated that long before there are clinical symptoms of a deficit there will be modifications in cell structures and sub-cellular structures. These will have functional consequences[534]. Moreover, as stated above, the term "nutritional deficit" is compared to some "normal" requirement, which was found hardly to exist[273]. This situation, however, creates a problem: How to find the personal requirements? Hopefully the next sections will give some assistance. Overall, often not even the recommended daily amounts of minerals are met[526].

4.1.5 There can be Selective Nutrient Deficiency

There can be selective nutrient deficiency in one cell line or one specific kind of tissues of a patient, without a deficiency in other cell lines or tissues[535]. Processes like this make it very difficult to diagnose local deficiencies that might contribute to (progressive) myopia, because e.g. an analysis of the blood serum might give no hint about a local deficiency in the eye.

4.1.6 Summary – the Balance

Here are some very general conclusions from the results of the following sections:

- Health is not best when some biochemical levels are highest or lowest, but when there is **appropriate balance**. The **balance of NO (cNOS vs. iNOS), TH1/TH2, blood sugar level / corresponding insulin level, sodium/potassium level,** and **cortisol** levels appear to be especially important for myopia.

- It appears likely that serious, progressive myopia is not a simple local process, but a rather **systemic process**, which involves multiple biochemical processes of the whole body.

- Most of the main factors affecting myopia **interact with each other**, i.e. a deviation of one of them can easily cause deviations of others. This refers to factors like immune system, neurotransmitter metabolism, NO balance, and last not least (psychical) stress.

  Therefore the apparently conflicting results of myopia research are not contradictory, but complementary.

- As myopia was not an issue some hundred years ago, **something must have been changed**. And this change offers the chance to counteract, i.e. to do something, which works to balance this change. This can be only:

- **Personal behavior and environment** – to balance the impact of modern life, as mentioned in the introduction to section 4.
- **Avoiding stress** – also related to modern life, sounds more easy than it is.
- **Nutrition** – to balance the impact of modern nutrition and migration to countries with different eating habits and less sunshine. Nutrition will be discussed in more detail in the following section.

There is just one change which cannot and should not be reversed: For the immune system the substantially reduced exposition to infections, and the introduction of vaccinations was a big change that might affect the vulnerability to autoimmune diseases which can involve the connective tissue, and for myopia autoimmune effects were found as well (see section 3.12). The price, however, to give up vaccinations is by far too high (in spite of the fact that some people are nowadays arguing against vaccinations).

4.2 Some Relevant Biochemical Key Issues

I have touched on some biochemical issues in previous chapters, like connective tissue, immune system etc. In the following sections some basic fact and explanations about these issues will be given in order to draw conclusions relevant to fighting myopia.

4.2.1 The Connective Tissue

From the results presented it can be concluded that the "health" of connective tissue is essential: even poor image quality resulted in degradation of connective tissue 3.3.3. Generally, sub optimal connective tissue includes:

- **A disturbed basic structure**, e.g. caused by inherited metabolic defects (see section 3.18). Berg et al. stated[536]: "Genetic diseases that result in mutations within the triple-helical region of type I collagen [which constitutes the sclera] that is also incapable of assuming a triple helix and is subject to this pathway of intracellular degradation of newly synthesized collagen."
- **Exaggerated feedback processes**, triggered by external influences like poor image quality, infections, elevated temperature, etc.
- **Deviations of individual nutritional needs.**

The various potential mechanisms which will be discussed in the following sections all end up with some impact on the connective tissue, even if they are starting at very different areas, like nutrition, immune system, mental stress, etc.

4.2.1.1 Connective Tissue in General

(General sources[537, 538, 539])

The connective tissue consists of fibers, ground substance, adhesive glycoproteins, and specialized connective tissue cells.

- The **fibers**: Collagen fibers consist of proteins, synthesized by various connective tissue cells (fibroblast, chondroblasts etc). In detail, there are 14 different kinds of collagen, and normally they are organized into long, dense, closely packed bundles of interlinked fibers, with very many cross-links between fibrils. Basic materials are various amino acids like lysine and proline, whereas the enzyme lysyl oxidase is important for the cross-linking – the types and the amounts of cross-links are largely responsible for the strength of the fibers. At least 25 different genes are encoding the 14 types of collagen[536].

    Elastin fibers are made of protein as well, and their elasticity is achieved by an arrangement of fibers in relaxed cross-linked coils.

- **Ground substance** is filling the space between fibers and cells, and consists of gel-like polymers, i.e. **proteoglycans** like hyaluronic acid etc.

- **Adhesive glycoproteins** play a part to hold the connective tissue structure together.

- The main **connective tissue cells** are the blood cells, fibroblasts (which build collagen and elastin), macrophages (scavenger cells to attack hostile microorganisms etc.), and mast cells (which are producing histamine and other agents that trigger responses of the immune system). These cells can therefore be considered as the control units of the connective tissue.

There is a **permanent and normal process of degradation and rebuilding of connective tissue, called turnover**. In case of inflammations, the rate of degradation is higher than the rate of synthesis (negative turnover balance). Typical turnover rates may be 2% – 5% per day [536, 540, 541, 542]. What is needed is a proper balance of degradation and synthesis of the connective tissue, i.e. the **appropriate turnover rate**. Various parameters influence the turnover rate, e.g. physical activity and exercise, dietary deficiencies, hypertension, increased heart rate etc.[288, 540].

Note:
Maybe strenuous accommodation is weakening the ciliary muscle structure of some people by an increased rate of turnover.

The strength of the connective tissue can therefore handicapped by two processes:

- **High rate of degradation**, negative turnover balance.
- **Low quality of collagen** fiber structure, including cross-links.

However, the two processes are interrelated. Volk et al. stated[540]: "Differences in amino acid composition of cross-links influence the stability and turnover of these fibers", i.e. low quality cross-links are chemically less stable.

Consequently, degraded connective tissue / degraded collagen fibers can be based on either:

> - **Poorly built fiber structure**, due to either a lack of necessary ingredients for building, or an (often inherited) enzymatic tendency for imperfectly building of fibers and cross-links.
> - **Too heavy, exaggerated influence of degrading agents**, like collagenase and cytokines, due to actions e.g. of the immune system or other controlling mechanisms.

Both alternatives are candidates for an elongated and sclera-weakened eyeball, i.e. myopia.

Numerous papers are describing the influence of nutrition on collagen [536, 288]. This will be discussed in more detail in the following sections.

There are very strong indications that the immune system plays a key role in maintaining the integrity of the connective tissue (see section 4.2.2).

Many **problems other than myopia** have been attributed to a sub-optimal connective tissue[539] (see also section 3.18).

4.2.1.2 The Connective Tissues of the Eye

(General source[537])

The sclera is the part of the eye that is designed to provide stability against expansion. Junqueira et al. stated[537]: "[the sclera]... consists of tough, dense connective tissue made up mainly of flat collagen bundles intersecting in various directions while remaining parallel to the surface...". The **collagen in the sclera is of type I**, and elastic tissue forms less than 2%[543, 544].

The ciliary muscle, which is responsible for accommodation, consists of smooth muscle fibers.

The vitreous body with a gel like structure consists of 99% of water, a minor amount of collagen, and heavily hydrated hyaluronic acid.

4.2.2 The Immune System

(General sources[545, 546])

Myopia and disturbances of the immune system were already connected with each other (see section 3.12), with most of the relevant research being done in Russia. The publications focus mainly on diagnosis, with few conclusions for a therapy for prevention of the progressing of myopia.

Note:
The following very short introduction is limited to a few facts and effects that might be important for our subject, and is far from being a complete tutorial about the immune system.

4.2.2.1 Natural (Innate) Immunity

This kind of immunity is already active at birth; it cannot distinguish between different foreign substances, and it cannot enhance its performance by learning.

A main reaction of natural immunity is **inflammation**. This inflammation consists of:

- Dilation and increased permeability of blood vessels, by which plasma can flow into surrounding tissues.

- Activation of blood and connective tissue cells that try to fight the enemy and to remove debris to set the basis for tissue repair. An example of these blood cells are lymphocytes, relevant connective tissue cells are macrophages, fibroblasts and especially mast cells.

Some of these inflammatory cells like the mast cells, neutrophils and macrophages produce agents that are ready to be released as soon as the cells are triggered. These agents are:

- **Histamine** causes dilation of small capillaries, increases the permeability of capillaries, causes contraction of smooth muscles[547, 548] (the ciliary muscle consists of smooth muscle fibers), and is involved in the generation of collagenase[549, 550], which attacks collagen in the connective tissue. It can, however, also stimulate the synthesis of collagen type I[551]. The sclera consists of collagen type I.

- **Serotonin** has also some effects on capillaries and smooth muscles.

- **Nitric Oxide (NO)** is produced by endothelium cells and phagocytic cells like macrophages. It has cytotoxic effects (i.e. it can destroy cells and tissue), and the effects of blood vessel dilation and smooth muscle relaxation, and can have neurotransmitter functions.

- **Prostaglandins** are hormone-like substances, which act on the tension of smooth muscles and on blood circulation.

- **Cytokines** are produced by lymphocytes and macrophages, and mediate communication between cells and coordination of activities of the immune system. Main cytokines are the various interleukines.

4.2.2.2 Acquired Immunity

The lymphocyte cells control acquired immunity. There is a differentiation between humoral immunity and cell-mediated immunity:

- **Humoral immunity** works against extracellular organisms and toxins by soluble proteins, the **immunoglobulins** also called antibodies. Cells called B-lymphocytes release these plasma cells. Each B lymphocyte is specialized by a specific immunoglobulin to recognize a particular enemy or antigen.

  There are five different classes of immunoglobulins: IgM, IgG, IgA, IgD and IgE; IgE are most relevant for our issue, and can **cause mast cells to release their vasoactive and chemotacic agents**.

- **Cellular immunity** uses **T lymphocytes**, which are specialized to recognize individual antigens by specific T cell receptors. Some of the T lymphocytes can become **cytolytic T lymphocytes**, which can destroy hostile cells; others, the **helper T lymphocytes** can release cytokines, the mediators of the immune system. T lymphocytes are built in the **thymus gland**. In detail, there are more sub-versions of helper cells, the TH1 cells and TH2 cells (see section 4.2.2.6).

4.2.2.3 Pathologic Immune Responses

There are two kinds of inadequate reactions of the immune system:

- **Autoimmunity:** Reactions of the immune system can lead to acute or chronic inflammation, which is directed against own cells and self-antigens. Reasons can be e.g. still overactive or mutated lymphocytes, which are left from an earlier immune reaction. Autoimmune diseases may include rheumatoid arthritis and diabetes type I. Genetics seems to play a role in autoimmune diseases.

  Autoimmune diseases may have arisen because in our evolutionary past very strong reaction of the immune system on a certain stimulus were very helpful[552]. The hypothetical threat no longer exists, but the negative side effect persists. For an example see section 4.2.3.12.

- **Hypersensitivity:** These are cases in which the immune system reacts in an uncontrolled, exaggerated or misdirected way. Examples are asthma, hay fever, etc.

- **Apoptosis**, or programmed cell death. Grodzicky stated[334] that apoptosis "is a physiological process of cell death that normally occurs when cells are damaged or no longer needed." Apoptosis is often strongly related to the immune system, and can lead to **autoimmunity** (for the impact of the immune system on myopia see section 3.12).

Common to both pathologic responses is that normally unaffected tissue and biochemical functions are negatively affected.

4.2.2.4 Effects of the Immune System on the Tissue

General principle of the immune system is that a sophisticated logic enables the body, to detect hostile substances or particles, and to eliminate them by very local application of toxic or dissolving agents. Clearly, an incompletely balanced mechanism can direct these toxic or dissolving agents also to body cells and tissues, causing unwanted effects and damage.

These effects of the immune system are:

- **Vasodilation**.

- **Contraction of smooth muscles** (can affect myopia via the ciliary muscle, see section 3.2).

- **Proteolytic destruction** (can affect myopia by a destruction of the connective tissue of the sclera, see section 3.3.3).

- **Release of cortisol**, normally stimulated by cytokines after actions of the immune system, reduces further actions of the immune system, causing it to return to an inactivated, normal status. The result is e.g. a decrease in collagenase activity[288] (myopia can be affected by exaggerated reactions of the immune system by proteolytic destruction and contraction of smooth muscles, see above; the cortisol level of myopes was mentioned in section 3.13).

- **Regulation of the level of extracellular superoxide dismutase (EC-SOD)**[553] (which is an antioxidant), in smooth muscle cells.

4.2.2.5 Turnover of Connective Tissue and the Immune System

Normally there is a proper balance between synthesis and degradation of connective tissue. Due to the effects of various degrading agents of the immune system, **an overactive immune system will result in a poor connective tissue**[540].

4.2.2.6 TH1/TH2 Balance

T helper type 1 (TH1) lymphocytes stimulate type 1 immunity, and cause intense phagocytic activity (and secrete etc. interleukin (IL)-2, interferon-gamma). Type 1 immunity is more cellular, and considered protective.

T helper type 2 (TH1) lymphocytes stimulate type 2 immunity, causes high levels of antibodies (and secrete IL-4, IL-5, IL-9, IL-10, IL-13)[554]. Type 2 immunity is more humoral.

An unbalance of the TH1/TH2 levels towards TH2 is responsible for autoimmune diseases, and considered to be negative[555].

The TH1/TH2 balance can be **shifted towards the negative TH2** side by the following events:

- **Lack of zinc, selenium, vitamins A, B, C, E**[555] (for the impact of zinc on myopia see section 3.16.5, for the impact of selenium see section 3.16.12.1).

- **Glutathione deficiency** (it determines whether T helper cells will develop into TH1 or TH2 cells)[555] (see also section 4.3.1.6).

- Lack of early **childhood infections**[556], and widespread use of **vaccinations,** which enforces the TH2 response[557].

    Note:
    This would explain the steep increase of myopia in populations, which have moved rapidly to the lifestyle of industrialized countries, where all children are vaccinated. The high death toll of serious infections and which is due to a lack of vaccinations, however, is no real alternative to myopia.

- Chronic **stress**[558] (for the impact of stress on myopia see section 3.13).

- Sufficient release of **melatonin** by the pineal gland[559]. (Melatonin release is activated by the day-/night-Rhythm; for the impact of the day-/night-rhythm on myopia see section 3.7.1).

- Sufficient availability of **nitric oxide (NO)**[555] (for the impact of No on myopia see section 3.12.4).

4.2.2.7 Neurotransmitters and the Immune System

For the impact of neurotransmitters on myopia see section 3.3.

Impact of **dopamine** on the **immune system:** There are contradictory results, but Williams et al. stated[469] that "the majority of evidence suggests that catecholamines [i.e. noradrenalin, dopamine, adrenaline] inhibit **histamine release** from mast cells." Moreover, dopamineric compounds had a pronounced effect on **T-cell dependent immunity**[560]. However, there is evidence for histamine enhancing mechanisms, too[561].

An explanation offered by Basu et al.[562]: "Direct effects of dopamine on the immune effector cells are also contradictory, it is suppressive in vitro, while in pharmacological doses, it is mostly stimulatory in vivo."

As dopamine can inhibit experimental myopia (see section 3.3.2), and as histamine can degrade collagen, the inhibition of histamine release would be an explanation.

Impact of the **immune system** on the **dopamine level**: Vice versa there are also reports about an influence on the dopamine level caused by the immune system: Experimental histamine receptor blockade produced a very significant increase in the level of dopamine[563].

Low concentrations of the **neurotransmitter acetylcholine** have been shown to induce histamine from mast cells, but atropine (which is used sometimes to treat myopia, see section 3.17) was shown to block this induced histamine release[469].

For the impact of **NO**, which can have neurotransmitter functions as well, see section 4.2.3.4.

4.2.2.8 Stress and the Immune System

For the impact of stress on myopia see section 3.13.

Some observations about interactions between stress and the immune system are:

- On one hand it is said that **stress increases cortisol** release, on the other hand **long-term** exposure to **stress** was said to **decrease cortisol release**[380] (for the consequences the cortisol level see section 4.2.3.3) and additionally Esch et al. stated[564]: "... it is widely accepted that acute stress tends to increase immune functioning, whereas chronic stress more likely suppresses it."

- Stress can cause a significant increase of **inflammatory cytokines**, or shift the relation of specific cytokines, or change the **TH1/TH2 balance** (see section 4.2.2.6)[565, 558].

- In experiments it was found that stress can increase the release of **histamine**[566] (with obvious negative consequences for the connective tissue), and significantly increased level of **interleukines** (which are a species of cytokines) and reduced **IgA** concentrations[567].

- Additionally, there appears to be a **stress related interaction between the immune system, the biosynthesis of neurotransmitters like dopamine, and the production of NO**[568]. More specific, immobilization stress increased the production of **iNOS**[569] (see section 4.2.3.4 about NO).

- Oishi et al. stated[570]: "A significant increase in plasma **TBARS** [thiobarbituric acid reactive substances, an indicator for the concentration of damaging reactive oxygen-containing molecules] was observed during and after the stress [of immobilization]. Dramatic increases of neutrophils and monocytes imply that **ROS** [reactive oxygen species] results from their activation.... These findings suggest that the **activation of immune cells** can be a source of the immobilization-induced ROS production..."
- There are **different kinds of stress**: Other experiments showed that stress, which is related to **active** participation at a task can **activate** the immune system, whereas stress which is related to **passive** watching can **weaken** the immune system[571].

4.2.2.9 Acupuncture and the Immune System

For the impact of acupuncture on myopia see section 3.19.3.

There are a few reports about an influence of acupuncture on the immune system. Their relevance for the connective tissue is, however, not clear.

4.2.2.10 Melatonin and the Immune System

For the impact of the day-/nigh-rhythm and melatonin on myopia see section 3.7.1, for the impact of oxidative processes see section 3.16.12.

Melatonin, which is produced by the pineal gland according to the day-/night rhythm, was found to stimulate the acquired and the natural immune system, and to have an impact on the zinc balance, and it can act as a counterbalance to corticosteroids (e.g. cortisol)[572]. Moreover melatonin is said to have a positive influence on autoimmune diseases (which may be related to myopia)[573,] via a shift of the TH1/TH2 balance towards TH1[559] (see section 4.2.2.6 for the implication of this shift).

Additionally, Melatonin has been shown to be an **antioxidant**, which is more effective than glutathione[572], and to improve **microcirculation**[574] (see section 3.11 for the impact of microcirculation on myopia).

4.2.2.11 The Eye and the Immune System

For some parts of the eye there exists attenuation against reactions of the immune system; this includes the anterior chamber, the vitreous body and the retina and is called immune privilege of the eye. This barrier, however, can break down, and this can result in excessive and exaggerated reactions of the immune system[524]. Among other factors the blood-retinal barrier is involved in this immune privilege.

4.2.2.12 Summary Immune System

Malfunctions of the immune system may lead towards myopia in several ways, described in section 3. The main effect is the tendency of the immune system to attack connective tissue.

The complexity of the immune system, however, makes it difficult to find the specific malfunctioning control mechanism.

Figure 16 schematically shows the effects of the immune system on connective tissue.

Note:
*It is a well-established fact that responses of the immune system that cause inflammations, are more common in females than in males. This matches with the result that **myopia is more common at females than at males** (see section 3.1).*

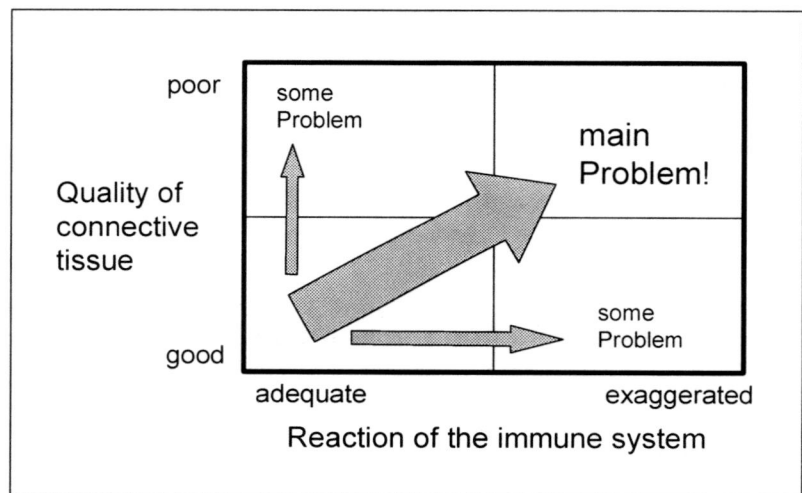

Figure 16 The interference between the immune system and the connective tissue

Immune reactions leading to pathological myopia may be blocked by the following basic means:

- **Reduce the over-reacting** of the immune system (e.g. by providing enough vitamin D (or sunlight) and avoiding nutrients which increase the level of iNOS).

- **Reduce the destructive effects** of the immune system by protective measures (e.g. by providing antioxidants like selenium).

- **Support the body in rebuilding** the attacked tissue (e.g. by providing enough copper which is needed for lysyl oxidase, a tissue repair agent).

4.2.3 Miscellaneous issues

Here I will discuss issues with an impact on myopia, either directly via the connective tissue or more indirectly, e.g. via the immune system or other biochemical processes.

4.2.3.1 The Metabolism of the Feedback Process Leading to Myopia via Degraded Image Quality

Section 3.3 already mentions details of biochemical processes involved in leading from a poor image quality to myopia.

Theses metabolic processes are – as all the other metabolic processes – under control of genetics, and under control of environmental processes, which includes nutrition. Genetics cannot be changed. However, nutrition and environmental conditions can be.

4.2.3.2 Oxidative Processes and Antioxidant Defense

(General source[575])

For the impact of oxidative processes and the antioxidant defense on myopia see section 3.12.2.

There are several names for the chemical compounds, which can cause severe damage to cells and tissues by oxidative processes: free radicals, ROS (reactive oxygen species), AOS (activated oxygen species) and sometimes TBARS (thiobarbituric acid reactive substances). Chemically they are, e.g., superoxide (O_2), hydrogen peroxide (H_2O_2), hydroxyl radical (HO), and singlet oxygen ($O_{2)}$.

Theses substances are created during every metabolic process in the body involving oxygen (e.g. all the muscular activities), and especially by reactions of the immune system and related inflammations. Moreover, they are created by air pollution, by chemicals in food and in our environment.

Oxidative processes have been implicated in numerous diseases, in spite of the fact that an effective immune system depends highly on oxidative agents to attack hostile invaders. Most dangerous is a situation, where abundant oxidative agents (like with an overactive immune system) are combined with a reduced antioxidant defense system. Many of the nutritional components which are discussed in section 4.3 were found to enforce the antioxidant defense system.

A summary of the effects of oxidative agents especially on the connective tissue, given by Henrotin et al.[576] says: "...review of the literature supports the concept that ROS are **not only deleterious agents involved in cartilage degradation**, but that they **also act as integral factors of intracellular signaling mechanisms**" and "ROS [reactive oxygen species] may cause damage to all matrix components, either by a direct attack or indirectly by reducing matrix components synthesis, by inducing apoptosis or by activating latent metalloproteinases."

There is also a connection between oxidative processes and the NO balance (see section 4.2.3.4 about NO). Thomas et al. stated[577]: "Growing evidence indicates that **impaired endothelium-derived NO bioactivity is due, in part, to excess vascular oxidative stress.**"

4.2.3.3 Cortisol and other Hormones

It has already been stated that cortisol inhibits inflammation initiated by the immune system (see section 4.2.2.4).

On the one hand it **inhibits the synthesis of fibers** by connective tissue cells[578] (which is negative), on the other hand cortisol and corticosterone **enhance the activity of** (copper containing) **lysyl oxidase and of cross-linking**[579, 580, 581], and **increases the synthesis of collagen**[582] (which is positive). There are controversial reports on whether cortisol increases[582] or inhibits[580] collagen synthesis.

Certain species of rats, which secrete high levels of the cortisol related corticosterone ("high activity of the hypothalamic-pituitary-adrenocortical axis", HPAC), were found to be very **resistant to the inflammatory disease** rheumatoid arthritis[583]. Deficient HPAC activity was brought into connection with depression, which reminds one of the introverted mentality of myopes (see section 3.13.2).

For the impact of stress on cortisol level see section 4.2.2.8, for the impact of carbohydrates on cortisol level see section 4.3.3.2.

Long-term treatment with **estrogen** increases the activity of the copper containing enzyme lysyl oxidase, which is essential for proper **cross-linking** of collagen[584]. There is no information whether estrogen-containing contraceptives have a positive effect on progressive myopia.

4.2.3.4 The Nitric Oxide (NO) Balance

General references about NO are[353, 585, 586].

Publications about the impact of the NO balance on myopia have been summarized in section 3.12.4. Moreover, NO was related to eye diseases like glaucoma, age-related macular degeneration, and cataract, as well as inflammatory diseases like rheumatoid arthritis, and autoimmune diseases like diabetes type I. NO can have positive effects on myopia, but an excess can be harmful.

NO is a gas, which is slightly soluble in water and diffuses easily across membranes, and it is a free radical, i.e. chemically very reactive.

4 A Synthesis – or how some Pieces might Fit together

The production of NO:

The production of NO requires nitric oxide synthetase (NOS), which exists in a few different versions: **nNOS** (neuronal NOS), **eNOS** (endothelial NOS), **cNOS** (collective name for nNOS and eNOS) are found in neuronal or endothelial cells, whereas **iNOS** (immunological or inducible NOS) is found in many cells and is activated **only in pathological conditions** by certain cytokines.

Normally, only a very small amount of NO is produced, mainly by the amino acid arginine and the n/b/cNOS enzyme. In special conditions, however, substantially higher levels of NO are produced by arginine and iNOS.

Note:
Arginine is an essential amino acid only during the period of growth, later it can be manufactured by the body[587]. If a nutritional lack of arginine proves to be a reason for the progressing of myopia in children, the NO balance would be an explanation.

Glutamate plays an essential role in NO metabolism. In section 3.12.7 it was mentioned that for **people with extreme myopia the concentration of the amino acid glutamate was increased 10-fold**[457].

Additionally, there appears to be a stress related interaction between the immune system, the biosynthesis of neurotransmitters like dopamine, and the production of (neuronal) NO[568, 588].

NO rapidly reacts with superoxide anions (i.e. free radicals) to produce **peroxynitrite, which is a toxic oxidant**. Zinc, magnesium, selenium, vitamin E, flavonoids/procyanidins, glutathione and possibly the vitamins B6 and B12 can **reduce or even prevent this damaging build-up of peroxynitrite**[361, 589, 590, 591, 592].

The effects of NO include:

- **Smooth muscle relaxation**[593] (the ciliary muscle is a smooth muscle, which is involved in accommodation; for the interconnection between accommodation and myopia see section 3.2).

- Maintaining **vessel tone** in blood vessels.

- **Vasodilation** (e.g. by antagonizing vasoconstriction caused by epinephrine and norepinephrine[910]).

- Increase of **ocular blood flow** (for the interconnection between ocular blood flow and myopia see section 3.11).

- Reduction of **intraocular pressure** (for the interconnection between intraocular pressure and myopia see section 3.6.2).

- Very strong interaction with the **immune system**: Decreases the release rate of **histamine**[594] and inhibits mast cell dependent **inflammatory processes**[595]. On the other hand, Bogdan stated[596]: "Protective and toxic effects of NO are frequently seen in parallel ... NO has been recognized as **one of the most versatile players in the immune system**." Coleman stated[597]: "It [NO] also regulates the functional activity, growth and death of many immune and inflammatory cell types..."

  Impact on **connective tissue**: NO often produced by **iNOS** plays an important role in **tissue destruction**, while NO produced by **eNOS** may be **protective and anti-inflammatory**. For the general effects of the immune system, which controls the release of histamine see section 4.2.2.

- **Signal transduction** of central and peripheral nervous system (for the interconnection between neurotransmitters and myopia see section 3.3.2).

- Regulation of **calcium concentrations** in cells (for the interconnection between calcium metabolism and myopia see section 3.16.3).

- Modulation of the release of **stress hormones and of cortisol**[598] (for the interconnection between stress and myopia see section 3.13).

- Modulation of **dopamine** metabolism[599, 600] - increases as well as reductions of dopamine were reported (for the interconnection between dopamine and myopia see section 3.3.2).

- Release of **zinc** ions from various proteins[601]. On the other hand, zinc can suppress the potentially harmful iNOS[602] (for the interconnection of zinc and myopia see section 3.16.5).

- Obviously NO has also some effect on the processing of **light signals in the retina**[568, 603]. For a summary of the effect of image processing on myopia see section 3.3.

- NO plays an essential role in the **regulation of the body temperature**[604, 605] (for the impact of the temperature on myopia see section 3.10).

- There is a close interaction between NO and **G6PD** (glucose-6-phosphate dehydrogenase, for the impact of G6PD on myopia see section 3.12.3, for details about G6PD see section 4.2.3.12).

- It appears that an **increased iNOS** level **decreases systolic blood pressure**, and **increases pulse rate**[606].

Therapeutic conclusions are hard to draw, according to Bogdan[596]: "**Protective and toxic effects of NO** are frequently seen in parallel. Its striking inter- and intracellular signaling capacity makes it extremely difficult to predict the effect of NOS inhibitors and NO donors, which still hampers therapeutic applications." Esch stated[564]: "Like stress, NO seems to be capable of principally exert-

4 A Synthesis – or how some Pieces might Fit together

ing **either beneficial/ameliorating or deleterious effects**. The actual distinction depends on a multitude of factors, such as duration of (an enhanced) NO release, amount of produced NO, and type of synthesis of NO molecules."

iNOS and eNOS may interact. Blantz et al. stated[607]: "...**iNOS transcription, and local inflammation can autoinhibit eNOS,** leading to selective renal and mesentric **vasoconstriction**..." This implies that with an **excess of NO producing iNOS, there is a lack of (also NO producing) eNOS**.

The term **endothelial dysfunction** describes a malfunction of the endothelium (the lining of vessels and cavities), which is strongly related to a reduced **synthesis of NO or an enhanced inactivation of NO**. Endothelial dysfunction appears to be reversible, e.g., by physical exercises, nutritional antioxidants, and by reducing cholesterol levels[608].

Notes:
- *Maybe **many of the harmful effects of NO** can be explained by the damaging effects of the oxidant peroxinitrate, which is built during degradation of NO. As mentioned above, extracellular zinc, magnesium, selenium, glutathione and possibly the vitamins B6 and B12 can help to **prevent this damaging built-up of peroxynitrite**.*

- *Frequent cold hands can be caused by a lack of NO.*

- In Table 9, Table 10 and Table 11 **The impact of some other nutrients on the NO metabolism**

the impact of some nutrients on the NO metabolism is shown.

Summary of the interaction of various nutrients on NO production[586]:

Vitamin	Reported direct effect on myopia (section)	Effect on constitutive NO synthesis (nNOS, eNOS collectively termed cNOS)	Effect on inducible NO synthesis (iNOS, substantially higher concentrations than cNOS, related to inflammatory processes)
		⬆ marks an increase of NO, ⬇ marks a decrease of produced NO	
Vitamin A	3.16.10	⬆ Increased eNOS activity	Depends on cell type
Vitamin B3	3.16.11		⬇ Reduced iNOS activity
Vitamin B6	3.16.11	⬆ Increased eNOS activity via reduction of homocysteine	⬇ Reduced iNOS activity (B6)[609]
Folic Acid	3.16.13	⬆ Increased eNOS activity (also via reduction of homocysteine)	
Vitamin C		⬆ Increased eNOS activity	
Vitamin D	3.16.3		⬇ Reduced iNOS activity in inflammatory brain cells ⬆ Increased iNOS activity in macrophage cell lines
Vitamin E	3.16.12.2	⬆ Increased eNOS activity	(⬇) Less formation of peroxynitrite[591]
Carotenoids	3.16.10		⬇ Reduced iNOS activity

Table 9 The impact of vitamins on the NO metabolism

4 A Synthesis – or how some Pieces might Fit together

Mineral	Reported direct effect on myopia (section)	Effect on constitutive NO synthesis (nNOS, eNOS collectively termed cNOS)	Effect on inducible NO synthesis (iNOS, substantially higher concentrations than cNOS, related to inflammatory processes)
		⬆ marks an increase of NO, ⬇ marks a decrease of produced NO	
Copper	3.16.5	⬇ Elevated copper inhibits nNOS	⬇ Inhibit iNOS activity
Iron		⬆ Deficiency of iron reduces nNOS	Depends on interaction between iron and other molecules, may enhance or reduce
Magnesium	3.16.4	⬆ Increased eNOS activity	
Manganese	3.16.7	⬆ Increased cNOS production	
Potassium	3.16.8	⬆ Increased eNOS production	
Sodium		⬇ Decreased eNOS production / activity	
Selenium	3.16.12.1	⬆ Increased eNOS activity[688]	⬇ Reduced iNOS activity[610, 611], reduced formation of peroxynitrite[591]
Zinc	3.16.5	⬇ Elevated doses decreases eNOS and nNOS activity	⬇ Reduced iNOS activity

Table 10 The impact of minerals on the NO metabolism

Other nutrients, biochemical agents and stress	Reported direct effect on myopia (section)	Effect on constitutive NO synthesis (nNOS, eNOS collectively termed cNOS)	Effect on inducible NO synthesis (iNOS, substantially higher concentrations than cNOS, related to inflammatory processes)
		⬆ marks an increase of NO, ⬇ marks a decrease of produced NO	
Arginine		⬆ Arginine rich diet increased cNOS	⬆ Arginine deficiency reduced iNOS activity in wounds
Carbohydrate fructose	3.16.1	⬇? Impairs vascular relaxation, but not necessarily via reduced NO	⬇ Sometimes elevated doses inhibit iNOS activity
Carbohydrate glucose	3.16.1	⬆ Deficiency reduces NO ⬇ Elevated doses decrease eNOS activity in large vessels ⬆ Elevated doses increase eNOS activity in microvascular vessels	⬇ Sometimes elevated doses inhibit iNOS activity
Flavonoids	3.16.12.2	⬆ Increased eNOS activity	⬇ Quercetin and hesperidin suppress iNOS activity in macrophages, procyanidins protect against peroxynitrite
Glutamate	3.12.7	⬆ Glutamate rich diet increased nNOS activity	⬆ Increased iNOS activity
Lysine		⬇ Lysine is an antagonist of Arginine	⬇ Decreased iNOS activity in macrophages
Proteins	3.16.15	⬆ Protein/casein rich diet increased cNOS activity	⬆ Arginine deficiency reduced iNOS activity in wounds
Fatty acids, saturated		⬇ Impaired eNOS activity	⬆ Increased iNOS activity
Fatty acids, unsaturated		Depends on the specific unsaturated fatty acid	Depends on the specific unsaturated fatty acid
Garlic		⬆ Increased eNOS activity[612]	No effect on iNOS activity[612]
Dopamine	3.3.1		⬇ Attenuated iNOS activity[613]
Estrogen		⬆ Increased eNOS activity[688]	⬆ Increased iNOS activity[614]
G6PD (see section 4.2.3.12)	3.12.3	⬆ Increased eNOS activity	⬇ Protection against iNOS induced cytotoxicity
Mental stress	3.13		⬆ Increased iNOS activity[569]

Table 11 The impact of some other nutrients on the NO metabolism

4.2.3.5 "The Nerves": Neurotransmitters, Stress and Personality

Interactions between stress and the immune system have been discussed in section 4.2.2.8, for the interconnection between stress and myopia see section 3.13.

Personality:

Myopes are considered to be more likely introverted (see section 3.13.2). Correspondingly, "social anxiety disorder" is said to be accompanied by **decreased dopamineric transmission**[615].

The contrary effect, "attention-deficit hyperactivity disorder", is often accompanied by an **increase in dopamine levels**[616].

Depression:

Depression has been linked to the metabolism of **NO**, neurotransmitter levels like the one of **dopamine**, the **immune system**[568, 617], and the status of **selenium**.

Stress (see also section 4.2.2.8):

- Generally it is assumed that stress increases **cortisol** release; long term stress, however, was found to decrease cortisol output[380], or decrease the utilization of dopamine in the brain. Pani et al. stated[618]: "There is enough preclinical evidence to support the view that stress, in both its acute and chronic form, may have a negative impact on the normal physiology of the dopamineric system." For the interconnection between dopamine and myopia see section 3.3.2.

- Overall, there appears to be a stress related interaction between **the immune system**, the biosynthesis of **neurotransmitters like dopamine**, and the **production of NO**[568].

- Stress can have an impact on **blood sugar level and insulin production** (see section 4.2.3.8), which in turn can have an impact on myopia (see section 3.16.1).

- Furthermore stress causes increased excretion of **vitamin C**[383], and corresponding negative effects for the connective tissue.

- **Mental stress increased the iNOS activity,** and Ghiadoni et al. stated[619] that "...findings suggest that brief episodes of mental stress, similar to those encountered in everyday life, may cause transient (up to 4 hours) endothelial dysfunction in healthy young individuals." Endothelial dysfunction is very strongly connected with a lack of endothelial-generated nitric oxide (NO) (see section 4.2.3.4 about NO).

- Experiments with rats showed that stress (in this case by prohibiting them from moving) leads to the formation of reactive oxygen species (ROS) and causes **oxidative damage** in various tissues[570]. For the interconnection between oxidative damage and myopia see section 3.16.12.

Note:
The stress of immobilization reminds of the stress of children and students in examinations and during difficult intellectual exercises, or just sitting in school.

- Even mild psychological stress can lead to increased levels of **homocysteine**[620]. For the interconnection between homocysteine and myopia, see section 3.16.13.

4.2.3.6 Homocysteine

Interrelations between homocysteine and myopia have been summarized in section 3.16.13, the impact of the related glutathione on myopia was mentioned in section 3.12.3.

The basic transformations between homocysteine and its metabolic partners are summarized in Figure 17.

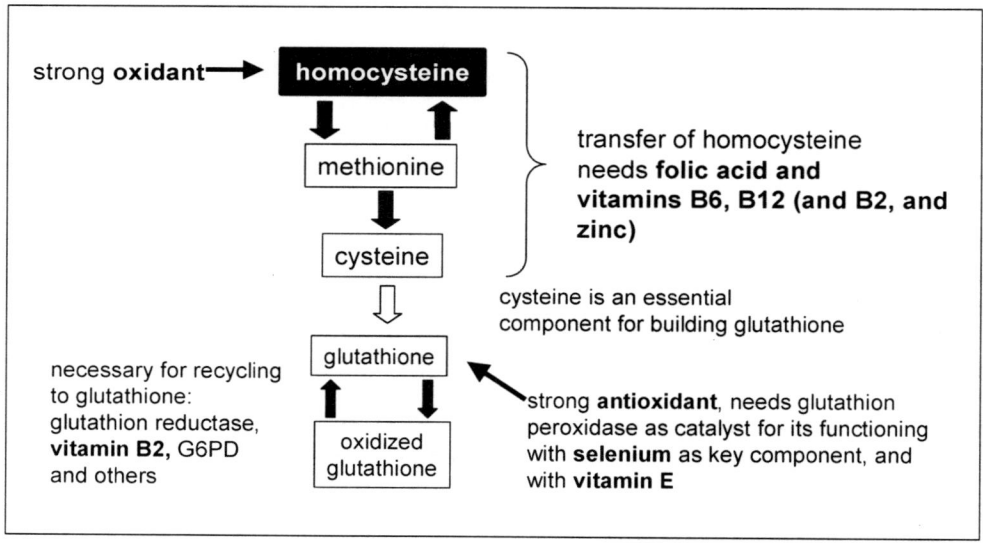

Figure 17 The metabolism of homocysteine

Additionally, an elevated level of homocysteine can be caused by a deficiency of **vitamin C**[621].

Homocysteine is essential for various methylation processes, i.e. processes where a methyl group (i.e. a configuration of one carbon atom and three hydrogen atoms) is transferred between organic molecules. Methylation is, among others, essential for the production of the neurotransmitters and of melatonin[622]. It is not poisonous in principle, but excess is harmful[623, 624].

In the case of homocystinuria, the transfer of homocysteine to methionine and cysteine is disturbed due to genetic defects (mostly a lack of the enzyme cystathionine synthase). Frequently a genetically caused, increased level of homocysteine can be lowered by extra vitamins B6 and B12, and folic acid.

The concentration of the amino acid **methionine** was 10-fold increased for people with extreme myopia (see section 3.16.13).

Even without this genetic defect there may be an elevated level of homocysteine, called hyperhomocysteinemia. This can be due to factors such as nutritional deficits, especially of vitamins B6 and B12, and folic acid).

An **excess level of homocysteine** can result in:

- Low levels of **copper**[625] (for consequences see section 4.3.1.3).
- Lowered activity of the copper dependent enzyme glutathione peroxidase and resulting **increase in reactive or pro-oxidative substances**[625, 626, 627].
- **Autoimmune** diseases[627, 628].
- Reduction or defective **cross-linking of collagen** in cases of homocystinuria[629, 630] or elevated levels of homocysteine[631] by suppression of lysyl oxidase activity.
- Long time effects on **connective tissue** even by chronic moderate hyperhomocysteinemia[632],
- Lowered levels of nitric oxide **NO**[633] by decreasing **eNOS** activity[586] or oxidative inactivation of NO[634, 635] (see section 4.2.3.4 for the effects of NO).

It was suggested that total plasma homocysteine is a more sensitive measure of folate (and vitamin B6, B12) deficiency[636]. Therefore, the sections on folic acid (4.3.2.3), vitamin B6 (4.3.2.2.2) and Vitamin B12 (4.3.2.2.4) are applicable to effects of homocysteine as well. There is a good chance that even in case of inherited homocystinuria high doses of the mentioned vitamins are effective[522].

Elevated levels of glutathione are reducing the **damaging effects of peroxynitrite**, which is built during the degradation of NO (see section 4.2.3.4).

4.2.3.7 The Day- / Night-Rhythm, Illumination, and Melatonin Metabolism

Interrelations between the day- / night-rhythm and myopia have been summarized in section 3.7.1, and between illumination and myopia in section 3.7.2.

The day- /night-rhythm of the body, called circadian rhythm is controlled by incident light, which triggers the pineal gland to release melatonin when it is dark. Consequently, melatonin activation decreases with light activation, while cortisol and dopamine levels increase.

Note:
This increase in dopamine with illumination[292] gives another justification for the recommendation to use good illumination (see section 3.8).

As modern life is largely independent of natural illumination and the corresponding rhythm (just think of watching TV late at night), any disturbance of this system, which was optimized by evolution for very different conditions, can have a negative impact.

What melatonin is doing: [573, 637]

- It stimulates and modulates both **acquired and natural immunity**[638, 639, 640], promoting TH1 immune activity[559] (see section 4.2.2.6); consequently permanent night-light hinders the immune system[572].

- It stimulates type I **collagen formation** (demonstrated so far for bone only; the sclera is, however, also built of collagen type I, see section 4.2.1.2)[641, 642].

- It is a very effective **antioxidant** / scavenger of free radicals[638, 643, 572].

- It can **modulate zinc** turnover[640, 572].

- It can **protect dopamine** neurons from oxidative damage[644].

- It can modulate **NO** levels[639, 645].

The effect of UV-light on the synthesis of vitamin D is well established.

Moreover, it was reported that light, and especially **specific colors of light** have an impact on numerous **biochemical and psychological effects**[302] (which are – again – correlated with biochemistry).

Note:
Many researchers consider these findings to be of dubious validity. That is not to say that the described processes are incorrect.

At animals the **NO** levels in serum were following a circadian rhythm as well[646]

4.2.3.8 Blood Sugar Level / Insulin Level

An interconnection between blood sugar level and myopia has been mentioned in section 3.16.1.

The impact of high blood sugar level (i.e. **hyperglycemia**) on mechanisms relevant to myopia, is:

- **Microcirculation** is disturbed[647, 648]: Glucose rich diet reduces **microcirculation** by reduction of the caliber of arterial microvessels, and vascular lesions as well, as microvasular aging was increased[649]. For the impact of microcirculation on myopia see section 3.11.

- Spanheimer stated[650]: "Diabetes mellitus is associated with a **generalized defect in connective tissue metabolism**." It appears to be very likely that similar effects exist at non-pathologic, but unusually high levels of blood sugar and insulin.

- Lien stated[651]: "**Glucose inhibits collagen fibril formation** in vitro."

- There are multiple negative effects of glucose and hyperglycemia on the **concentration of free radicals and on the antioxidant defense system.** Maritim et al. stated[652] that "Glucose oxidation is believed to be a main source of free radicals.". **Oxidative stress** is created, and, e.g., the level of the antioxidant glutathione is decreased[653, 654, 655, 656]. Furthermore, a diet high in fructose weakens the free radical / **antioxidant defense system**, e.g. by lowering the Cu/Zn-SOD activity[657]. Koska et al. stated[658] that "...glucose already in the low dose was an important triggering factor for oxidative stress." For the impact of oxidative processes on myopia see section 3.16.12, for the general impact of glutathione see section 4.2.3.6.

- **NO (nitric oxide)** formation is depressed, or the balance between synthesis and degradation of NO is disturbed[659, 660, 661, 662, 688] (for the impact of NO on myopia see section 3.12.4).

- **Cytokine production and inflammatory response** of the immune system is increased[648, 663] (for the impact of the immune system on myopia see section 3.3.3).

- Carbohydrate consumption during exercise and stress was found to **attenuate the cortisol level**[664, 665]. This matches with the findings that myopes are consuming above average carbohydrates (see section 3.16.1), and that cortisol attenuates inflammatory reactions, which are involved at least in higher grades of myopia (see section 3.12): More carbohydrates results in lower cortisol, which results in more inflammatory reactions.

- Elevation of **insulin** increases the levels of the insulin growth factor-1 (**IGF-1**), "a potent stimulator of growth in all tissues" according to Cordain et al.[405]. Additionally Cordain et al. stated[405]: "Reduced levels of the insulin like growth factor binding protein-1 (**IG"FBP-1**) may reduce the effectiveness of the body's natural **retinoids** in activating genes that would normally limit scleral cell proliferation." (For the role of retinoic acid on myopia see section 3.3.1). The glycaemic load factors of carbohydrates were shown to be significantly higher than in other nutrients.

- The level of **insulin** can influence the **central nervous system (CNS)** and the transport of **dopamine** significantly[666].

- Schaffer et al. stated[667] that artificially induced hyperglycemia "markedly impaired wound breaking strength and **collagen deposition**" of type I collagen (the sclera consists of type I collagen as well). Glucose was found to alter the structure of **cross-linking** in type IV collagen, and to lead to significantly reduced strength[668].

- High **glucose inhibits G6PD**. It was concluded by Zhang et al.[669] "that these changes in G6PD activity play an important role in high **glucose-induced cell damage/death**." Vice versa a G6PD deficiency **causes hyperglycemia**[670]. Via its effect on G6PD hyperglycemia has also an impact on the **NO** metabolism. For more information about G6PD see section 4.2.3.12.

- **Vitamin C deficiency** can be created[671], and high levels of plasma glucose reduce the positive effect of **vitamin C** on proteoglycan and **collagen** synthesis[672] (for the impact of vitamin C on the connective tissue see section 4.3.2.5).

- Sugar (sucrose, fructose, glucose) as a source of carbohydrates has profound effects on **copper** metabolism, and symptoms of copper deficiency are enhanced[288, 673]. For the impact of copper see sections 3.16.5 and 4.3.1.3.

- Fructose as a source of carbohydrates has negative effects on **magnesium** metabolism of individuals whose magnesium status is sub optimal[674]. For the impact of magnesium see sections 3.16.3 and 4.3.1.4.

- Increased levels of insulin (e.g. caused by "high-glycemic-index" starches and white wheat flour) tend to increase **homocysteine** levels[675] (see section 3.16.13 about the impact of homocysteine on myopia).

Blood sugar level and insulin production are also affected by:

- A **lack (moderate) of exercise** and physical activity[676, 677].
  Note:
  Myopia has been attributed to an excess of reading – maybe the lack of physical activity is relevant too. Vice versa, many children may be relatively inactive because they wear glasses, and so drift into sedentary activities.

- **Stress**[678, 679].
  Note:
  In section 3.13 a transient pseudomyopia was reported after an earthquake. Maybe the biochemical reason was hyperglycemia caused by stress.

Sugar consumption in the USA was increasing by 30% between 1983 and 1999, reaching 158 pound per person[680].

4.2.3.9 The Sodium / Potassium Balance

An interconnection between the electrolyte balance and myopia has been mentioned in section 3.3.1. An interconnection between potassium and myopia was mentioned in section 3.16.8.

- The sodium / potassium balance has a significant impact on the NO balance:

    A shift of the sodium / potassium balance towards sodium leads to an **inhibition of eNOS**[681, 682, 683] (see section 4.2.3.4 about NO) and correspondingly reduced vasodilation (see section 3.11 about the impact of blood circulation on myopia), and to a **loss of calcium** (see section 4.3.1.1 about calcium, and section 3.16.3 about the impact of calcium on myopia).
    A high salt diet can impair **microcirculation and vasodilation**[684]. For the impact of microcirculation on myopia see section 3.11. Microcirculation and vasodilation are frequently related to NO metabolism.
    There are indications that a high salt diet leads to a reduced activity of the **antioxidant Cu/Zn SOD**, which contributes to a loss of **NO** in arteries[685, 686] (see sections 3.12.2 and 3.16.12 about the impact of oxidative effects, and section 3.12.4 about the effect of NO on myopia).

- Additionally, **low potassium** diets can increase **superoxide production** (see sections 3.12.2 and 3.16.12 for the correlation of oxidative damage and myopia), and **high sodium** diets can induce **insulin resistance**[687] (see section 3.16.1 about the impact of insulin metabolism on myopia).

- McCarty stated[688]: "The unsalted, whole-food diets consumed by our paleolithic ancestors were **remarkably higher in potassium and lower in sodium** (and salt) than our current 'civilized' diet...". Manufactured foods contribute about 65%-70% of dietary sodium[689], which should result in substantially increased sodium consumption.

- Weber[579] postulated the hypothesis that **a potassium deficiency is causing lysyl oxidase and other copper enzymes to decline**, on the basis of "a mechanism which may have evolved to help fight potassium wasting infections".. For the impact of copper deficiency see section 4.3.1.3.

Note:
Maybe the finding that myopia is hardly found in some Pacific islands (see section 3.16.1) can not only be explained by the low carbohydrate diet, but also by their diet with a balanced sodium / potassium ratio.

4.2.3.10 Hormones

Estrogen increases **endothelial nitric oxide**[688, 690] (see section 3.12.4 about the impact of NO on myopia, and section 4.2.3.4 about NO metabolism), and extended **estrogen treatment** increases the activity of lysyl oxidase, an enzyme which is essential for the cross linking of collagen the structure of the collagen of the sclera is degraded in myopia[375].

4.2.3.11 Physical Exercises

Summary: Moderate exercising is very healthy, excessive exercising is very dangerous.

The more detailed results are:

- All forms of physical exercise **reduce the intraocular pressure (IOP)**[395]. For the impact of the IOP and myopia see section 3.6.2.

- General exercising may have a positive impact on myopia by its impact on the metabolism of insulin and **hyperglycemia**[676, 677]. For the impact of the blood sugar metabolism on myopia see section 3.16.1.

- Kuiper et al. stated[691]: "...a **higher exposure [to physical workload]** was associated with **higher effective type I collagen synthesis...**"

  Note:
  Reduced collagen Type I synthesis was found to be related to artificial myopia (see section 3.3.3).

- During **very extensive** exercises the generation of **reactive oxygen species (ROS)** is highly increased[692]. Myopia was brought into connection with oxidative damage (section 3.16.12); whether a very strenuous load of the ciliary muscle during near work can be made partially responsible for this damage is unknown. Moderate exercise increased, however, the activity of the antioxidant enzymes superoxide dismutase (SOD) and glutathione peroxidase.[658] Conclusion: **Excessive exercise is as harmful as a lack of exercise.**

  Accordingly, however, Oishi et al. stated[570]: "A significant increase in plasma **TBARS** [thiobarbituric acid reactive substances, an indicator for the concentration of damaging reactive oxygen-containing molecules] was observed during and **after the stress [of immobilization]**. Dramatic increases of neutrophils and monocytes imply that **ROS** [reactive oxygen species] results from their activation.... These findings suggest that the **activation of immune cells** can be a source of the immobilization-induced ROS production..."

Note:
This reminds one of the stress, which school kids, and students are having during classes and especially during examinations.

- Physical exercise appears to be able to reverse endothelial dysfunction, i.e. to increase endothelial nitric oxide (NO) synthesis[608] (see section 4.2.3.4 about NO).

4.2.3.12 G6PD (Glucose-6-Phospahate Dehydrogenase) Deficiency – an Example

An interconnection between glucose-6-phospahate dehydrogenase and myopia has been mentioned in section 3.12.3.

Glucose-6-phospahate dehydrogenase deficiency is inherited, and is the most common enzyme deficiency in the world; it **involves between 200 to 400 million people**, and can exist in over 400 different variants. Therefore, e.g. in Brunei and Singapore newborns are routinely screened for G6PD deficiency (especially high rates are found in the Chinese population – there is a high prevalence for myopia among the Chinese as well). Its effect is, simplified that **the reduction of oxidized glutathione to glutathione is hindered** (see the figure in section 4.2.3.6). This results in a limited antioxidant defense capability, because the level of glutathione is reduced. G6PD exists in all human cells, but its effect is especially important in red blood cells, where a breakdown of the antioxidant defense can lead to severe anemic crisis (frequently the number or reticulocytes, i.e. of newly built red blood cells is elevated). G6PD deficiency can range from an almost total lack to nearly full activity.

People with this defect may have a better chance at surviving malaria.

The reason that this defect is mentioned here in some more detail is to give an impression about the existence of a tremendous amount of biochemical individuality, which might have been useful in the past, but has new disadvantages in the modern life, but can be influenced by nutrition (see section 4.3).

Additionally, it was found in one study that there is more G6PD in patients with progressive myopia than in people with stable myopia[345], which is a hint of abnormal oxidative processes.

Although the traditionally known effect of G6PD is on red blood cells, new research showed that:

- Ho et al. stated[693] that "... results show that G6PD deficiency **predisposes human fibroblasts to retarded growth** and accelerated cellular senescence."

    Fibroblasts decrease during increasing myopia, and fibroblasts are building collagen, and they are the only cell type in the sclera[88].

- G6PD deficiency **decreases eNOS bioavailability**[694]. Moreover, the G6PD status determines how fibroblast cells (which are part of the connective tissue) are reacting on **NO** – either with cell death or with cell growth[695].

  An elevated activity of **G6PD increased the resistance against NO-mediated apoptosis** (i.e. programmed cell death) of neuronal cells[696], and protected against **iNOS mediated reactive, damaging agents.**[697]

  For the impact of NO on Myopia see section 3.12.4. For more information about NO see section 4.2.3.4.

- G6PD deficiency **promotes endothelial oxidant stress**[694, 698].

- The vascular endothelium **responds to local oxidant stress by increasing the activity** of the antioxidant enzyme **G6PD**[698].
  Note:
  *This can explain the result that in cases of **progressing myopia the level of G6PD was found to be elevated**: apparently the myopia was caused or accompanied by an attack by oxidative or reactive substances.*

- G6PD deficiency **causes hyperglycemia**[670], and vice versa Zhang et al. stated[669]: "High **glucose-induced inhibition of G6PD** predisposed cells to cell death". The impact of hyperglycemia on myopia was described in section 3.16.1.

Table 12 summarizes how nutritional components can influence the G6PD level or the G6PD activity. Several of these nutrients were already mentioned in direct connection with myopia (see section 3).

Nutrient	Effect on G6PD deficiency
Vitamin B1	People with a lack of G6PD were found frequently to have a lack of vitamin B1[699].
Vitamin B2	• For rats G6PD activity was decreased significantly by vitamin B2 deficiency[700, 701]. • If rats are treated with ethanol, those with a deficiency in vitamin B2 show a decrease in G6PD[702]. • At G6PD deficiency, vitamin B2 supplementation increases substantially pyridoxine phosphate oxidase (essential for the glutathione cycle)[701]. *Note: A deficiency of vitamin B2 can result in a deficiency of vitamin B6; for consequences of vitamin B6 deficiency see section 4.3.2.2.2.*
Vitamin B3	High doses of vitamin B3 can have a positive effect on inherited G6PD deficiency[522].
Vitamin B6	Deficiency of vitamin B6 caused marked reduction on G6PD activity[703, 704, 705, 706]. Vitamin B6 deficiency is common - see section 4.3.2.2.2.
Vitamin D	Vitamin D treatment caused a significant increase in G6PD activity[707, 708]. Vitamin D deficiency is rather common - see section 4.3.2.6.
Vitamin E	Some authors found a significant protection against a lack of G6PD; others could not confirm this[709].
Folic acid	Rats with folic acid deficiency showed G6PD deficiency[710]
Magnesium and copper	Serum magnesium and copper were found to be significantly lower in G6PD deficient people; it was concluded that the demand for these elements is higher for people with G6PD deficiency to compensate for the loss during the shortened life span of red blood cells[711]. *Notes: For effects of magnesium and copper on myopia see section 3.16, for general impact on related topics see section 4.3.1.* *Low content of copper in the serum exists in cases of rather substantial deficiency only.*
Selenium	Improved erythrocyte survival in G6PD deficiency by selenium and vitamin E supplementation (better than vitamin E alone)[712]
Polyunsaturated fatty acids	The activity of G6PD is reduced by the addition of polyunsaturated fatty acids to a high carbohydrate diet[713]. For information on fatty acids see section 4.3.3.3.
Sugar, carbohydrates	Increased glucose inhibits G6PD. It was concluded by Zhang et al.[669] "that these changes in G6PD activity play an important role in high glucose-induced cell damage/death." For information on blood sugar level see section 4.2.3.8.

Table 12 The effect of some nutrients on G6PD deficiency

4.2.3.13 Is there an Analogy between Structural Heart Problems and Progressive Myopia?

For the heart, which consists of smooth muscle cells like the ciliary muscle, numerous reports have been published about structural **connective tissue defects** as a result of dietary copper deficiency[714,715,716,717].

Among others, the **enlargement of the heart** (hypertrophic cardiomyopathy)[718],[719] reminds one of the **enlargement of the eye** in myopia. Hypertrophia is caused not by an increase in the number of cells, but an **enlargement of the size of the cells** – which results in a weakened structure. **Other effects** of copper deficiency on the heart, which remind of myopic effects, are:

- decreased **stiffness of muscle cells** (myocytes),
- decreased **tensile strength**, reduced cross-linking,
- reduced **amount of connective** tissue,
- reduced **ability to contract** (reminds of the accommodation deficit of myopes), and
- increased **inflammation**.

These effects could already be observed by Wildman et al.[720] at **marginal deficiencies of copper**: "This study suggests that abnormalities in cardiac ultrastructure occurred in rats chronically fed diets marginally low in Cu, despite minimal changes in conventional biochemical indicators of Cu status."

The negative effect of a copper-deficiency was substantially increased if the diet was **high in fructose**[721].

For the reported impact of copper on myopia see section 3.16.5, for the more general impact of copper see section 4.3.1.3.

4.2.3.14 Is there an Analogy between Arthritis and Progressive Myopia?

Arthritis is an inflammation of the connective tissue of the joints.

It was found that people suffering from this disease had a diet containing **less copper** than the typical American diet (TAD) and less **vitamin B6, zinc, and magnesium** than the recommended dietary allowance (RDA)[722]. Moreover, arthritis was connected with a lack of **sunlight or vitamin D**[723].

All these nutrients have been brought into connection with myopia as well (see section 3).

Nevertheless, arthritis is associated with an increased level of copper in the serum (and a reduced level of copper in the liver which is serving as a storage for copper): more copper is made available because of the abnormally high destruction of connective tissue, and the increased need for the copper-containing enzyme lysyl oxidase[579].

4.3 The Impact of Nutritional Components

We have heard already about the impact of connective tissue on myopia. There are not too many publications about myopia and nutritional components (see section 3.16), but about nutrition and health[724, 725, 461] and nutritional components and their impact on the connective tissue and related issues. Therefore, some of these results will be presented here.

One author of a medical textbook expressed the significance of the impact of nutritional components:

"A lack of trace elements is stimulating primarily the destruction of tissues and secondarily the production of cytokines" [translated from Biesalski[726]].

There are four different mechanisms by which metabolism and quality of connective tissue can be improved:

a) Higher rate of the synthesis of collagen

b) **Improved strength** of the synthesized collagen, e.g. by improving the cross-linking between the fibers

c) **Better protection** by improving the stability of the collagen against attacking enzymes (like collagenase), oxidants (like free radicals), and solving agents (like acids).

d) **Fewer attacks from potentially damaging agents**, e.g. by reducing overreactions of the immune system (autoimmune reactions).

The segmentation between b) and c) is fluent, as an improved structure may result in an improved resistance as well[727].

Due to the long replacement time (i.e. turnover) of collagen in the sclera, improvements via b) (improved strength) will show results rather slowly, whereas improvements via c) (protection) can show quick results. On the other hand, without degradation of collagen of poor quality, no new formation of improved collagen would take place.

The situation is clearly expressed by Tinker et al.[288]: "Often there is a strong genetic interaction between diet and the expression of connective tissue lesions".

It has to be emphasized – again! – that all the people affected by myopia are not necessarily suffering from a lack of a certain nutrient, but there is a chance to counterbalance certain handicaps by optimally adjusted nutrition.

Many of the following results were obtained by experiments with animals, very often with rats. This procedure, however, is common due to their metabolic similarity.

> **The conclusion from the following sub-sections should not be to get mega-doses from the mentioned nutrients, but to gain the insight that an unbalanced lack of any one of them, compared with the inherited and individual needs, can have very significant consequences for the health, and in our context for myopia as well.**

4.3.1 Minerals

4.3.1.1 Calcium

Publications about the impact of calcium on myopia have been summarized in section 3.16.3.

Table 13 describes the impact of some components on the calcium metabolism, and some relevant effects of calcium on the connective tissue. The effects of deficiencies are obviously opposite to the benefits.

Sunlight and nutrition	Vitamin B6			Sodium (in salt)	Proteins and sulfur containing amino acids in nutrition
⬇	⬇	⬇	⬇	⬇	⬇
Vitamin D is necessary for calcium metabolism.	Improved efficiency of vitamin D[728].	Reduced loss of Calcium with the urine[729] and reduced loss of calcium by creation of oxalic.	A lack of vitamin B6 produced increased levels of calcium in the serum[730] *(note: maybe by releasing calcium from body tissue?)*.	Increased loss of calcium with the urine[731, 732].	Increased loss of calcium with the urine and the feces[731, 733].

Effects of calcium

⬇

- Calcium is essential for an optimal **collagenase** activity[288].
- Calcium reduces the release of histamine, a mediator of the **immune system**[734], which appears to be involved in the release of (collagen attacking[549, 550]) collagenase and which increases the permeability of capillaries[561]. Histamine is closely related to allergies. (For the impact of the immune system on myopia see section 3.12).
- Calcium reduces the losses of **copper**, which is essential for the connective tissue[735] (see section 4.3.1.3).
- cNOS is **calcium dependent**[564, 586, 736] (see section 4.2.3.4)
- Calcium plays a rather complex role in **muscle tone and muscle relaxation** (relevant for the accommodation anomalies, which were found at myopes – see section 3.2.1?)

Table 13 Nutrition, calcium and the connective tissue

Elevated levels of calcium in the hair can be seen frequently in case of allergies and chronic stress[737] (in section 3.16.3 it was reported that increased levels of calcium were found for people with increasing myopia).

Calcium absorption from food is promoted by the amino acid lysine in food and is hindered by sulfur containing amino acids in food (e.g. protein from soy)[725].

4.3.1.2 Chromium

Publications about the impact of chromium on myopia have been summarized in section 3.16.6.

Some general aspects of the effect of chromium are:

- **Oxidative processes** were found in the **retina** of rats fed a diet high in polyunsaturated fatty acids and deficient in vitamin E, selenium, sulfur-containing amino acids, and chromium. Dietary supplementation with methionine and chromium significantly reduced the indicators of oxidative processes[738]. For the impact of oxidative processes on myopia see section 3.16.12.

- People with diabetes type 2 showed a significant reduction of plasma **TBARS** after supplementation with Chromium[813]. TBARS (thiobarbituric acid reactive substances) is an indicator for the concentration of damaging reactive oxygen-containing molecules. Persons with high myopia have elevated levels of TBARS (see section 3.12.2).

- The **antioxidative effect** of chromium appears to be responsible for its effect of increasing **insulin sensitivity**. Jain et al. stated[739]: "...chromium inhibits the secretion of TNF-alpha, a cytokine known to inhibit the sensitivity and action of insulin." For the impact of the insulin metabolism on myopia see section 3.16.1.

- Chromium deficiency caused abnormal reactions of the **immune system** in the retina of rats[432], and chromium has a strong impact on the immune system in general[740]. For the impact of the immune system on myopia see section 3.12.1.

- Some experiments with animals showed a decrease in serum **cortisol** after chromium supplementation. For the impact of cortisol on myopia see section 3.13.

- Chromium potentiates the action of **insulin**, and **reduces peripheral vascular resistance**[741] (see section 3.11 on blood circulation) in insulin resistant states. Chromium-deficient rats had significantly **higher blood sugar levels**[431]. For the impact of the insulin metabolism on myopia see section 3.16.1.

- The structure of the **retinal pigment epithelium** was showing more damage for Chromium deficient rats[431].

Note:
*Retinal **dopamine** is located mainly in the retinal pigment epithelium[742] and is assumed to be involved in the lens induced and the deprivation myopia (see section 3.3.2).*

4.3.1.3 Copper

Publications about the impact of copper on myopia have been summarized in section 3.16.5.

Table 14 describes the impact of some nutritional components on the copper metabolism, and some relevant effects of copper on the connective tissue. The effects of deficiencies are obviously opposite to the benefits.

Lack of **copper** in the nutrition	Too much of these nutrients can result in a deficit of copper[288, 743, 744, 745]:	**Vitamin B6** deficit		
		↓	↓	↓
		Increased level of **homocysteine** (see section 4.2.3.6)	Reduced absorption of **copper**[746]	Reduced activity of the enzyme **G6PD**[703]
	zinc, sucrose, fructose, glucose, soybean protein, iron			
↓	↓	↓	↓	↓
Copper deficit	Copper absorption and metabolism disturbed	Copper deficit[625]	Copper deficit	Copper deficit in serum[711]

↓

- Copper deficit causes **poor collagen** (and elastin) **cross-linking**[288, 747, 584, 748, 540], because copper is part of **lysyl oxidase**, which important for this cross-linking. Moreover, the **stability of tissue** is impaired[749]. Vice versa, **copper can increase collagen synthesis**[750, 751].
- Copper reduces the release of **histamine**, a mediator of the immune system[752], which appears to be involved in the release of (collagen attacking[549, 550]) collagenase and which increases the permeability of capillaries[561]. Histamine is closely related to allergies.
  The histamine is released by mast cells, and copper deficient animals have more mast cells[748] (for the impact of the immune system on myopia see section 3.12).
- Copper deficiency reduces (**NO-mediated**) **smooth muscle relaxation and vasodilation**, depending **exponentially** on the copper dose in the diet[753, 754, 748] *(note: this may have an impact on the smooth ciliary muscle which is active in accommodation, see section 3.2; on the impact of NO see section 3.12.4, on the impact of blood circulation see section 3.11).*
- Copper can **inhibit iNOS activity** (see section 3.12.4 and 4.2.3.4).
- Copper deficiency reduces the **antioxidant Cu/Zn-SOD activity**[753], and increases the activities of oxidizing agencies[755, 756] (for the impact of oxidative processes on myopia see section 3.16.12).
- Copper deficiency can cause **reduced microcirculation** in capillaries[748] (for the impact of blood circulation on myopia see section 3.11).
- Copper deficiency during gestation and lactation resulted in **lower dopamine levels** in the brains of the post-weaning rats[66], and low dopamine was never observed when copper was supplemented[757] (for the impact of dopamine on myopia see section 3.3.2).
- Copper depletion experiments with men and women have revealed impaired **glucose metabolism**[758, 759].
- Copper deficiency causes a **loss of photoreceptor cells** in the retina[432].
- Miesel et al. stated[760]: "The concentrations of **Cu-thionein** [a copper protein] were **significantly diminished** in patients with **connective tissue diseases**."
- The rate of **apoptosis** (programmed cell death, see section 4.2.2.3) can be increased at copper deficiency[761]. For the impact of apoptosis on myopia see section 3.12.2.

Table 14 Nutrition, copper and the connective tissue

Moreover, there is the hypothesis that a **lack of potassium is blocking** the building of the copper containing enzyme **lysyl oxidase**[579], which is essential for the connective tissue.

It does not need clinical deficiencies to have an impact on the connective tissue. Wildman et al. stated[762]: "...study suggests that **abnormalities in cardiac ultrastructure** occurred in rats chronically fed diets marginally low in Cu, **despite minimal changes in conventional biochemical indicators of Cu status**." It was suggested that there is a **threshold effect** of copper deficiency; under this threshold lesions are developing.[763]

In general, a deficit in copper can be caused by five different mechanisms:

- **Deficit in nutrition:** Frequently the content of copper in the nutrition is insufficient[526, 764]. The daily need is about 1.5 to 3.0 mg, for Europe and the USA, however, in 30% of the cases the supply is under 1.0 mg per day[765].

- **Deficit in early childhood:** If the nutritional deficit in copper was experienced in early childhood, e.g. during gestation and lactation, metabolic anomalies can be established which cannot be reversed any more later[66].

- **Bioavailability:** In spite of a sufficient supply with copper the bioavailability can be reduced because of other ingredients in the nutrition; copper was described as a "victim" nutrient, because its absorption can be easily inhibited, e.g. by the (increasing) consumption of sugar[743] (see table above).

- **Genetic metabolic effects,** which had advantages in the history of evolution in one respect, but which have a negative impact on the connective tissue (like increased usage of copper for other biochemical functions, e.g. within the immune system)[579].

- **Genetic metabolic defects** like the copper related Menke's disease, which affects the connective tissue.

- **Increased demand** of copper can be caused by activities of the immune system. These activities increase the level of cortisol, which increases the level of copper-containing lysyl oxidase that is needed for tissue repair (see section 4.2.3.3). Milanino et al. stated[766] that "...during **acute inflammation**, the organism **increases its requirement for copper and zinc**..."

An **examination of the serum is not reliable** for the assessment of copper status, as the serum level is homeostatically controlled until there are already serious deficits. More suitable is the evaluation of copper containing enzymes[765], and some authors recommend hair analysis[737].

The antioxidant properties of the copper containing Cu/Zn-SOD are well published[767], and traditionally wearing copper bangles treated arthritis, another problem of the connective tissue[768]. Furthermore contact with copper was found to have positive effects on other connective tissue problems[579]. Large quantities, however, may be toxic.

Interesting connections: In section 3.13.2 the findings have been mentioned that statistically myopes were showing a higher intelligence. Other studies indicate that newborns into lower socioeconomic level families show higher concentrations of copper serum.

Notes:

- *There are serious effects of copper deficiency on the heart[758], which remind strongly of myopia related problems:*

    - *cardiac enlargement - reminds of the extension of the sclera,*
    - *smooth muscle problems - reminds of the smooth ciliary muscle,*
    - *aortic fissures - reminds of fissures of the retina, and*
    - *arrhythmias - reminds of accommodation problems.*

- *Moderate* **dietary copper supplements appear to be highly recommendable for prevention of myopia progression**, *in spite of the fact that this has not been explicitly recommended by the scientific world so far.*

4.3.1.4   Magnesium

Publications about the impact of magnesium on myopia have been summarized in section 3.16.3 (hypomagnesemia).

The following mechanisms might explain the impact of magnesium on the connective tissue:

- Galland et al. stated[769]: "...Magnesium deficit hinders the mechanism by which fibroblasts degrade defective collagen...", i.e. a **deficit in magnesium results in a degraded quality of the connective tissue**.

- **Vitamin B6** requires magnesium for its metabolic processes[770, 523]. (For the impact of vitamin B6 on myopia see sections 3.16.11 and 3.16.13, for the impact of vitamin B6 on the connective tissue see section 4.3.2.2.2).

- The activity of reactive, **oxidative agents of the immune system** is increased in case of a deficit of magnesium[771, 772], e.g. the level of histamine (which appears to be involved in the release of collagen attacking[549, 550] collagenase, and which increases the permeability of capillaries[561]) and of inflammatory cytokines. For the impact of the immune system on myopia see section 3.12, for the impact of the immune system on the connective tissue see section 4.2.2.

- The **NO balance** is disturbed by a deficit of magnesium[618,] and Magnesium can **increase eNOS activity** [586, 773]. For the impact of NO on myopia see section 3.12.4, for the impact of NO on the connective tissue see section 4.2.3.4.

- Magnesium can help to prevent a **damage of the retina**, caused by peroxynitrite, which is built during degradation of NO[361].

- **Spasms of smooth muscles** can be caused by a deficit of magnesium[774] - maybe via a disturbed NO-balance. In section 3.2 the often handicapped smooth ciliary muscle of myopes was discussed.

- Magnesium supplementation can reduce the **bone turnover rate**[775]. Bone consists of type I collagen. The sclera consists of type I collagen as well.

- Magnesium deficiency can cause **deficiency of potassium**[776]. For the interrelation between potassium and myopia see section 3.16.8, general information about the sodium / potassium balance is given in section 4.2.3.9.

- McCoy et al. stated[772]: "... **statuses** of both vitamin D and **magnesium** are less than optimum due to inadequate dietary intakes of the nutrients and to environmental, biological and disease factors..." where **the following nutrients or items can cause a deficiency of magnesium**[777, 773]:

    - **Lack of** vitamin D
    - Lack of vitamin B6
    - Lack of selenium
    - Lack of parathyroid hormone

    - **Excess of** alcohol/ethanol
    - Excess of salt
    - Excess of phosphoric acid (sodas)
    - Excess of coffee
    - Excess of sweating
    - Excess of stress.

4.3.1.5   Manganese

Publications about the impact of chromium on myopia were already summarized in section 3.16.7.

Individual results about the effects of manganese deficiency on related issues are:

- Deficiency of manganese is associated with defects in the **synthesis of proteoglycans** of the connective tissue[288].

- Manganese is a critical **cofactor for collagen synthesis** and metabolism[540].

- Manganese is an important **cofactor for cross-linking** of matrix proteins[778].

- Manganese Superoxide-Dismutase (**Mn-SOD**) **is an effective antioxidant** and very effective in prohibiting damages of structures caused by oxidation[779, 780]. For the impact of oxidative processes on myopia see section 3.16.12.

- Experimentally initiated deficits of manganese caused an increase of the calcium level in the serum[781] (i.e. a disturbance of the calcium metabolism, see section 4.3.1.1).

- Manganese helps to **control the release of histamines**[780], a mediator of the immune system[752], which appears to be involved in the release of (collagen attacking[549, 550]) collagenase and which increases the permeability of capillaries[561]. Histamine is closely related to allergies.

- A direct correlation between manganese and **dopamine** concentrations in the brain of mice was found[782]. For the impact of dopamine on myopia see section 3.3.2.

- Highest concentrations of manganese were found in the pineal gland[783], which, produces **melatonin**, and was brought already in connection with myopia (see section 3.7.1).

- For the maintenance of its cell structure the **cornea needs manganese**[784].

- Low levels of manganese appear to increase plasma **glucose** levels[785]. For the impact of insulin on myopia see section 3.16.1.

- A deficiency in manganese results in a **loss of photoreceptor cells** and capillary anomalies in the retina[433].

- Manganese can **increase cNOS activity** (see section 4.2.3.4).

4.3.1.6 Selenium

Publications about the impact of selenium on myopia were already summarized in section 3.16.12.1.

A simplified biochemical explanation of the functioning of selenium as an **antioxidant**[786] is shown in Figure 18.

4 A Synthesis – or how some Pieces might Fit together

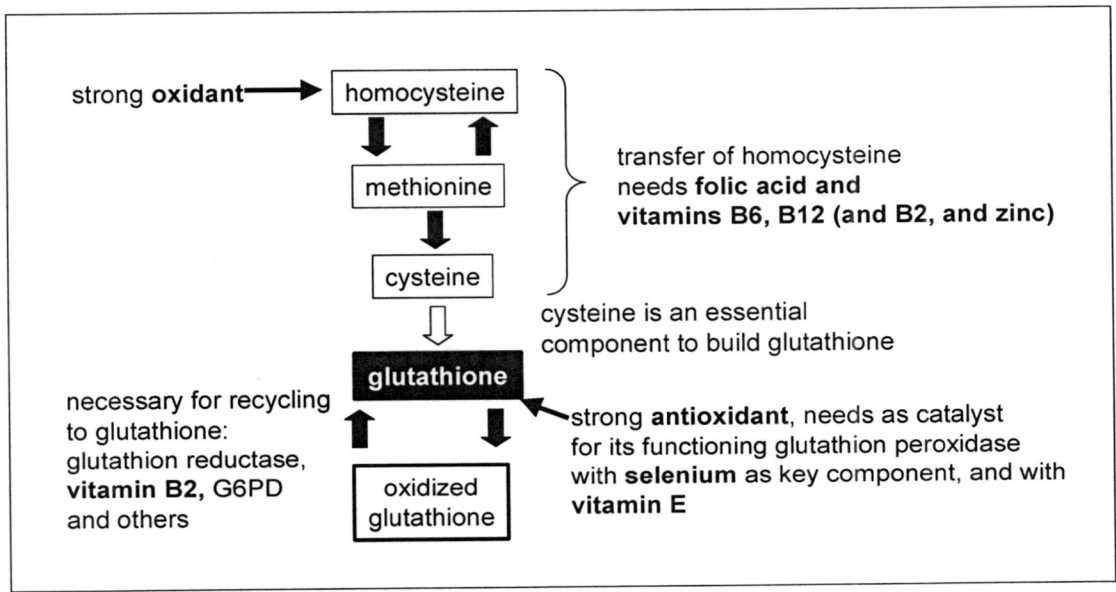

Figure 18 The glutathione metabolism

There are several genetic defects that may have a negative impact on the gluathione cycle: **G6PD deficiency**, glutathione reductase deficiency, glutathione peroxidase deficiency.

Even harmless painkillers like paracetamol need gluathione for metabolism, and damaging agents may be created if there is a lack of glutathione[787].

Individual results about the effects of selenium or selenium deficiency are[788]:

- A **deficiency** of selenium decreases the activities of all versions of glutathione peroxidase[789], and therefore **increase the risk of oxidative damage.**

- Selenium can **increase cNOS** and **lower the (potentially dangerous) iNOS** activity and **reduce the formation of highly reactive peroxynitrite**, with selenium deficiency having the adverse effect[586, 688, 790, 610, 611, 591, 791] (see section 4.2.3.4 about NO balance).

- Elevated levels of glutathione are reducing the **damaging effects of peroxynitrite**, which is built during the degradation of NO. Selenoproteins can help to protect against peroxynitrite (see section 4.2.3.4).

- Dietary deficiency of selenium (half the adequate content), as well as excess selenium (a factor of 20 above normal) caused considerable **alterations in tissue**s of rabbits[792]. Within four days of exposure to deficiency ducklings showed major pathologic changes in collagen and muscle cells[793].

- **Dopamine** turnover was increased when rats were fed selenium deficient diet. The decrease in brain antioxidant protection caused by a nutritional deficit of selenium and a following decrease in glutathione peroxidase activity was made responsible for this effect[794]. Interrelations between myopia and dopamine were discussed in section 3.3.2.

- McCarty et al. stated[795]: "Adequate selenium nutrition may down-regulate **cytokine signaling [of the immune system]**", i.e. selenium is expected to have a balancing effect on the actions of the immune system[796], or has acute anti-inflammatory effects[797]. Interrelations between myopia and the immune system were discussed in section 3.12, the immune system was discussed in more detail in section 4.2.2.

- A selenium-enriched diet decreased **glucose levels** in the capillaries of patients with Type 2 diabetes[798].

  The protection of retinal capillaries by selenium against sucrose induced injuries, however, was found to be independent of glutathione peroxidase activity[799].

  Interrelations between the glucose level and myopia were discussed in section 3.16.1.

- Long-term deficits of selenium can create disturbances of the **functioning of muscles**[796]. Interrelations between the functioning of the ciliary muscle and myopia were discussed in section 3.2.

- Selenium was found to be required for proper functioning of the **thyroid gland**, via glutathione peroxidase, which has selenium as a component[437]. Interrelations between myopia and the thyroid gland were discussed in section 3.16.9.

- Rats fed a diet higher in selenium (200 µg/kg diet) had **fewer cellular degenerating capillaries in the retina and a higher central choroid**[442].

- The enrichment of wheat with selenium leads to decreased **concentrations of TBARS** (thiobarbituric acid reactive substances)[800], which is an indicator of the concentration of damaging reactive oxygen-containing molecules. Persons with high myopia have elevated levels of TBARS (see section 3.12.2).

- Severe selenium deficiency can lead to **heart enlargement, a cardiomyopathy** called Keshan disease[801].

  Note:
  This enlargement reminds one of the myopic effects of the eyeball enlargement and reduced or lagging accommodation.

- Low selenium diet was associated with greater incidence of **depression and anxiety, and an altered turnover rate of some neurotransmitters** (see section 3.13 about mental issues and myopia). The dietary selenium intake of this low-selenium diet was **similar to, e.g., the current average intake** in many European countries[788].

- The rate of **apoptosis** (programmed cell death, see section 4.2.2.3) can be reduced by selenium supplementation[802] or increased by selenium (and vitamin E) deficiency[342]. For the impact of apoptosis on myopia see section 3.12.2.
- A lack of selenium can cause a **lack of magnesium** (see section 4.3.1.4).
- A lack of sympathetic innervation was made responsible for myopia (see section 3.2.1.5), and selenium is necessary for the **survival of sympathetic neurons**[803].

Note:
These effects of selenium seem to be widely diverse. Many of them are, however, based on the antioxidant effect of glutathione peroxidase, which has selenium as a component.

4.3.1.7 Silicon

So far, there are no publications linking the metabolism of silicon and myopia.

Some observations about silicon are:

- It has been proposed that silicon may have a role in protein **cross-linking** or in the structure of proteoglycans of the ground substance of the connective tissue[288].
- Seaborn et al. stated[804]: "Silicon deprivation also decreased femoral **calcium, copper, potassium and zinc concentrations...**". This means that silicon is not necessarily effective by itself, but by its impact on other elements and nutrients.
- Seaborn et al. stated[804]: "Both arginine and silicon affect **collagen formation** and bone mineralization."
- Seaborn et al. stated[805]: "[Results] suggest that silicon is a nutrient of concern in **wound healing** as well as bone formation."
- Refitt et al. stated[806]: "...orthosilicic acid [which contains silicon] at physiological concentrations stimulates **collagen type 1** synthesis in human oseoblast-like cells and enhances osteoblastic differentiation."

Notes:
- Most of these results were obtained by research on bone formation, which is not directly related to the structure of the sclera of the myopic eye. Some of the results are, however, explicitly mentioning the effect on collagen type 1 – and collagen type 1 is the main type of collagen, which constitutes the sclera.

- It can be expected that the "modern", more clean and refined nutrition contains less sandy components, i.e. less silicon.

4.3.1.8 Zinc

Publications about the impact of zinc on myopia have been summarized in section 3.16.5.

Zinc plays several different roles in the biochemistry of the connective tissue, but detailed established knowledge about the participation of zinc in the growth process is still missing[807]. Some observations are:

- Zinc deficiency impairs wound healing and **wound breaking strength**[808] (there is an increased concentration of zinc in healing wounds).

- Milanino et al. stated[766] that "...during **acute inflammation**, the organism **increases its requirement for copper and zinc**..."

- Zinc deficiency probably causes a **decreased rate of collagen synthesis** in connection with a decreased turnover rate[288].

- High doses of **zinc hinder copper absorption, but low doses of zinc are bad for the copper metabolism as well**[809, 810] (see section 4.3.1.3 for the effects of copper deficiency).

- Zinc is a component of the efficient **antioxidant Cu/Zn-SOD** (the relationship between myopia and oxidants was discussed in section 3.16.12). An overexpression of **Cu/Zn-SOD can reduce oxidative stress, protecting neurons** against ischemic damage[811].

- Rats fed zinc deficient diet showed enhanced lipid peroxidation and **increased TBARS**[812]. TBARS (thiobarbituric acid reactive substances) is an indicator of the concentration of damaging reactive oxygen-containing molecules. Correspondingly, people with diabetes type 2 showed a significant reduction of plasma TBARS after supplementation with Zinc[813]. Persons with high myopia have elevated levels of TBARS (see section 3.12.2).

- Zinc is an essential component of the **immune system**[814], especially in cooperation with **NO** (a deficiency of zinc enhances **iNOS activity**, see section 4.2.3.4) and a shifted **TH1/TH2 balance**[555] (see section 4.2.2.6). The relationship between myopia and the immune system was discussed in section 3.12.

- Zinc is an essential component of the biochemical circle, which recycles **homocysteine**[815] (the relationship between myopia and homocysteine was discussed in section 3.16.13).

- There is evidence that **melatonin can modulate zinc turnover.** Melatonin production is related to the night/day rhythm, whose relevance to myopia was discussed in section 3.7.1.

- Zinc deficiency causes a **loss of photoreceptor cells** in the retina[432].
- Zinc can help to prevent a **damage of the retina**, caused by peroxynitrite, which is built during degradation of NO[361].

4.3.2 Vitamins

4.3.2.1 Vitamin A

For vitamin A no direct connection with myopia has been published so far. The impact of the Vitamin A - related retinoic acid, however, has been mentioned in section 3.3.2.

On the one hand, a deficit of vitamin A can have the consequence that collagen attacking **collagenase** is abundant [816]. On the other hand, high (i.e. nonphysiological) doses of vitamin A can inhibit **collagen synthesis**[536].

Additionally there is the result that in experiments retinoic acid administered in the dark mimics the **effect of light** for some proteins expressed in the eye[196], which offers a link to the results presented in section 3.7.2.

Moreover, vitamin A deficiency causes a **loss of photoreceptor cells** in the retina[432].

Vitamin A can **increase eNOS activity**, and its precursor, the carotenoids can **decrease iNOS activity**[586] (see section 4.2.3.4).

Where **rice is the main food, the diet is deficient in vitamin A**[817]. This can have an effect not only on the connective tissue, but can as well result in poor night vision.

Note:
The last statement refers especially to Asia, where the highest incidence of myopia exists; moreover, among the Eskimos is an especially significant increase in myopia, and a significant switch off from a very vitamin A rich traditional diet characterizes their change in nutrition.

4.3.2.2 B-Vitamins

4.3.2.2.1 Vitamin B2 (Riboflavin)

For vitamin B2 no connection with myopia was published so far.

Individual results about the effects of vitamin B2 deficiency on related issues are:

- Vitamin B2 deficiency creates **oxidative stress in tissues**[702], and lenses of animals fed vitamin B2 deficient diets had reduced levels of the antioxidant glutathione[818]. Moreover a lack of vitamin B2 reduces the glutathione reductase activity[819] and the activity of G6PD (for the effect of this reduced activity see figure in section 4.3.1.6). For the impact of oxidative processes on myopia see section 3.16.12.

- **Solubility of collagen** was increased and the proportion of insoluble collagen was reduced in the skin of both vitamin B2 as well as vitamin B6 deficient rats[820].

  Note:
  The increase in the soluble fraction of collagen makes it easily degradable.

- The **mechanical stability of corneas** was improved by treatment with vitamin B2 (and UV irradiation), introducing additional cross-links[821].

- Deficiencies in vitamin B2 produce irregularities in the **cell-mediated immune response**[822]. Interrelations between myopia and the immune system were discussed in section 3.12, the immune system was discussed in more detail in section 4.2.2.

- It was concluded that vitamin B2 is essential for a pigment in the retina, which controls the circadian clock, i.e. the **day-/night-rhythm**[823]. Interrelations between myopia and the day-/night-rhythm were discussed in section 3.7.1.

- Vitamin B2 deficiency has a negative impact of the metabolism of **vitamin B6**[824], and of folic acid in relation with the **homocysteine cycle**[825].

- Vitamin B2 deficiency results in **poor bioavailability of zinc** (and iron)[826].

- Vitamin B2 deficiency was found to be **widespread in Asia**[827, 819]. As discussed in section 3.1 myopia a especially significant problem in Asia.

A deficiency in vitamin B2 can cause deficiencies in vitamin B6[828] and reduced levels of an active form of folic acid[825].

If a therapy with vitamin B2 is indicated, 5 to 10 times the recommended daily allowance (RDA) is sufficient[829]. An excess of vitamin B2 can damage of the photoreceptor layer of retinas[830].

4.3.2.2.2 Vitamin B5 (Pantothenic Acid)

Supplementation with vitamin B5 resulted in **greater strength of newly built collagen tissue** after wound healing than supplementation with vitamins C (ascorbic acid); this result was explained by its effect on the metabolism of copper, magnesium and manganese (which are increased), and Iron (which is decreased)[831].

4   A SYNTHESIS – OR HOW SOME PIECES MIGHT FIT TOGETHER

4.3.2.2.3   Vitamin B6 (Pyridoxine, but also Pyridoxal or Pyridoxamine)

The few publications about the impact of vitamin B6 on myopia have been summarized in section 3.16.11.

To become effective as a coenzyme, vitamin B6 has to be transferred into its phosphate version.

A lack of pyridoxine in the nutrition is quite frequent[832, 833], and Gregory stated[833] that "current understanding of the factors that govern vitamin B6 bioavailability is incomplete".

Table 15 describes the impact of some nutritional components on the vitamin B6 metabolism, and some relevant effects of vitamin B6 on the connective tissue. The effects of deficiencies are obviously opposite to the benefits.

Cause		Effect		Vitamin B6 deficit		Consequences
Magnesium deficit	→	Magnesium is needed for the absorption of pyridoxal phosphate by tissues[770].				• Defective **collagen and elastin cross-linking**[288, 630]. Increased **solubility** of collagen[820].
Substantial intake of **protein**, especially meat	→	Increased demand of vitamin B6 creates deficiency[850, 459].				• **Peroxidative stress** (measured via TBARS content)[834, 835]. Reduced synthesis of cysteine, a precursor of the **antioxidant glutathione**[836] and reduced activity of G6PD[824], which is important for the glutathione cycle. For the impact of oxidative processes on myopia see section 3.16.12.
Vitamin B2 deficiency	→	Affected conversion of vitamin B6 to its effective coenzyme version[851, 824].	→	Vitamin B6 deficit	→	• Increased release of **histamine**[837], a mediator of the **immune system**[734], which appears to be involved in the release of (collagen attacking[549, 550]) collagenase and which increases the permeability of capillaries[561]. Histamine is closely related to allergies. Moreover vitamin B6 was found to be essential for histamine degradation[838], and vitamin B6 deficiency led to increased levels of IgE, which is often involved in allergic reactions[839], and reduced **thymus weight**[840]. For the impact of the immune system on myopia see section 3.12.
Zinc deficiency	→	Affected conversion of vitamin B6 to its effective coenzyme version[852].				• Increased level of oxalic acid[841], which hinders **calcium absorption**[842]. For the impact of calcium see section 4.3.1.1.
Use of **oral contraceptives**	→	Increased demand of vitamin B6 creates deficiency[853].				• Lack of **dopamine** in the brain[843, 844]. Inherited lack of dopamine may respond to high doses of vitamin B6[522]. The impact of dopamine on myopia was discussed in section 3.3.2.
Physical **inactivity**	→	Reduced storage of vitamin B6[854].				• Decreased/shifted level of **melatonin**[845, 846, 847, 848] (**insomnia**[849]) which has not only an impact on the day-/night rhythm (see section 3.7.1), but which is also an effective antioxidant[638]. Most effective was an administration of vitamin B6 at nighttime[845].
Increased intake of **vitamin C**	→	Increases excretion of metabolite of vitamin B6[828].				• The **NO balance** is disturbed by a deficit of vitamin B6[618, 773]. Vitamin B6 can **increase cNOS** and **lower the iNOS** activity[586, 609] (for the impact of NO on myopia see section 3.12.4, for the impact of NO on the connective tissue see section 4.2.3.4).
Elevated **blood sugar** level	→	Reduced level of vitamin B6[855].				• Altered **zinc** metabolism, reduced **copper** absorption[746].
Genetically based malabsorption causes vitamin B6 deficiency, which can be treated by daily doses which are 5 to 50 times the normal dose[523, 856].						• The level of **homocysteine**, an oxidant, is increased (see figure in section 4.3.1.6). An elevated level of homocysteine can lower the level of copper (see section 4.3.1.3 for the impact of copper).
						• Reduced absorption of **vitamin B12**[828], see section 4.3.2.2.4.
						• Most likely vitamin B6 can help to prevent a **damage of the retina**, caused by excessive NO[361].

Table 15 Nutrition, vitamin B6 and the connective tissue

4.3.2.2.4 Vitamin B12 (Cobalamin)

For vitamin B12 no connection with myopia was published so far.

Individual results about the effects of vitamin B2 on related issues are:

- Vitamin B12 was found to be related to the circadian rhythm, i.e. the **day-/night-rhythm** in the retina[857, 432]. The day-/night-rhythm was found to be related to myopia, see section 3.7.1.

- It was concluded that vitamin B12 acts as an **immunomodulator** for cellular immunity[858]. The immune system was found to be related to myopia, see section 3.12.

- Vitamin B12 deficiency can cause inadequate usage of **folic acid**[859], and an increased level of the **oxidant homocysteine**. Folic acid and homocysteine were found to be related to myopia, see section 3.16.13.

- Most likely vitamin B12 can help to prevent excessive NO from **damaging the retina**[361].

A deficiency in vitamin B12 can cause deficiencies in folic acid [859]. Due to genetic heredity, an increased daily dose may be necessary[523].

4.3.2.3 Folic acid (member of the family of B-vitamins)

Publications about the impact of folic acid on myopia have been summarized in section 3.16.13.

Individual results about the effects of folic acid on related issues are:

- Folic acid supports the **biosynthesis of collagen** in muscles[860].

- Folate analogues are used in the treatment of **autoimmune** diseases[861]. For the impact of the immune system on myopia see section 3.12.

- Lower levels of **dopamine** accompany folic acid deficiency[636, 862, 863]. The impact of dopamine on myopia was discussed in section 3.3.2.

- Fournier et al. stated[864] that "...findings indicate that folate deficiency dramatically alters **melatonin** secretion in rats." The impact of melatonin and the day-/night rhythm was discussed in section 3.7.

- Folic acid is essential to keep the level of the **oxidant homocysteine** low. By this effect it can help to reach normal levels of nitric oxide **NO**[586, 633]. Both homocysteine and NO were found to be related to myopia, see the section 3.16.13 and 3.12.4.

- Levels of the **antioxidants glutathione peroxidase, glutathione and superoxide dismutase** significantly increased after folate treatment[865]. A deficiency of glutathione peroxidase reduces the **vasodilator** function, most likely due to a decrease in bioavailability of **NO** and to increased vascular oxidant stress[866]. The impact of blood circulation on myopia was discussed in section 3.11.
- The rate of **apoptosis** (programmed cell death, see section 4.2.2.3) can be increased[867]. For the impact of apoptosis on myopia see section 3.12.2.

Due to genetic heredity, an increased daily dose may be necessary[523]. Too much **UV radiation** on a skin with light pigmentation can destroy folates[868], and high **alcohol** consumption has a strong antifolate effect as well[869]. Antagonists to folate dependent enzymes are anti-inflammatory drugs like ibuprofen, salicylic acid and aspirin (which is converted to salicylic acid)[870].

A mild folate deficiency results in some protection against **malaria**[871].

Note:
Maybe a genetically induced, reduced bioavailability of folic acid in Asia offered an advantage against malaria before, but plays a role in myopia prevalence (see section 3.16.13) in Asia today.

4.3.2.4 Interactions between B Vitamins

It has been mentioned above that a deficiency of one B-vitamin could cause the deficiency of another B-vitamin (B2 / B6, B6 / B12, B2 / folic acid, B12 folic acid). Due to this reason, and because most B vitamins are found in similar food making the deficiency of multiple B vitamins more likely, it is recommended to take multiple vitamin B supplements[872].

An interesting observation: Supplements of elevated doses of vitamins B1, B6 and B12 have been found to **improve target shooting in marksmen**. This was explained by an influence on the physiological tremor[873]. Maybe there is an analogy with the ciliary muscle (section 3.2) and the saccades for focusing (section 3.5).

4.3.2.5 Vitamin C

So far, there are no publications, which are linking vitamin C and myopia directly.

Individual results about the effects of vitamin C on related issues are:

- Vitamin C improves the **synthesis of collagen**[288, 536], and can there for be **expected to be essential** especially for cases of malignant myopia.
- An elevated level of **homocysteine** can be caused by a deficiency of **vitamin C**[621] (see section 4.2.3.6).

- Vitamin C can **increase eNOS** activity[586] (see section 4.2.3.4).
- Neal et al. stated[367]: "Ascorbate release in the retina may have an important physiological role in **prolonging the life of dopamine...**" (dopamine is related to myopia, see section 3.3.1).

Note:
Many animals are able to build vitamin C by themselves, and it is said that humans lost this ability due to genetic mutations. The resulting increased vulnerability of the connective tissue, together with the substantially changes environment (e.g. near work) might have contributed to the spreading of myopia as well.

4.3.2.6   Vitamin D – or Sunlight

Publications about the impact of vitamin D on myopia have been summarized in section 3.16.3.

Individual results about the effects of vitamin D on related issues are:

- Vitamin D balances the **calcium metabolism** (for the impact of calcium see section 4.3.1.1) and is necessary for **magnesium absorption** (for the impact of magnesium see section 4.3.1.4).

- Vitamin D **suppresses various overreactions of the immune system** and related autoimmune effects[874, 875, 876, 877], and decreases immunoglobulin production[878]. Quite logically, the same effect was described for ultraviolet radiation or sunlight[879]. Additionally Vitamin D can **reduce iNOS** activity in brain cells[586] (see section 4.2.3.4).

- For the impact of the immune system on myopia see section 3.12.

- Vitamin D is essential for normal **insulin secretion, thereby preventing hyperglycemia**[880] (for the impact of hyperglycemia on myopia see section 3.16.1).

- Excessive (pharmacological!) doses of vitamin D have a **negative influence on bone collagen** formation; vitamin D deficiency influences bone collagen cross-linking[288].

The physiological status of vitamin D in human populations was found to be less than optimum[772, 881, 882]. A lack of vitamin D is more common in women[883], even with supplementation[884], and women are more affected by myopia (see section 3.1).

Few nutrients (mainly just fish and liver) contain vitamin D[885], most of it has to be generated by sunlight hitting the skin, which is frequently not enough because of indoor working and because of a skin pigmentation, which was originally adjusted by heredity for more sunny regions[886].

Notes:

- Especially persons whose ancestors are coming from regions with plenty of sun are advised to take care to get enough vitamin D.

- Furthermore, changed lifestyle and changed working conditions have reduced the exposure to sunlight in many countries significantly – this might contribute to the steep increase of myopia in Asia.

4.3.2.7 Vitamin E

Publications about the impact of vitamin E on myopia have been summarized in section 3.16.12.2. Individual results about the effects of vitamin E on related issues are:

- Vitamin E deficiency causes an increase in salt-soluble **collagen** in skin, and an increase in degradation by proteinases, and additionally structural changes in muscular fibers. Extremely high doses of vitamin E, however, caused a decreased accumulation of collagen, and collagen of lower tensile strength[288].

- Vitamin E decreases immunoglobulin production by the **immune system**, and related allergic reactions[887]. For the impact of the immune system on myopia see section 3.12.

- Supplementation with vitamin E resulted in a significant release of **dopamine**[888]. The impact of dopamine on myopia was discussed in section 3.3.2.

- The enzyme glutathione peroxidase, which is important for **antioxidant defense**, requires vitamin E as well as selenium[889], see figure in section 4.3.1.6. Generally vitamin E protects lipids of membranes from damage by oxidants[890]. For the impact of oxidative processes on myopia see section 3.16.12.

- The **activity of a protease called caspase**, which causes oxidative stress, is significantly increased by vitamin E (and selenium) deficiency[342].

- Vitamin E deficiency causes a **loss of photoreceptor cells** in the retina[432]. Bhutto et al. stated[451] that "...findings indicate that the **decrease in retinal capillaries** in vitamin E-deficient rats is secondary to retinal degeneration."

- Du et al. stated[403] that "...vitamin E for 2 months significantly inhibited the diabetes-induced increase in production of **superoxide in the retinas**."

- Vitamin E has some modulating effects on **NO** metabolism[891, 892], can **reduce the formation of highly reactive peroxynitrite**[591] and can **increase eNOS activity**[586] (see section 4.2.3.4).

4.3.3 Other Components of Nutrition, and some Facts about Nutrition

4.3.3.1 Flavonoids

Publications about the impact of flavonoids on myopia have been summarized in section 3.16.12.2.

There are about 4000 different types of flavonoids[893], and therefore from individual results of one species it is hard to draw conclusions about the effect of other species. In fact the magnitude of specific effects of individual flavonoids was found to be quite different. This makes it hard to give recommendations for any specific flavonoid. Some names of individual flavonoids are quercetin, hesperidin, rutin, anthocyanidin, pycnogenol and catechin. Flavonoids can be found in many vegetables and fruits.

Individual results about the effects of flavonoids on related issues are:

- Flavonoid catechin made **collagen** more resistant to collagenase[894], and from a decreased solubility of collagen it was concluded that flavonoids improve the cross-linking[727].

- Numerous publications reported the **antioxidant** properties of flavonoids[288, 893, 895, 896, 897, 898] and even specific antioxidant effects on the retina were found[899]. For the impact of oxidative processes on myopia see section 3.16.12.

- Flavonoids have antiinflammatory effects on the **immune system**[900, 901, 902, 903], sometimes including reduction of the release of histamines from mast cells[904, 905, 906]. For the impact of the immune system on myopia see section 3.12.

- Flavonoids can improve the **microcirculation**[897]. For the impact of the blood circulation on myopia see section 3.11.

- Flavonoids were reported to promote **relaxation**[907] and **contractile function**[908] of the cardiovascular **smooth muscle**; maybe this effect exists for the smooth ciliary muscle, which provides accommodation as well. In section 3.2 the often impaired accommodation via the smooth ciliary muscle of myopes was discussed.

- One flavonoid was found to reduce the oxidant **homocysteine**[909]. Homocysteine was found to be related to myopia, see section 3.16.13.

- Flavonoids Pycnogenol, quercetin, hesperidin and procyanidins suppress the activity of (negative) **iNOS**[586, 592, 910, 911, 912] or protect against peroxynitrite, but flavonoids increased (positive) **eNOS** activity[913] (see section 4.2.3.4 about NO balance). NO was found to be related to myopia, see section 3.12.4).

- **Tea** with its ingredient theaflavin was found to down-regulate the synthesis of the **iNOS and reactive oxygen, and to scavenge NO**[790, 914, 915]. Oxidants and iNOS can have negative effects on myopia (see sections 3.12.4 and 4.2.3.4).

  Note:
  Is the switch from tea to soft drinks among the younger Asian population connected to the increasing prevalence of myopia in Asia?

- **Red wine** and **purple grape juice** can increase platelet derived **NO** release (not via iNOS!) and decrease **superoxide** production[916]. NO can have positive effects on myopia (see sections 3.12.4 and 4.2.3.4).

- **Quercetin**, and to a lesser degree **rutin** were found to suppress **iNOS** production[917]. INOS can have negative effects on myopia (see sections 3.12.4 and 4.2.3.4).

- Flavonoids were found to suppress **hyperglycemia**[918]. Hyperglycemia was found to be related to myopia, see section 3.16.1.

4.3.3.2 Carbohydrates

Publications about the impact of refined carbohydrates / sugar on myopia have been summarized in section 3.16.1, and the impact of an elevated blood sugar level was described in section 4.2.3.8.

Apparently there are metabolic effects of glucose beyond its influence on the level of insulin. Valikangas et al. stated[919]: "... **results indicate that high levels of glucose, but not insulin, directly down-regulate the type I collagen synthesis...**" Myopia is mainly caused by defect in collagen Type I (see section 3.3.3).

Moreover, a high blood sugar level causes a reduced level of **vitamin B6** (see section 4.3.2.2.2), and Lien et al. stated[651] that "**glucose inhibits collagen fibril formation** in vitro."

The negative effects of sugar have been questioned by referring to the rather similar metabolism of other carbohydrates. It should be undisputed, however that substantial consumption of sugar or empty carbohydrates results in a reduced amount of essential nutritional components like e.g. minerals, vitamins, amino acids and fatty acids. This lack of essential nutritional components will be harmful, even if the sugar or the empty carbohydrates might not be harmful by themselves.

Additionally it is emphasized in the literature that it is very important to keep a diet **avoiding steep increases in blood sugar level**, i.e. to have a "low-glycaemic index-low-fat-high-protein" diet[411, 412]. Very frequently these steep increases in blood sugar (Hyperglycemia) result in a later drop in blood sugar to low levels (hypoglycemia).

A problem might still occur even when blood sugar level is low: this low blood sugar level might be achieved only with a **high production of insulin,** and this may have other negative effects (see section 4.2.3.8).

If carbohydrates are consumed substantially in the form of sugar (i.e. sucrose and fructose) instead of starch, the **symptoms of a deficiency of copper are worsened** (see section 4.3.1.3).

Finally it has to be emphasized that sugar and carbohydrates like white wheat flour were **not part of the nutrition, to which we are genetically adjusted** via our ancestors (see introduction to section 4).

4.3.3.3 Lipids and Fatty Acids

So far, there are no publications, which are linking lipids or fatty acids and myopia.

There are different types of fats[920, 921]:

- **Saturated fats**, which have no double bonds between the carbon atoms in the fatty acid chains. Fats from animals are mostly saturated.

- **Mono- and polyunsaturated fats**, which have one or several double bonds between the carbon atoms in the fatty acid chains.

- **Trans fatty acids** are created during hydrogenation of unsaturated fats, when plant oils are exposed to hydrogen at high temperature, and the configuration of their molecules is changed (there are "cis" and "trans" configurations of the remaining double bonds). This results in a hardening of the fat. They are marketed because of the availability of very cheap and abundant plant oils, but solid fats are needed for many cooking applications. They are rare in nature and not part of a healthy nutrition.

- **Omega fatty acids** are described by a nomination where the position of the first double bond of an unsaturated fatty acid is given: e.g. an omega–3 fatty acid is an unsaturated fatty acid with its first double bond after carbon atom number 3. Fish oils are rich in omega-3 fatty acids. One problem is storage, which has led to reduction in usage.

Individual results about the effects of lipids and fatty acids on related issues are:

- Effects on the **immune system:** Polyunsaturated vegetable omega-6 fat (e.g. corn oil) and hydrogenated trans fatty acids with omega-6 fatty acids are found to be pro-inflammatory and immune function enhancing (higher production of cytokines and immunoglobulin). In contrast, highly polyunsaturated omega-3 (e.g. fish oil) is anti-inflammatory and immune function suppressive and works positive against autoimmune diseases[922, 923, 924, 925, 926, 927]. Results about olive oil are contradictory[927, 922]. For the impact of the immune system on myopia see section 3.12.

A typical western diet was said to contain, however, almost 10 times more omega-6 than omega-3 fatty acids[928], and the usage of omega-6 fatty acids is said to have increased dramatically[923].

Note:
This may contribute to the highly increasing rate of myopia among Eskimos, whose traditional diet was very high in fish oil.

- Effects on the **antioxidant system**: Increased antioxidant enzyme levels accompanied feeding with omega-3 lipids[923]. For the impact of oxidative processes on myopia, see section 3.16.12.

- Saturated fatty acids **impair (positive) eNOS activity**, but **increase (negative) iNOS activity**. For the impact of NO on myopia see section 3.12.4, for general information about NO see section 4.2.3.4.

4.3.3.4   Amino Acids

Amino acids (especially essential amino acids, which cannot be synthesized by the body) can be expected to have significant impact on the issues, which are related to myopia. There is, however, by far less information available for amino acids compared to vitamins and minerals. Moreover, interrelations are very complex. An example: **Lysine is an essential** component for the synthesis of connective tissue, but it is competing with arginine for absorption[459, 586], and the antioxidant[929] **arginine is essential** for proper levels of NO[930], and is used to lower intraocular pressure and to increase ocular blood flow. High levels of NO, however, are toxic[353]. Consequently, a diet that differs significantly from the diet of the ancestors (and to which the evolution adjusted the ancestors) can have substantial impact on the NO balance (see section 4.2.3.4 about NO balance).

Consequence: Supplements are hardly recommended, until the right targeted balance is known – which is hardly ever the case. In this respect, there is no replacement for a properly balanced nutrition with a lot of variety (e.g. vegetables, fruits, fish, meat).

4.3.3.5   Proteins

Experiments with cats, which were exposed to stress, showed that animals fed with **casein** (the main protein found in cheese, and other milk products) **instead of soya** as the protein source were showing a **greater resistance to stress**. The animals fed with soya had significantly increased levels of **insulin** and **dopamine-beta-hydroxylase**, and a significantly reduced level of **vitamin B6**[679].

Moreover, a **casein** rich diet increased (positive) **cNOS activity** (see section 4.2.3.4).

Note:
The enzyme dopamine-beta-hydroxylase mentioned above is converting dopamine into norepinephrine, which might reduce dopamine levels. **Reduced dopamine and reduced vitamin B6 levels can be connected with myopia.**

Moreover, the norepinephrine causes **vasoconstriction**[910], and reduced blood circulation in the eye was connected with myopia (see section 3.11).

4.3.3.6 Some Other Nutrients

- Other plant derived **antioxidants** are the large group of various **carotenoids** including lutein[931], which can be found in many vegetables, and the less common plant **sterols and sterolins**, which are said to be very effective against autoimmune diseases[932, 933], and to keep a balance between **TH1 and TH2** cell types[934] (about TH1 and TH2 see section 4.2.2.6). The strong antioxidant **coenzyme Q10** can be synthesized by the body, and can be found mainly in meat and fish.

- **Caffeine** can increase blood vessel resistance and **decrease blood flow** in the eye[935]. For the impact of microcirculation on myopia see section 3.11. Resulting consequence: Avoid coffee. On the other hand, Trier et al. stated[476]: "Methylxanthine, a metabolite of caffeine, **increases collagen concentration and the diameter of collagen fibrils in the posterior sclera**, and may be useful for treatment or prevention of conditions ... such as **axial myopia** ..." which means coffee can have positive effects as well.

- **Ethanol** can reduce blood vessel resistance and **increase blood flow** in the eye[936]. For the impact of microcirculation on myopia see section 3.11. Consequence: Moderate consumption of alcohol might be not too bad (not for children).

- Soy based products significantly **inhibited the production of inducible nitric oxide (iNOS)**[937]. For the negative effects of iNOS on myopia see section 3.12.6 and 4.2.3.4.

    Note:
    Maybe the essential dietary changes in Asia, off from the traditional diet, which was rich in soy products, is contributing substantially to the increased number of myopes in Asia.

- Suzuki et al. stated[938]: "In conclusion, intake of vegetables and fruits rich in **carotenoids might be a protective factor against hyperglycemia**." For the negative effect of hyperglycemia on myopia see section 3.16.1.

4.4 Nutrition, some General Facts

As mentioned before, the nutritional mix of today is rather different from the diet to which we have been adjusted by heredity in ancient times.

Some of these changes are:

- **Food processing** causes many of these changes. By the preparation of Wheat flour the following losses were reported[939, 940]:

Vitamin B1	80%:
Vitamin B2	60%
Vitamin B3	75%
Vitamin B5	50%
Vitamin B6	50%
Calcium	50%
Magnesium	98%
Manganese	75% / 91%
Copper	65% / 70-90%
Chromium	87%
Iron	81%
Selenium	11-75%
Zinc	83%

- The ingestion of **proteins** and **sugar/carbohydrates** has increased very substantially; the mixture of dietary **lipids** has changed largely as well (for the negative consequences see sections 4.3.2.2.2, 4.3.3.2, and 4.3.3.3).

- Mainly due to **depletion of soils,** the concentration of nutrients in individual fruits and vegetables has changed substantially[528], as detailed charts show, which compare 1963 and 1992 data. The average reductions in content are:

Calcium	30%
Iron	32%
Magnesium	21%
Potassium	6%

    The decline in content of calcium, magnesium and iron compared to data from 1914 are still larger.

    Comparisons of trace minerals in 1948 and 1992 show large reductions in manganese and copper.

- The diets in all industrialized countries (and in some other countries as well) have been changed very substantially towards higher consumption of empty carbohydrates.

4 A Synthesis – or how some Pieces might Fit together

E.g., the consumption of **sucrose** per head has risen e.g. in **England** from 6.6 kg in 1815 to 54.5 kg in 1979[404].

An **example for Eskimos**, who are especially affected by an increase in myopia:

Their traditional diet contained, compared with the diet of today these additional contents[528]:

Calcium	540%
Magnesium	790%
Fat-soluble vitamins	1000%

- The different eating habits in different countries can explain at least partially the dramatic increase of myopia among various populations:

    E.g., **copper** plays a key role for the metabolism of the connective tissue (see sections 3.16.5 and 4.3.1.3). The content in copper of some nutrients is (per 100 g)[941]:

unpolished rice	240 µg
polished rice	130 µg
wheat bread, full grain	420 µg
white bread	220 µg

    Result:
    - Industrial processing has led to a reduction in copper by about 50%.
    - Rice, the main nutrient in Asia, where myopia is most common, is especially low in copper.

Some other important issues are:

- **Absorption:** Bergner stated[528] that "Perhaps the most widespread cause of indigestion in the United States today is the habit of eating in **stressful** or hurried situations. Stress inhibits the secretions of stomach acid and other enzymes that are necessary to digest foods and release their mineral content". Additionally, often the content of one nutrient is hindering the absorption of another nutrient (e.g. oxalic acid hinders the absorption of calcium).

- **Metabolic competition and metabolic linkage:** Frequently nutritional components are influencing each other in specific biochemical pathways, e.g. execration of abundant sodium pulls out calcium as well.

As a consequence, even if the personally appropriate amount of a nutrient is ingested, **there can be still a deficit of this nutrient** .

4.5 Impact of Nutrition and Behavior– Summary

The following table gives a rough summary of the results of the impact of some nutritional components on functions found to be related to myopia.

Certainly, there are many people who believe that the impact of a deficiency of nutritional components can be neglected, because of self-regulating biochemical mechanisms. The contrary opinion as worded by a professor for nutritional sciences is:

"... as we know about various nutrients that **long before there are visible clinical symptoms of a deficiency, there are changes in cell structures and sub cellular structures which can degrade their function.**" [Translated from Biesalski[534]]

"A lack of trace elements primarily stimulates the destruction of tissues and secondarily the production of cytokines" [translated from Biesalski[942]].

On the other hand, it was found that in many cases of inherited enzyme defects, high doses of the vitamin component of the corresponding coenzyme can at least partially restore enzymatic activity. This was especially verified for the B vitamins, where very high tolerances for high doses exist[522].

4 A Synthesis – or how some Pieces might Fit together

Nutritional component	Immune system	Antioxidant defense	Dopamine metabolism	Quality of connective tissue	NO balance	Homo-cysteine cycle	Day-/night-rhythm	Blood sugar level etc.	Strong synergy with
Calcium	X			X	X				
Magnesium	X			X	X				Se, K, vit. B6,
Copper	X	X	X	X	X				
Zinc	X	X		X	X	X			
Manganese	X	X	X	X	X			X	
Chromium	X	X						X	
Silicon				X					
Selenium	X	X	X	X	X			X	Mg, vit. E
Vitamin A				X					
Vitamin B2	X	X		X		X	X		Vitamin B6
Vitamin B6	X	X	X	X	X	X	X		Vitamin B12
Vitamin B12	X				X	X	X		
Folic acid	X		X	X	X	X	X		
Vitamin C		X			X	X	X		
Vitamin D	X			X	X			X	Ca, Mg
Vitamin E	X	X	X	X	X				
Flavonoids	X	X		X	X	X		X	
Carbohydrates	X	X	X	X	X			X	
Behavior									
Stress	X	X			X	X		X	

Columns grouped under: **Function with a reported impact on myopia**

Table 16 Impact of nutrients and of stress on functions with a reported impact on myopia

The table above gives an impression of the very high complexity of the potential interrelationships, and of the large variety of biochemical individualities, which might, among other results, lead to myopia.

Note:
The large variety of nutrients that can have an impact makes it rather unlikely that a single gene or very few genes are responsible for myopia.

Additionally, the table shows the very substantial impact, which a healthy and balanced nutrition must have.

It should be noted that some functions, which are represented as columns, are very strongly interrelated with each other. This makes it plausible that they are influenced by the same nutrients.

Note:
A very personal view:
NO (produced by iNOS or eNOS/nNOS, see section 4.2.3.4) appears to be a central issue for the development of myopia and its severe complications. **Nutritional control of iNOS should have, therefore, a very high priority.**

Some information about the general supply status of some nutrients is given in the sections about the individual nutrients, and in section 4.6.

4.6 The "Right" Supply with Vitamins and Minerals, and the Supply Status

There are many different recommendations for the daily dose, sometimes called recommended dietary allowance (RDA): In different countries the respective organizations publish different numbers, and the numbers are different for males and females, and they are age dependent[943]. Additionally there are different definitions like "minimum dose" and recommended dose".

Last, but not least it has to be emphasized again that there is a very substantial biochemical individuality, which means that individual persons have very different needs for an optimum supply with nutritional components[273].

Table 17 shows the daily doses which the respective organizations in the USA and in Germany recommended. The deviations result from different concepts of estimations.

4 A Synthesis – or how some Pieces might Fit together

	Recommended daily dose for age 19 to 25 in Germany[944] (differences between age 10 to 65 not very significant)		United States recommended dietary allowances for age 31 to 50[945]		Maximum dose[946]	
	Male	Female	Male	Female	No adverse effect level	Lowest adverse effect level
Vitamin A	3300 IU / 1.0 mg	3000 IU / 0.8 mg	1.0 mg	0.8 mg	10,000 IU	21,600 IU
Vitamin D	200 IU / 5µg		200 IU / 5µg		800 IU	2000 IU
Vitamin E	15 mg	12 mg	10 mg	8 mg		
Vitamin C	100 mg		60 mg		1000 mg	
Vitamin B1 (Thiamine)	1.3 mg	1.0 mg	1.2 mg	1.1 mg	50 mg	
Vitamin B2 (Riboflavin)	1.5 mg	1.2 mg	1.3 mg	1.1 mg	200 mg	
Vitamin B6 (Pyridoxine)	1.5 mg	1.2 mg	1.3 mg		200 mg	500 mg
Vitamin B12 (Cobalamin)	3 µg	2 µg	2.4 mg		3000 µg	
Folic acid	400 µg (recently increased)		400 µg		1000 µg	
Calcium	1000 mg		1000 mg		1500 mg	2500 mg
Magnesium	400 mg	310 mg	420 mg	320 mg	700 mg	
Chromium	30 - 100 µg		50 - 200 µg		1000 µg	
Copper	1 – 1.5 mg		1.5 – 3 mg		9 mg	
Manganese	2 - 5 mg		2 - 5 mg		10 mg	
Selenium	30 - 70 µg		70 µg	55 µg	200 µg	910 µg
Zinc	10 mg	7 mg	15 mg	12 mg	30 mg	60 mg

Table 17 Appropriate doses of various nutrients

Remark about vitamin D: It was reported that the vitamin D supply of sunlight-deprived persons should be at least 600 IU per day[881, 882].

Generally for safety reasons it appears to be wise, not to go beyond the "**no adverse effect level**" with supplements.

The bioavailability of the respective minerals is often very different, e.g. depending whether they are in organic or inorganic form. Generally **the inorganic form has a higher bioavailability**.

The "Nutrition Almanac"[958] is an excellent reference for answering the question, which natural food contains which components.

Note:
The content of a specific nutrient can vary not only due to a different processing, but to a different content of minerals in the soil where the plants have been growing.

Table 18 about the supply status is just a snapshot of a few publications. The variety in individual diets of individual persons is very large, making the selection of appropriate samples very difficult – not mentioning the already discussed biochemical individuality.

4 A Synthesis – or how some Pieces might Fit together

	Supply Status
Vitamin A	At rice eating populations 42% of RDA[817].
Vitamin D	Without sufficient sunlight no sufficient supply[882, 881, 947].
Vitamin B1 (Thiamine)	Marginal lack for 15-30% of population of USA[948]. Supply below RDA for Chinese[949].
Vitamin B2 (Riboflavin)	At rice eating populations only 70% of RDA[817]. In Germany lack for 10-20% of young people[950]. Supply below RDA for Chinese[949]. Subclinical deficiency leading to low glutathione reductase in Malaysia[819].
Vitamin B6 (Pyridoxine)	Inadequate status in 10-20% of population[951]. 20-70% of women had inadequate level even at intake of 1.33 mg/day[952]. In Germany insufficient supply for about 10% of population[832]. Chinese women in childbearing age: 26% are deficient[953].
Folic acid	Chinese women in childbearing age: 23% are deficient[953]. Pregnant women in South East Asia: 30-50% deficient[954].
Calcium	The average American diet contains 40 to 50 % of the RDA of calcium.[955]
Chromium	90% of diets lack sufficient chromium intake[955].
Copper	The average diet contains 50% of the RDA[955].
Magnesium	The average diet contains 50 to 60% of the RDA.[955]
Selenium	The average diet contains only 50% of the RDA[955]. There are large variations according to large variations in the content of the soil in the respective area.
Zinc	68% of Americans do not consume the RDA[955].

Table 18 Supply status of some vitamins and minerals

An anecdotal result reported by Dollhite et al.[956]: "Forty-three menus that were to be used in a diet manual were designed to meet the requirements of a specific diet ... only 11% of the menus met the RDA for zinc, half of the menus did not meet the RDA for vitamin B6 and one third did not meet the RDA for Iron."

"23% of Americans only are consuming two thirds of those [RDAs]."[957]

Additionally, there is the impact of individually different requirements[273].

It should be mentioned, however that some people deny that there is a nutritional problem, and that "you simply have to keep a balanced diet". True, but who is in a position to invest this much energy in getting the appropriate food, and to resist all these sweet and empty snacks and drinks?

Additionally, please look at the table in the introduction of section 4. It **compares the amount of selected nutrients in our diet and in the diet of our ancestors.**

> It is very important to realize, however that **all these supplements can never be a substitute for a healthy diet – they can only be add-ons:**
> A tremendous amount of nutrients in natural food are not analyzed yet (and maybe will never be analyzed completely), and therefore are not available as supplements. However, they certainly have important effects.

4.7 The Speed of Nutritional Effects

Often there are expectations that a change in nutrition will show rather immediate effects. Biochemical imbalances, which might have been developed over many years, can hardly be corrected within a short time. And in any case the quality of the connective tissue cannot be expected to improve significantly before the turnover time of this tissue has elapsed. And a reduction of myopia, i.e. a shortening of the eyeball cannot be reached by improving the quality of the connective tissue. Stopping the progression of myopia is worth, however, many and extensive efforts!

4.8 Overall Recommendations

There is a multiplicity of potential reasons for myopia, with most of these reasons having close interactions with each other (e.g. neurotransmitters influencing the immune system, and the day-/night rhythm influencing the NO balance), as was mentioned above. This is summarized in Figure 19.

4 A Synthesis – or how some Pieces might Fit together

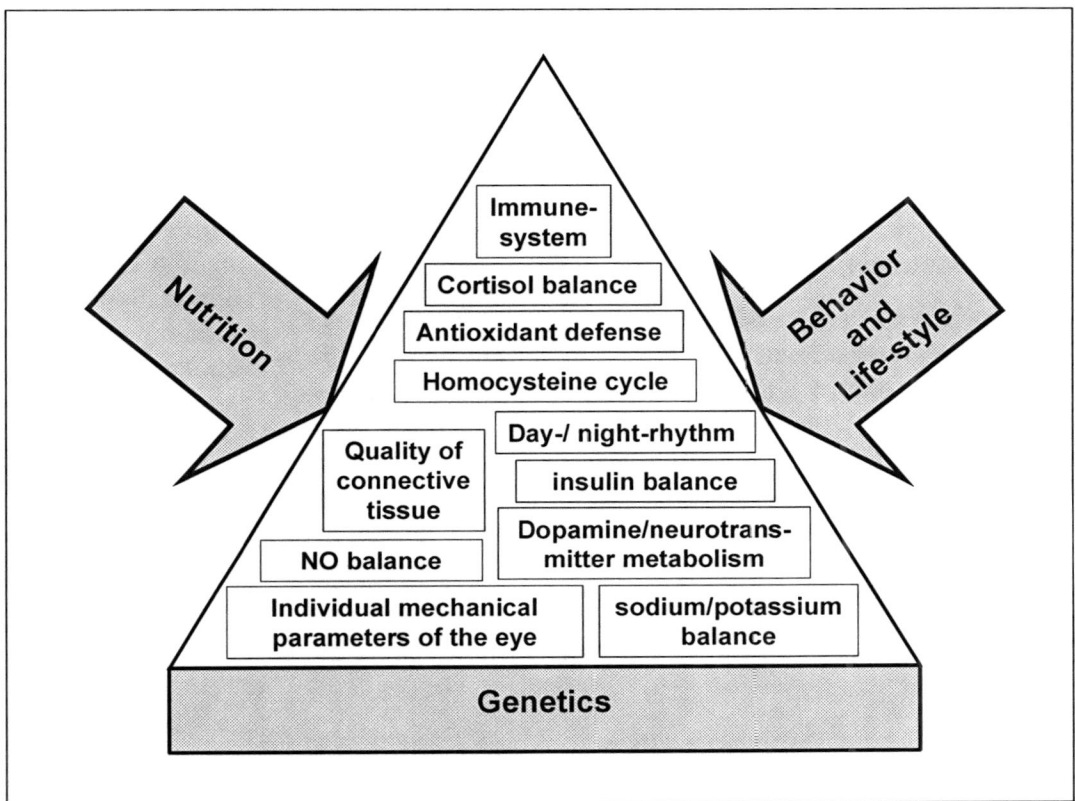

Figure 19 Some biochemical issues which can have an impact on myopia

Consequently it will be extremely hard to find out for individual patients, where exactly the unbalance of their biochemistry is located. Moreover, a specific and individual therapy can hardly be given in any case. What can be done, however, is to follow overall recommendations to eliminate potential weak points with respect to myopia and related issues.

The decision to follow these recommendations is made easier by the fact that hardly any risk accompanied them.

There is no guarantee that following these recommendations will stop the progression of your myopia. However, you can have the confidence that you did the best you could do.

The overall recommendations are summarized in Table 19 and Table 20.

Recommendations for preventing, or inhibiting the progression of myopia	
Recommendations from the **optical side**	**Potential risks**
• **Interrupt your near work** every 30 minutes by focusing on distant objects and maybe by wearing **plus glasses**, and relax your eyes especially in the evening. • For near work keep a reasonably large distance to your book / paper / computer screen, or better use **under-correcting or bifocal glasses** (not for driving a car! And general under correction can result in a blur picture on the retina, which will result in deprivation myopia, too). **Plus glasses** for extensive near work should be of advantage especially for people who are not myopic yet, but are at risk, and for people, who wear contact lenses. *Note:* *Reading in bed leads mostly to an insufficiently long reading distance.* • Better, read printings with **large letters.** • Do not read at bad light, **300 Lux** are the minimum. • Some **exercising of the accommodation** by alternating focusing near and far objects can be helpful (but don't expect miracles from classes which are offered about this issue). • **Do not keep a light switched on in the kid's room at night** (there is a controversy in the literature about this issue, but better be on the safe side). Additionally, take care to have **enough sleep** at the proper time and in darkness[309]. • Regular **physical exercises** can help to reduce the intraocular pressure and the mental stress, and regulate blood sugar level.	No risk, but avoid a permanent and substantial undercorrection without the consultation of an optometrist, as an inappropriate undercorrection or inappropriate bifocals may create, e.g., a deprivation effect[120].
Use **rigid gas permeable contact lenses** (RGP). Soft contact lenses don't show this positive effect.	None if properly fitted and maintained.

Table 19 Optical recommendations for preventing myopia or inhibiting the progression of myopia

4 A Synthesis – or how some Pieces might Fit together

Recommendations for preventing, or inhibiting the progression of myopia	
Recommendations from the **behavioral and the nutritional side**	**Potential risks**
Reduce negative mental **stress**, possibly by appropriate physical and mental exercises.	Potential risk for your professional career.
Keep a **healthy and balanced diet**, which is **low in sugar and low in refined carbohydrates** (incl. white wheat), **low in sodium**, low in fat except omega-3 (fish) oil, and have **plenty of (if possible unprocessed) vegetables and fruits.** There are many books for a healthy diet on the market, with tables showing the contents in specific nutrients[958].	None
If the progression of your myopia is worrying you, **additional supplements** of **multiple vitamins** (especially the vitamins E, B2, B6, folic acid), **minerals** (especially of **calcium, selenium, copper and zinc**) and especially also of **flavonoids** are recommended. Only for the **B vitamins** doses substantially higher than the recommended daily doses may be helpful[522, 523] (for flavonoids no recommended doses are available). Especially if your ancestors came from regions with plenty of sun, you may easily have an individual lack of **vitamin D** – and in general our ancestors spent by far more time outdoors, which gave them plenty of vitamin D. Therefore supplements are recommended.	Do not take higher doses of **vitamin A** than the recommended daily allowance for it and keep the appropriate balance between **copper and zinc**, and **calcium and magnesium**. See section 4.6 for **maximum amounts**.

Table 20 Behavioral and nutritional recommendations for preventing myopia or inhibiting the progression of myopia

5 Additional Information

This section contains numerous hopefully helpful hints and explanations dealing with the myopia issue. These hints and explanations cover the correction of myopia by glasses, contact lenses or surgical operation, as well as the dosage of dietary supplements.

5.1 Optical Correction

5.1.1 Glasses

Often the customer is not aware of the big variety in the quality of optical glasses. This section should help to ask the optician the right questions when ordering new glasses (even if you are wearing contact lenses you need spare glasses).

5.1.2 The Material of the Glass

The refractive index of the lens material determines the thickness of the lens: The higher the index, the thinner the lens (which is important for higher degrees of myopia). For mineral ("real") glasses the index is between 1.5 and 1.9, for organic ("plastic") glasses the index is between 1.5 and 1.7. Generally the rule is, the higher the refractive index, the higher the price of the glasses. Therefore highly myopic people who generally need thick glasses have to spend more money to get thinner (better looking) glasses.

Often not only the thickness of the lens is important, but also the weight: Organic lenses are lighter than mineral lenses, and for the mineral lenses the rule is, the higher the refractive index, the higher the specific weight.

A few numbers for comparison:

The Edge **thickness** for a lens with 65 mm diameter, a power of $D = -10.00$ and a refractive index 1.5 is 13.3 mm, and for a refractive index 1.9 the edge thickness is 7.4 mm.

The **weight** of a lens with 65 mm diameter, a power of $D = -10.00$ and a refractive index 1.5, made of a mineral glass is 56 gram, whereas the weight for an organic glass is only 33 gram.

5 ADDITIONAL INFORMATION

A few typical numbers for the specific weight are shown in Table 21:

Material	Refractive index	Specific weight in gram/cm^3
Organic glass	1.5	1.32
	1.6	1.34
Mineral glass	1.5	2.55
	1.6	2.67
	1.7	3.19
	1.8	3.62
	1.9	4.02

Table 21 Data of some materials used for glasses

Another parameter of the lens material is the dispersion, i.e. the difference of the refractive index for various color components, which can result in disturbing color effects on the edge of the lens. Generally, the higher the refractive index, the higher the problem of dispersion.

Additionally, the glass should have a high absorption of UV light.

5.1.3 The Coating of the Glass

Without a coating, there would be very disturbing reflections on the surface of the glass, for example making the eyes "invisible" to other people, and which create reflections of light which are very disturbing during night driving.

For organic glasses there is another reason for coating: The relatively soft surface has to be protected from getting scratched too easily.

Overall, up to ten layers have to be brought to the lens, and significant differences in quality (and price) can be found for lenses from different manufacturers, and for different product lines of the same manufacturer.

5.2 Contact Lenses

(General sources[959, 960, 961, 485])

Already in 1999 it was reported that worldwide about 80 million people wore contact lenses, with about 33 million people in the USA at this time.

A person who is switching from glasses to contact lenses experiences a magnification of the image on the retina. Table 22 compares the image size on the retina for people with glasses and for people with contact lenses[962] (image size for contact lenses are rather similar to emmetropic people).

Myopia in D	Increase of image size by contact lenses compared to glasses
- 5.00	7 %
- 7.50	10 %
- 10.00	14 %
- 15.00	23 %

Table 22 The image size when using contact lenses compared to glasses

As the **accuracy of vision** is, among others, determined by the "granularity" of the retina (see section 1.11) for higher grades of myopia a smaller image results in poorer vision.

Additionally it was found that contact lenses improved the **contrast sensitivity** for high myopes (more than - 6.25D)[214].

Contact lenses have some general advantages, e.g., no dimming by condensed water or rain. Features greatly depend on the type of lens.

5.2.1 Basic Types of Lenses – Soft Lenses versus Hard Lenses

The different types of contact lenses are:

- **Hard lenses** (this type of contact lenses was developed first):
  - Rigid gas permeable (**RGP**) lenses, which allow substantial oxygen supply for the cornea through the lens.
  - Lenses with low or no transmission of oxygen, type **PMMA or CAB** (obsolete, should not be used any more).
- **Soft lenses**, which are containing between 35% and 85% water, and which are soft and flexible when they are wet:
  - **Conventional soft lenses**, with no specific time schedule for replacement.
  - **Planned-replacement lenses**, which are regularly replaced typically every month (depending on the instructions of the practitioner and the lens manufacturer).
  - **Disposable lenses**, which are used once and then discarded (no maintenance for cleaning).

5 Additional Information

For hard lenses the shape remains the same after being put on to the cornea. For **soft lenses the shape is modified**, because the lens adjusts to a great extent to the shape of the cornea. This can be expected to result in spherical aberrations, which decrease the image quality.

Typical features of the individual types of lenses are shown in Table 23 and Table 24:

Hard RGP contact lenses	
Advantage	Disadvantage
• Suitable for stabilization of myopia? • Can correct some astigmatism without toric lens design. • Excellent optical quality and quality of the surface. • Little absorption of chemicals. • Less frequently serious eye infections than with soft lenses. • Fewer deposits on the lens. • Can be polished if scratched; edges and power can be manually optimized. • Additional oxygen supply by exchange of tears during blinking. • Average lifetime of the lens several years • Easier maintenance. • Lenses for very high grades of myopia available. • Normally all lenses with an accuracy of 0.25 D available.	• Needs highly qualified professional for proper fitting (especially difficult to fit when the lid tension is high). • Longer time for getting used to the lens (up to 3 weeks). • Occasionally less comfortable (depends largely on quality of fitting). • Dust may be more disturbing than with soft lenses (because of smaller size). • Loss of the lens is more likely than with soft lenses (because of smaller size). • Not suitable in cases of highly fragile epithelium of the cornea. • Not so suitable if worn occasionally only. • Few types of lens have a scratch sensitive coating.

Table 23 Features of hard (RGP) contact lenses

	Soft contact lenses	
	Advantage	**Disadvantage**
General and conventional type (i.e. no specific time schedule for replacement)	• Better compatibility, often immediately comfortable. • Easier to fit (but maybe only because a miss-fitting is not realized in the short term) • Less sensitivity to dust. • Rarely any dislocation or loss of the lens, e.g. during sport activities. • Suitable for frequent changes between contact lenses and glasses.	• Easy absorption of chemicals, e.g. from cleaning. • Badly fitted lenses stay unnoticed for a longer period, which may create long-term damages. • Higher rate of complications were reported (maybe caused by unprofessional fitting). • Less crisp vision than with hard lens. • Average lifetime of the lens less than 1 year. • Gets damaged easily. • No oxygen supply by exchange of tears during blinking. • More accumulation of surface deposits. • More complicated/expensive maintenance. • Frequently not available for high grades of myopia, and sometimes with an accuracy of 0,50 D only. • Difficult to verify lens parameters. • Correction of astigmatism requires toric lens.
Planned replacement	• Less lens degradation. • Easy to have spare lenses.	• Less variety of lens parameters available.
Disposable	• No cleaning of lenses. • Less lens degradation. • Easy to have spare lenses.	• Still less variety of lens parameters available. • Potential edge and surface problems depending on manufacturing process.

Table 24 Features of soft contact lenses

It was estimated that the probability for microbial keratitis (disease of the cornea) is about 3-fold for daily-wear soft lenses, and about 20 fold for extended wear soft lenses, compared with daily-wear hard RGP lenses[963]. Other authors claim that this rate is mainly a matter of proper fitting and maintenance[485]. Additionally, the time for recovery was reported to be substantially shorter for incidents with hard RGP lenses than for soft lenses[964].

Those who wear the lenses overnight have a risk of eye infection 10 to 15 times that of users who insert and remove the lenses daily[965].

People, who use lenses for continuous wear should do so under the strict control of an experienced practitioner, who follows established guidelines[966].

> Therefore the tradeoff appears to be to choose between a
> - More healthy, but maybe a little bit less comfortable lens – the hard RGP lens, and a
> - More comfortable, but maybe somewhat less healthy lens – the soft lens.

Interestingly, a report from USA says that higher education makes hard lenses more popular than lower education, where wearers of hard lenses had a higher average income, and among soft lenses people with lower education favor disposable lenses[967].

There are by far more soft lenses sold than hard lenses – which creates, by the way, more revenues for the industry, and allows individual opticians to enter the business, who are hardly qualified for the more demanding fitting of hard lenses.

5.2.2 How about Lenses for Permanent Wear?

Generally, it is differentiated between:
- **Daily wear**, for usage up to about 18 hours, and
- **Extended wear**, for overnight use, e.g. for several days, and
- **Continuous wear** for up to 30 days and nights.

It was claimed that lenses made of silicone hydrogel are already completely safe for 30-day extended wear[968, 969]. There are, however, still reports about increased amounts of deposits on the lens and dehydration of the lens[970], and an increased amount of metaplasia (abnormal cell structures) of the cornea[971].

5.2.3 Potential Complications

When getting contact lenses fitted, and for daily care extra cleanliness and accuracy are necessary. The following list of a few of the numerous potential incidents should not prevent anybody from wearing contact lenses. It should be, however, a good reason to be sensitive, to handle the maintenance with great care and to see the ophthalmologist (or optometrist) without any delay, if something unusual is noticed.

- The practitioner can **check the status of the cornea** by the application of fluorescein to the eye. Damages to the cornea appear as stains. From the location of the stains conclusions about the fitting or corneal damages (e.g. caused by dust particles) can be drawn.

- Frequent **deposits on the lens** (or even a blurred lens) are an indication that something is wrong, either with the mechanical properties of the lens, with some chemical toxication of the lens, or with too long wearing. A visit to your practitioner is strongly recommended.

- If the lens cannot be removed as usual, there might be a **tight lens syndrome**. Do not apply force, better apply some saline solution or wetting drops, or see your practitioner.

- The lack of oxygen generally (e.g. at night) causes a swelling of the cornea, an **edema**. Depending on the transmission of oxygen by the lens, edemas occur to various degrees even when wearing at daytime only. It is not just a mechanical swelling, but a shift in various biochemical processes.

- Extended lack of oxygen in the cornea can lead to the building of new blood vessels from the conjunctiva to the cornea, called **vascularization**.

- A chronic inflammation of the conjunctiva may become **giant papillary conjunctivitis (GPC)**, with papillae developing on the conjunctiva up to a size of 2 mm.

- Small wounds in the cornea can become an **ulceration** of the cornea.

- More generally, **bacterial and fungal infections** caused by dirty lenses, as well **as residual toxic or allergic traces of agents for lens care** can cause serious damage to the eye, especially if they are taken care of rather late.

5.2.4 Parameters of the Material for Contact Lenses

So far, the selection of the ideal material for contact lenses has often been a compromise, e.g. best oxygen transmission may be accompanied by limited wettability, or increased fragility. The art of fitting the lenses consists in selecting the best lens type for the specific needs of the individual customer. Individual characteristics of a patient are e.g. duration of wearing every day, quantity and quality of tears (there may be above average lipids), tension and geometry of the lids, quality of the cornea, sensitivity of the cornea, and working environment (like dust).

For hard RGP lenses there is a rather small number of manufacturers of the basic material for the lenses, and they often leave the cutting of the final lens to a large number of final distributors. All the lenses are cut from bulk material.

For soft lenses the complete manufacturing of the lenses is in one hand, and a few large companies are covering almost the whole market. The lenses are either cut from bulk material, molded, or spin cast.

5.2.4.1 Oxygen Transmission

Limited oxygen supply for the cornea (hypoxia) is a central problem for all contact lenses. These hypoxic effects include corneal swelling, endothelial blebs, epithelial desquamation, change of epithelium cell structure, and biochemical changes like the release of intracellular enzymes (like lactate dehydrogenase) into the tear fluid. The swelling of the cornea occurs at night even without any lens, because of the coverage by the lid. Clearly, these tiny damages are making the cornea more vulnerable to bacterial and fungal infections.

Due to this hypoxia at night it is recommended, to wait in the morning some 15 minutes before putting the lenses in to the eye to allow the cornea to recover from the lack of oxygen.

The units, in which the transmissibility of oxygen is measured is called **Dk**, with the following dimension:

$$10^{-11} \cdot \frac{ml\, O_2 \cdot cm^2}{ml \cdot sec \cdot mmHg}$$

The data for Dk can be obtained by two different ways for measuring, one is called "gas to gas", the other one is called "ISO/FATT", sometimes called polarographic method.

Typical values for ISO/FATT-Dk are between about 10 and 200, where the gas to gas numbers are between 40% and 100% higher than the ISO/FATT numbers. Mostly the data are given in ISO/FATT units. Clearly, the higher the number, the better the oxygen transmission.

It appears that for the lenses currently on the market the average Dk/L numbers of hard RGP lenses are somewhat higher than that of the soft lenses. The leading manufacturers of soft lenses, however, have a very broad portfolio of lenses with very different Dk/L numbers – a good reason to ask your practitioner carefully what lenses you are supposed to get.

As Dk describes the properties of the material only, it does not take into account the thickness of the lens. Therefore a number **Dk/L** is defined, where L relates to the thickness of the lens. The dimension of Dk/L is:

$$10^{-9} \cdot \frac{mlO_2 \cdot cm}{ml \cdot sec \cdot mmHg}$$

The thickness of the lenses in the center is between about 0.08 mm and 0.15 mm for hard RGP lenses and between about 0.04 mm and 0.15 for soft lenses (in reality the fact that the thickness varies over the surface of the lens, and is smallest in the center, has to be considered for the Dk/L calculation as well).

Table 25 shows a summary of a few reports about the impact of various Dk/L numbers, not taking into account additional oxygen supply by the exchange of tears for hard lenses:

Dk/L	Impact on the cornea
23	Required for minimum oxygen supply to the basal epithelium of the cornea of the open eye[972].
24	Required for daily wear without cornea swelling[973].
35	Required for minimum oxygen supply for the whole thickness of the cornea of the open eye[972].
87	Required for wearing at night without any additional swelling[973].
89	Required for minimum oxygen supply to the basal epithelium of the cornea of the closed eye[972].
125	• Required for minimum oxygen supply for the whole thickness of the cornea of the closed eye[972]. • No increase in epithelial lactate levels[974]. • Still no normal oxygen supply[975]. • Decreased thickness of the cornea after 3 months, but no change after 1 month of extended wear[976].

Table 25 The impact of the oxygen transmission Dk/L of contact lenses

As a summary, and considering the state of the art of currently available lenses, **Dk/L numbers should be over 25 for daily wear in any case**, but lenses with numbers **over 35** are widely available and are **clearly more recommended.**

Another way to measure the oxygen supply to the cornea is the **EOP** (equivalent oxygen percentage) number, which indicates the percentage of oxygen directly at the cornea. At sea level and without a lens EOP equals about 21%.

For **extended wear** a minimum EOP of about 18% (corresponds to about Dk/L 85) is recommended, for **daily wear** a minimum EOP of about 10% (corresponds to about Dk/L 25) is recommended.

During sleeping, the EOP is only 7.7%, which explains the swelling of the cornea at night. The exchange of tears by blinking when wearing hard lenses can contribute an additional EOP of about 3% to 4% (for the old hard lenses made of PMMA material this was the only one way of oxygen supply).

The higher the Dk of a lens, the shorter is generally the life expectancy of the lens[977], and for soft lenses there is a general relation: The higher the water content, the higher the oxygen transmission.

As result of a study it was concluded: "High-Dk silicone hydrogel lenses can be worn for up to 3 years with virtual elimination of the hypoxic consequences observed with low-Dk lenses made from conventional lens materials."[978]

There is evidence that the lower the Dk/L of the lens is, the larger the thinning of the epithelium of the cornea is[979]. This thinning of the epithelium was still observed with lenses with Dk=140 (continuous wear), and the thinning was still evident after 3 months with no contact lenses[980]. This thinning is sometimes primarily attributed to a lack of oxygen, sometimes primarily to the mechanical pressure which is applied by the lens.

5.2.4.2 Wettability and Resistance against Deposits

A lens with excellent oxygen transmission, but poor wettability and poor resistance against deposits is not acceptable.

There is a scale for the **wetting capability**, the wetting angle. It can be measured by two procedures (with different resulting numbers):

- The "**captive bubble**" method measures the angle between the edge of an air bubble and the lens surface, with the lens immersed in water or saline.
- The "**sessile drop**" method measures the angle between the edge on a drop of water and the lens surface.

For both numbers the rule is: The lower the angle, the better the wettability.

There exists no measurement procedure for the **resistance against deposits**, which consist of tear mucin and protein (and bacteria). Whether there is a problem with deposits, depends heavily on the consistency of the tears of the individual person. If there are irritations of the eye due to a lack of oxygen or mechanical stress of the lens on the cornea, deposits will increase substantially.

Different lens types can have significantly different resistance against deposits, and it is up to the practitioner to select the proper material – and it is up to the user to be very careful about daily cleaning. Mainly the deposit problem is the reason for the recommendation to change regularly to new lenses – especially for lenses with a very high Dk.

5.2.4.3 Hardness and Stability

The hardness of lens materials is only specified for hard lenses. It is measured in Rockwell (a sharp sample is pressed onto the material, and the remaining depth of the damage is measured) and in Shore (a hard ball is dropped onto the material, and the height to which the sample is bouncing back is measured). The Rockwell numbers give more of an indication for the resistance against scratches; the Shore numbers describe more the elasticity. The higher the oxygen transmission of the lens is, the softer the material in many cases.

A soft lens does may not be more comfortable, as blinking may cause a deformation of the lens and a transient edge lifting, which interacts with the upper eyelid[981].

A hard, rather inflexible lens will be more suitable for masking astigmatism of the cornea than a flexible lens, which will just take the shape of the cornea.

Warping of the lens may be an issue for the longer term: It is the capability of the lens to keep exactly its shape, and not to become distorted. Very thin, hard lenses are more likely at risk for warping or even for breaking.

5.2.4.4 Specific Weight and Refractive Index

These two parameters are sometimes expected to be important - mainly for contact lenses of higher grades of Diopter because of a higher volume of the optical part: A heavier lens (i.e. of higher specific weight and lower refractive index) might have more a tendency to move downward, i.e. centration is more likely to become a problem.

Detailed analysis and experiments, however, have shown that "the lens **mass is not a significant predictor of lens dynamics.**" More important is the **center of gravity** of the lens. Carney et al. stated[982] that "... lenses with a center of gravity location further behind the lens vertex show better stability." The center of gravity is shifted into this direction by an increasing diameter, decreasing lens thickness (and increasing negative power and increasing lens curvature, but these two are determined already for other reasons).

Anyway, a lower weight of the lens can be achieved by manufacturing it with minimal center thickness (depending on the specific material), or by a specific lens cut called lenticulation[983].

5.2.4.5 UV Blocking

Most lenses are coming with a substantial UV blocking capability; this should never be considered, however, as a substitute for wearing sunglasses.

5.2.5 Parameters of the Geometry of Contact Lenses

In principle hard and soft lenses are described by the same set of parameters. For hard lenses, however, these parameters are by far more important, and the lenses are available with by far more detailed numbers of these parameters. Because of this large variety of hard lenses, the final lenses for an individual customer are custom made, and the practitioner is working with a set of trial lenses only, which is normally do not match with the final required refractive power. Soft lenses, however, are generally "ready to go" because of their rather limited spread of parameters – sometimes the refractive power is the only parameter.

The geometrical parameters are:

- **Diameter of the Lens (TD, Total Diameter)**

  Typical diameters of hard RGP lenses are between 9.00 mm and 10.50 mm; the selected size depends e.g. on the diameter of the iris, and the position of the upper eyelid. Generally, lens diameters above 9.5 mm were found to be more comfortable[984].

  Typical diameters of soft lenses are between 13 mm and 15 mm.

  Astonishingly, a report found that oxygen uptake increased with increasing diameter of hard lenses (and their typical diameter)[985]. A really large diameter of a hard lens may create, however, problems for fitting, if no aspheric design is used (see "Aspheric Design", below).

- **Base Curve Radius (BCR, or Back Optic Zone Radius BOZR)**

  This very important number determines the fit of the lens on the cornea, and it is for hard RGP lenses between 6.50 mm and 9.00 mm; this radius is available with a granularity of 0.1 mm or better of 0.05 mm.

  For soft lenses, the exact fit to the cornea is by far less important, because due to their flexibility they can adjust to the radius of the cornea. Very often soft lenses are coming with one radius of about 8.6 mm only; sometimes there is a choice between numbers like 8.4 mm, 8.7 mm, and 9.00 mm.

- **Aspheric Design, Secondary Curve Radius (or Back Peripheral Radius BPR)**

  When contact lenses were first introduced, both sides of the lens were spherical. However, this matches the shape of the cornea only for very small lenses. In reality the cross section of the cornea looks more like an ellipsoid or a paraboloid. Carney et al. stated[219]: "A tendency for the cornea to flatten less rapidly in the periphery with increasing myopia was shown, however."

Consequently, there were other back surfaces developed, created by one of these methods:

- An aspherical outer curve is joined to the inner spherical curve, i.e. the lens becomes progressively flatter towards the edge. As the cornea itself is aspheric, a closer fit to the cornea can be achieved.

- Mathematically, the aspherical part of the lens follows the shape of a conic section, where a parameter e describes the eccentricity of the selected conic section: for spheres e equals zero, for ellipsoids e is between 0 and less than 1, for paraboloids e equals 1. Typically, the cornea corresponds with a value for e between 0.4 and 0.6.

- A disadvantage is that it is more difficult to verify the parameters of a lens, or to compare lenses from different manufacturers – and they are often more expensive.

- Various spherical curves are joined onto each other, with the curves with the larger radius towards the edge of the lens. This lens design is normally used for very special cases and custom design only.

Most common (and cheaper) lenses are, however, still simple spherical designs.

- **Shape of the Edge, Edge Lift**

    The shape of the edge of the lens, where the outer surface is meeting the inner surface, is primarily important for hard lenses only. This shape is mathematically hard to describe and usually at least partly hand made at the manufacturer's laboratory. Nevertheless, the specific shape of the edge is very important to feel comfortable with the lens, as well as for an efficient tear exchange.

    A larger axial edge lift (up to 0.3 mm) was found to be less comfortable than a lower axial edge lift (around 0.1 mm), which gave a better-centered lens as well[986].

    More experienced practitioners are able to modify the edge of a lens according to the specific needs of a customer.

- **Center Thickness**

    The thickness of the lenses in the center is between about 0.08 mm and 0.15 mm for hard lenses and between about 0.04 mm and 0.15 for soft lenses. The thickness of the lens has not only an impact on the oxygen transmission, but also on the flexibility of the lens: To avoid in certain cases a warping of the hard lens, a lens with increased thickness is provided.

- **Back Optic Zone Diameter (BOZD or OZ)**

    The back optic zone is the area, which has the "right" optic without any disturbing optical effect of the aspheric design, or a secondary curve. This diameter should be not too small for good vision.

- **The Power of the Contact Lenses**

    The numbers for the refraction of the glasses and for the refraction of the contact lenses are different, especially for higher grades of myopia. The formula is:

$$D_{lens} = \frac{D_{glasses}}{1 - d \cdot D_{glasses}}$$

where d is the distance between the cornea and the glasses in m.

An example:

With $D_{glasses}$ = - 10.00, and d = 16 mm the power of the contact lenses D_{lens} = - 8.62

5.2.6 Surface and Edge Finishing

A few big companies make the basic material of the lenses, but numerous smaller vendors do the final manufacturing especially of the RGP lenses. Different materials are requiring different surface finishing processes, and different manufacturers of the lenses may achieve different qualities. This should be considered when switching to a new material or another optometrist who is buying from a different vendor.

Frequently the edges of RGP lenses are still finished manually. Consequently, this process depends on the skill of individual people and appropriate quality control.

5.2.7 The Fitting of Contact Lenses

A description of the fitting process is beyond the scope of this book, and there are very good sources about this issue available[959]. Therefore just a few remarks:

There are several successful strategies of how to fit the best lens (especially for hard RGP lenses). Basis of each fitting process is a measurement of the topography of the eye, especially the various radii of the cornea, measured in different directions, and in the center as well as in the periphery.

A general differentiation is between a more flat fitting and a steeper fitting: Flat fitting means that the base curve radius (BCR / BOZR) is clearly larger than the radius of the cornea. This results in some edge clearance, which allows for enhanced exchange of tears and oxygen, and good mobility of the lens, but the lens may become more off-centered (which may have unwanted long-term effects on the shape of the cornea). Steep fitting means that the base curve radius closely matches the radius of the cornea. This results in a good central position, but if the lens is sitting too tight (i.e. too steep fitting) a "tight lens syndrome" may develop.

Fitting of hard lenses is more demanding than the fitting of soft lenses, but a bad fitting of a hard lens is noticed earlier, generally before some damage happens to the eye.

Special harm can be done by overly tight lenses, i.e. which don't move during blinking.

An irritation can be caused not only by a lens that was fitted too steep (most uncomfortable) or too flat, but also by the sliding of the upper lid over the edge of a rather small lens[984]. A larger lens might help in these cases.

When changing from older, non-gas-permeable lenses (PMMA-type) to highly gas permeable lenses the fitting should be done either without any break in between, or with a break of several weeks[959].

It is very helpful for the fitting practitioner, if the patient can describe the problem very clearly. Therefore it is helpful, to get the basic knowledge about the fitting process by yourself. This also enables you to ask the right questions (and to find out whether you are at the right practitioner).

Experience is a key issue to become an expert for fitting. Therefore an ophthalmologist or an optometrist who is really focusing on contact lenses as the main job is most likely a better choice than somebody who is doing this task only occasionally.

5.2.8 Determining the Refraction after Wearing Contact Lenses

When the refraction of contact lens wearers is determined – e.g. to fit spare glasses – it has to be considered:

- Flat fitted lenses flatten the cornea (see section 3.20.1.1), herewith reducing the Diopter of myopia.

- If lenses of low oxygen transmission (i.e. PMMA material) had been used, it takes 3 weeks until an accurate refraction could be determined. Rengstorff stated[987]: "...myopia decreases over the first 3 days after stopping PMMA wear and then increases over several weeks until it stabilizes." Therefore the transition to a material with high oxygen transmission can be accompanied by a wrong refraction and improper fitting

If the determination of the refraction, however, serves only the purpose of fitting spare glasses, these effects can be ignored, as these glasses are used in general immediately after wearing the contact lenses.

5.2.9 Maintenance of the Lenses

The maintenance procedure is different for hard RGP and soft lenses, but there are some general recommendations:

- Generally, follow the routine recommended by the manufacturer of your lenses, and by your practitioner.
- If you are not satisfied with your lenses, talk to your practitioner and ask him what other brands of lens care products, or what other procedures would be compatible with your lens type, and try them. There is a very big variety of lens care products, made by the manufacturer of the lens as well as products made by independent suppliers. There is always the possibility that you are sensitive against a preservative or tensides, which is used in a lens care agent.

5.2.9.1 Maintenance of Hard RGP Lenses

Essential for the maintenance of hard RGP lenses is the fact that they contain less than 1% of water, i.e. absorption of agents into the lens material is by far less a problem than for soft lenses. The steps of treatment are (not considering the necessary rinsing between individual steps):

a) Cleaning after the use to remove surface deposits.
b) Disinfecting over night.
c) Wetting before inserting into the eye.
d) Occasional enzyme cleaning to remove proteins, if necessary.

- The cleaning solution for step a) contains tensides and, depending on the brand, some abrasive particles (a few lens types do not like abrasive agents!)
- Normally the steps b) and c) are performed with the same type of agent, but this might not be the best for you: There are solutions which are very effective for disinfecting[988], but which can be somehow irritating for wetting, when they come in direct contact with the eye[989, 990], and vice versa[991].
- There are also solutions on the market that combine the steps a), b) and c), but do not be astonished if this compromise does not satisfy you; anyway, it is good that these products exist for the emergency case, e.g. for traveling.
- As the solutions for b) and c) have to use preservatives, there is a possibility that you are sensitive to any one of them, and that a switch to a different brand would help.

- It could be very helpful for you to use **different solutions for step b) and for step c)**, even though most solutions are claimed to work for both b) and c.

- Occasional enzyme cleaning is efficient, but if heavy deposits build up frequently there might be something wrong with the lens. Enzyme cleaners can be based on either animal- or plant-enzymes, maybe you are more sensitive to one of them (there is always a chance that traces are left on the surface).

- Special care has to be taken when cleaning the lenses by hand to avoid **warping** them – therefore some practitioners are recommending to put the lens into the palm of the hand for cleaning, and not to rub it between the tips of two fingers.

- A **change of the lens parameters is not necessarily visible to the patient**: the lens can become **flatter in fitting**, and/or **stronger in power**. Both changes work like "stronger glasses", and are give no immediate cause for complaint to myopes. Nevertheless, the resulting **overcorrection** can increase the myopia further as outlined before. Resulting **advice**: insist that your practitioner checks the parameters of the lens at least annually.

5.2.9.2   Maintenance of Soft Lenses

Essential for the maintenance of soft lenses is the fact that they contain a very substantial amount of water (35% to 85%), i.e. absorption of agents into the lens material is a problem. The steps of treatment are (not considering the necessary rinsing between individual steps):

a) Cleaning after the use to remove surface deposits.

b) Disinfecting by the chemical method, or by hydrogen peroxide, or by heat, or by UV-light, or by microwave radiation (depending on the individual lens).

c) Disinfecting is especially important for soft lenses, as some types of fungi can grow within 20 hours through a soft lens; bacteria and virus, however, cannot get inside a undamaged soft lens.

d) Storing, and wetting before inserting into the eye.

e) Occasional enzyme cleaning to remove proteins, if necessary.

For soft lenses the variety of lens care systems, which often combine steps mentioned above, is substantially higher than for hard lenses. The requirements are more dependent on the individual lens type. There are also "all in one" solutions on the market, similarly as for hard lenses.

The fact that proper lens care is more difficult for soft lenses than for hard RGP lenses is one of the reasons for the trend towards disposable soft lenses.

In any case, the specified intervals for renewing the lens should not be ignored.

5.2.10 "I Cannot Wear Contact Lenses"

This conclusion "I cannot wear contact lenses" might be not generally valid, but based on

- specific lens care liquids which you cannot tolerate
- a specific lens material which is not suitable for you (this might be influenced by the manufacturing process of the specific vendor)
- the geometry of your lenses.

Therefore, before you take more serious and final steps like surgery, ask your contact lens practitioner for different liquids, different materials, or, finally, go to a different practitioner.

5.2.11 Presbyopia

For presbyopia, the contact lenses are required to replace the accommodation of the human lens, i.e. to offer focus as well for near objects as well as for distant objects, as with bifocal glasses.

There are some different concepts to handle presbyopia with contact lenses. Generally there are two groups of systems, i.e. for alternating vision, where an image is produced either for distant view or near view, and simultaneous vision, where the evaluation of the different images is done in the brain. In any case, it will take a while until the patient is used to the new vision.

The individual methods are:

- The optical zone of the lens is split into an upper section for distant focusing and a lower section for near focusing (alternating vision).

  A problem is that the lens has to be kept in the right rotational and vertical position. The lens is difficult to fit, and is normally fitted flat.

- The optical zone of the lens is split into a center section for distant focusing and a peripheral section for near focusing (simultaneous vision).

- This lens is fitted more on the steeper side to have the lens properly centered. When the aperture of the iris is small, e.g. at bright light, near focusing may be a problem. As with all methods which are using simultaneous vision, the contrast of the images is reduced.

- Into the optical zone of the lens fine microscopic steps are inserted. These steps create via diffraction two focus points – one for distant vision and one for near vision (simultaneous vision).

  An exactly centered position, and the aperture of the iris is not as important as in the method described on top. The reduction of the contrast, however, is similar.

- Monovision: The lens of one eye is adjusted for distant vision; the lens of the other eye is adjusted for near vision.

  This method is less expensive, and easier to fit than the previous methods. Good success rates have been reported for this method. For driving (especially night driving) the use of additional glasses, which compensate for the undercorrection of one eye, is recommended. Especially for reading additions that were not greater than 2.50 D the visual results were reported to be quite satisfying[992].

- Good results were also reported for the combinations of monovision and LASIK[993].

- Permanent undercorrection to allow reading, use additional glasses for distant vision, e.g. for driving.

  This method, however, can satisfy only in the early stages of presbyopia, when the resulting uncorrected distant vision is still acceptable for daily life (except driving), i.e. when it is around 1.00 D only. Moreover, this method can be expected to delay the total presbyopia, because the permanent accommodative effort keeps the own lens longer elastic.

- Intraocular lenses which can accommodate.

  In the trial status are intraocular lenses for people undergoing cataract surgery (i.e. whose lens was removed), which can accommodate via the ciliary muscle. While this sounds very promising for cataract patients, the risk of this operation for normal presbyopes without a cataract problem appears to be large, but this may change within a few years[994].

  Note:
  Because of their shorter remaining life expectancy long-term effects of surgery might be less important for patients with presbyopia than for young myopes.

5.2.12 Contact Lenses and Nutrition

Some nutritional components are especially supporting a healthy cornea, which is important when wearing contact lenses:

- **Vitamin A** is generally necessary for the metabolism of mucous membranes, and a long-term nutritional deficiency causes severe damages of the cornea, which can lead to blindness.

- Local, lesions of the cornea are often treated with eye drops containing **pantothenic acid (vitamin B5) or retinoic acid (vitamin A)**.

- The mechanical stability of corneas was improved by treatment with **vitamin B2 (riboflavin) and UV irradiation**, introducing additional cross-links[821].

Therefore, and as vitamin B2 was shown to have a positive effect on the connective tissue in general (see section 4.3.2.2.1) it is advised to have sufficient vitamin B2 in the diet.

Note:
From this point of view, contact lenses, which are blocking UV light almost completely, are not of benefit in every respect.

- The cornea needs manganese for the maintenance of its cell structure[784].
- The stability of the tear film on the cornea is essential for comfortably wearing contact lenses. It was found that taking a **standard supplement** containing the recommended daily dose of vitamins (e.g. A, B1, B2, B6, E) and trace elements (e.g. calcium, manganese) improved tear stability[995].

5.3 Refractive Surgery

Refractive surgeries like PRK, LASIK and LASEK (the basic principle was outlined in section 3.20.1) have become a big industry, and estimates for the USA were 1,900 000 procedures in 2002, up from 465 000 in 1998[996].

In the USA, "at least" several hundred ophthalmologists had LASIK or PRK for themselves – of about 20.000 ophthalmologists in practice[997].

Nevertheless, people who are expecting that they are getting rid of glasses or contact lenses by refractive surgery forever should consider:

- The rate of **complications** at LASIK was estimated to be at 7.2%[998], and for 11.6% of the eyes were re-treatment was found to be necessary[999].

- Some data about the **probability that no more glasses or contact lenses are necessary**: A report states that for -4.25 D up to -8.00 D 86.5% of the patients stayed within 1.00 D of intended correction, and for above -8.25 D 82.9% of the patients stayed within 1.00 D of intended correction.

  The **regression** was -0.5 D for patients between -0.5 D and -4.0 D (only during 1st to 3rd month), -0.8 D for patients between -4.25 D and -8.0 D (1st to 6th month), and -1.2 D for patients above -8.25 (1st to 9th month)[506].

  For **follow-up LASIK procedures** to eliminate residual myopia the rate of complications is substantially elevated[1000].

  This means, you have a **good chance, to need still some glasses or contact lenses** – which you wanted to get rid of forever.

Additionally, even if myopia is (rather) stable, there are often some moderate changes during the lifetime, which are easy to correct with glasses or contact lenses. And for your presbyopia you need some glasses or contact lenses anyway.

- For a group of 1308 patients the one-year **re-treatment incidence** was 12.1% for myopic eyes, with an increase to 14% for patients older than 40 years[1001].

- Barclay stated[1001]: "In most cases, LASIK flaps could be lifted using manual technique up to three years after the initial surgery."

   Note:
   This means the stability of the LASIK-flap is rather limited for quite a long time.

- There is a serious risk to develop **dry eyes** after the LASIK surgery[1002].

- Machet stated[507]: "Just as the good can be very good, the bad can be very bad."

Some questions you should ask before getting surgery done, are[1003]:

- What is your success rate for achieved visual acuity (that is, 20/40 or better)?
- How many operations have you performed personally?
- May I speak with any of the patients on whom you have done this procedure?
- How many of them have required second operations? (It should be under 10%.)
- What is the best correction I can expect?
- How much will the operation cost me?
- What are the chances I may not see as well as with glasses or contact lenses?
- Do you operate on both eyes the same day?
- What are the possible complications?
- What anesthesia will I receive during the operation?
- How long will the procedure take?
- What is the recovery period?
- When will I be able to return to work?
- If the operation fails to correct my vision, will I be able to go back to contact lenses?
- What if, years from now, I develop cataracts? Will this operation prohibit or interfere with later cataract surgery?
- What are the long-term risks of this surgery?

5 ADDITIONAL INFORMATION

Most refractive surgeons prefer an undercorrection instead of an overcorrection, because this leaves room for later corrections[1004] (maybe you prefer a slight undercorrection because of the presbyopia you might face later, see section 5.2.10).

Generally it is recommended that only **one eye at a time** is operated, to preserve at least the vision of one eye in the worst case of complications.

Refractive surgery is not recommended for people with diabetes, or rheumatic diseases[1005].

For people who had photorefractive surgery like PRK it was found that high dose of vitamin A and E supplementation may accelerate the healing of the cornea and may reduce corneal haze formation[1006].

More information about LASIK can be found in the "Official Patient's Sourcebook on Myopia"[1007], and in the "Official Patient's Sourcebook on LASIK Surgery"[1008].

5.4 Useful Links

- **Scientific publications**

    The United States National Library of Medicine (NLM) maintains a database called MEDLINE of 11 million indexed journal citations and abstracts now covering nearly 4,500 journals published in the United States and more than 70 other countries. MEDLINE includes references to articles indexed from 1966 to the present.

    Abstracts of the respective publications can be searched and retrieved via the address:

    http://www.ncbi.nlm.nih.gov/entrez/query.fcgi?CMD=search&DB=PubMed

    Full text articles can be bought from a library in your country (sometimes articles can be bought directly by accessing a link which is sometimes shown together with the abstract). Addresses of the respective libraries can be found at:

    http://www.nlm.nih.gov/ild/main.cfm (outside United States)

    http://nnlm.gov/members/ (United States)

    Numerous sources of information about all kind of issues which are related to myopia can be found in: Parker JN, Parker PM (editors), The 2002 Official Patient's Sourcebook on Myopia ("A reference manual for self-directed patient research"), ICON Health Publications, http://www.icongrouponline.com/health

- **Other sites about myopia and related issues, which are especially worth visiting**

    http://www.nb.net/~sparrow/myopia.html

    http://www.chinamyopia.org/mainenglish.htm

    http://www.i-see.org

    http://dmoz.org/Health/Conditions_and_Diseases/Eye_Disorders/Refractive_Errors/Myopia/

    http://www.zeal.com/category/preview.jhtml?cid=273952

    http://members.aol.com/myopiaprev/index.htm

- **Connective tissue disorder site**

    http://www.ctds.info/

- **Organizations in the field of myopia**

    A record of vision science research institutes worldwide can be found at

    http://www.visionscience.com/vsInstitutes.html

- **Eyes and contact lenses in general**

    http://www.eyemdlink.com/Condition.asp?ConditionID=131

- **Some manufacturers of contact lenses or material for contact lenses**

    Bausch & Lomb: http://www.bausch.com/us/resource/visioncare/

    Ciba Vision: http://www.cibavision.com/ and

    http://www.cibavision.co.uk

    Johnson & Johnson: http://www.jnjvision.com/

    Menicon: http://www.menicon.co.jp/english/

- **Some manufacturers of care products for contact lenses**

    http://www.allergan.com/sitemap/index.htm

    http://www.alconlabs.com/

- **Refractive surgery**

    http://drmcdonald.eyemdlink.com/EyeProcedures.asp

6 References

[1] Srinivas C., Various etiopathological studies of simple myopia in Myopia Updates, Proceedings of the 6th International Conference on Myopia, Springer, Tokyo 1998

[2] Shih Y.-F., Relationship between choroidal blood flow and myopia in Myopia Updates, Proceedings of the 6th International Conference on Myopia, Springer, Tokyo 1998

[3] Sardi B. Personal information

[4] Eaton SB, Konner M, Shostak M, Stone agers in the fast lane: chronic degenerative diseases in evolutionary perspective. Am J Med 1988 Apr;84(4):739-49

[5] Grosvenor T., Goss D. A., Clinical management of myopia, Butterworth-Heinemann, Boston 1999

[6] Trichtel F., Zur Enstehung und Therapie der Myopie, Enke, Stuttgart 1986

[7] Cassel G. H., Billig M. D., Randall H. G. , The eye book, The Johns Hopkins University Press, Baltimore 1998

[8] Lang G. K., Ophthalmology: A short textbook, Thieme Medical Pub., New York 2000

[9] Tokoro T. (Ed.), Myopia Updates, Proceedings of the 6th International Conference on Myopia, Springer, Tokyo 1998

[10] Lin L.L.-K., Shih Y,-F., Hung P.T. (Eds.), Myopia Updates II, Proceedings of the 7th International Conference on Myopia, Springer, Tokyo 2000

[11] Hollwich F., Ophthalmology, Thieme Medical Pub., New York 1985

[12] Reim M., Augenheilkunde, Enke, Stuttgart 1990

[13] Optometric Clinical Practice Guideline, Care Of The Patient With Myopia, Reference Guide for Clinicians, Prepared by the American Optometric Association, Consensus Panel on Care of the Patient with Myopia. http://www.aoa.org/conditions/docs/CPG15%20Myopia.doc

[14] Goss DA, Grosvenor TP, Keller JT, Marsh-Tootle, Norton TT, Zadnik K. Optometric clinical practice guideline, Care of the patient with myopia, American Optometric Association, 1997, http://www.aoanet.org/clincare/pdf/CPG-15.pdf

[15] Weale RA. Epidemiology of refractive errors and presbyopia. Surv Ophthalmol. 2003 Sep-Oct;48(5):515-43

[16] Chen JC, Schmid KL, Brown B. The autonomic control of accommodation and implications for human myopia development: a review. Ophthalmic Physiol Opt. 2003 Sep;23(5):401-22

[17] McCollim, On the nature of myopia and the mechanism of accommodation. Med Hypothesis 1989;28:197-211

[18] Drexler W, Findl O, Schmetterer L, Hitzenberger CK, Fercher AF, Eye elongation during accommodation in humans: differences between emmetropes and myopes, Invest Ophthalmol Vis Sci 1998 Oct; 39(11): 2140-7

[19] Shum PJ, Ko LS, Ng CL, Lin SL. A biometric study of ocular changes during accommodation. Am J Ophthalmol. 1993 Jan;115(1):76-81

[20] Hope G.M. et al., Night myopia, Survey of Ophthalmology 1984 Sept, Oct; 29(2): 129-136

[21] Epstein D., Accomodation as the primary cause of night myopia, Klin Monatsbl Augenheilkd 1982 Nov; 181(5): 400-1

[22] Leibowitz H.W. et al., New evidence for the intermediate position of relaxed accommodation, Doc Ophthalmol 1978 Oct 16; 46(1): 133-47

[23] Charman W.N., Night myopia and driving, Ophthalmic Physiol Opt 1996 Nov; 16(6): 474-85

[24] Fejer T.P. et al., Night myopia: implications for the young driver, Can J Ophthalmol 1992 Jun; 27(4): 172-6

[25] http://webvision.med.utah.edu/light_dark.html

[26] Berman E.L., Clues in the eye: Ocular signs of metabolic and nutritional disorders, Geriatrics 1995 July; 50(7): 34-44

[27] Coats DK (editor), Acute transient myopia in a child. Medscape Ophthalmology 3(2), 2002

[28] Zhou X.-D. et al., A computed tomographic study of the relation between ocular axial biometry and refraction in Myopia Updates, Proceedings of the 6th International Conference on Myopia, Springer, Tokyo 1998

[29] Kusakari T., Scleral changes and melatonin in form-deprivation myopia in Myopia Updates, Proceedings of the 6th International Conference on Myopia, Springer, Tokyo 1998

[30] Krumpaszky H.G. et al., Cause of blindness in Bavaria. Evaluation of a representative sample from blindness compensation records of Upper Bavaria, Klin Monatsbl Augenheilkd 1992 Feb; 200(2): 142-6

[31] Ho T.-C. et al., Longitudinal followup of lacquer cracks in myopic maculapathy using digitized indocyanine green angiography and scanning laser ophthalmology in Myopia Updates II, Proceedings of the 7th International Conference on Myopia, Springer, Tokyo 2000

[32] Rosenberg T, Klie F. Current trends in newly registered blindness in Denmark. Acta Ophthalmol Scand 1996 Aug;74(4):395-8

[33] Noorani HZ. Scleral support surgery for pathologic myopia. Issues Emerg Health technol 2002 Sep;(39):1-4

[34] Il'nitskii V.V. et al., Peripheral vitreochorioretinal dystrophies in myopia patients; Vestn Oftalmol 1993 Jul-Sep; 109(4): 18-20

[35] Tano Y. Patholgic myopia: where are we now? Am J Ophthalmol 2002 Nov;134(5):645-60

[36] Chen W.-C. et al., Retinal lattice degeneration and traction tear of myopia in high school students in Myopia Updates II, Proceedings of the 7th International Conference on Myopia, Springer, Tokyo 2000

[37] Fledelius H.C., Myopia and significant visual impairment: Global aspects in Myopia Updates II, Proceedings of the 7th International Conference on Myopia, Springer, Tokyo 2000

[38] Lane B.C., Dietary risk factors for fibrillar and non-fibrillar vitreous degeneration in myopia, Myopia: Pathogenesis, Prophylaxis of Progression and Complications: Proceedings of International Symposium Moscow, 1988

[39] Hosaka A, Acta Ophthalmol Suppl 1988; 185: 95-9

[40] Novartis Ophthalmics press release Atlanta 2/5/2001

[41] Yeo TC, et al. Clinical and echocardiographic features of mitral valve prolapse patients in a local population. Singapore Med J 1996 Apr;37(2):143-6

[42] Goldschmidt E., Can myopia progression be controlled? in Myopia Updates II, Proceedings of the 7th International Conference on Myopia, Springer, Tokyo 2000

[43] Friberg TR, Lace JW. A comparison of the elastic properties of human choroid and sclera. Exp Eye Res. 1988 Sep;47(3):429-36

[44] Garner LF, Yap MK, Kinnear RF, Frith MJ. Ocular dimensions and refraction in Tibetan children. Optom Vis Sci. 1995 Apr;72(4):266-71

[45] Zhao J, et al. Accuracy of noncycloplegic autorefraction in school-age children in China. Optom Vis Sci. 2004 Jan;81(1):49-55

[46] http://www.lpf.com/source/rk/20something.html

[47] http://orgap.py.ruhr-uni-bochum.de/euphoria/container/uFile116.pdf

[48] http://www.vision-training.com/Vision%20test/Myopia%20test.htm

[49] http://www.smbs.buffalo.edu/oph/ped/IVAC/IVAC.html

[50] Schaeffel F, et al. Molecular biology of myopia. Clin Exp Optom. 2003 Sep;86(5):295-307

[51] Saw SM. A synopsis of the prevalence rates and environmental risk factors for myopia. Clin Exp Optom. 2003 Sep;86(5):289-94

[52] Goldschmidt E., Epidemiology of myopia: Scandinavian and Hong Kong experiences in Myopia Updates, Proceedings of the 6th International Conference on Myopia, Springer, Tokyo 1998

[53] Hu D.-N., studies of genetic and environmental factors in the occurence of myopia based on epidemiologic Data in Myopia Updates, Proceedings of the 6th International Conference on Myopia, Springer, Tokyo 1998

6 REFERENCES

[54] Schaeffel F. et al., Myopia development as a result of visual deprivation? System analysis and possible biochemical correlates in Myopia Updates, Proceedings of the 6th International Conference on Myopia, Springer, Tokyo 1998

[55] Daubs J.G., Some geographic, environmental and nutritive concomitants of malignant myopia, Ophthal. Physiol. Opt., 1984, 4(2): 143-149

[56] Schaeffel E, Das Raetsel der Myopie, Ophthalmologie 2002; 99: 120-141

[57] Goldschmidt E. The mystery of myopia. Acta Ophthalmol Scand. 2003 Oct;81(5):431-6

[58] Morgan IG. The biological basis of myopic refractive error. Clin Exp Optom Sep;86(5):276-88

[59] Lyhne N. et al., The importance of genes and environment for ocular refraction and its determiners: a population based study among 20-45 year old twins; Br. J. Ophthalmol 2001 Dec; 85(12): 1470-6

[60] Trachtman D, personal information

[61] Young T.L. et al., Evidence that a locus for familial high myopia maps to chromosome 18p, Am. J. Hum. Genet. 1988 Jul; 63(1): 109-19

[62] Naiglin L. et al., Familial high myopia: evidence of an autosomal dominant mode of inheritance and genetic heterogeneity, Ann. Genet 1999; 42(3): 140-6

[63] Thorn F, Grice K, Held R, Gwiazda J. Myopia: Nature, nurture, and the blur hypothesis in Myopia Updates II, Proceedings of the 7th International Conference on Myopia, Springer, Tokyo 2000

[64] Grosvenor T., Goss D. A., Clinical management of myopia, Butterworth-Heinemann, Boston 1999 p. 49

[65] Chien-Jen Chen et al., Epidemiological studies on multiple risk factors for myopia in Taiwan: Gene-environment interaction in Myopia Updates II, Proceedings of the 7th International Conference on Myopia, Springer, Tokyo 2000

[66] Feller D.J. et al., Dopamine and norepinephrine in discrete areas of the copper-deficient rat brain, J. of Neurochemistry 1980 May; 34(5): 1259-1263

[67] Keen C.L. et al., Effect of copper deficiency on prenatal development and pregnancy outcome, Am. J. Clin. Nutr. 1998 May; 67(5 Suppl): 1003S-1011S

[68] Cousins R.J., Nutritional regulation of gene expression in Shils M.E. et al. (Eds.), Modern nutrition in health and disease, Lippincott Williams & Wilkins, Baltimore 1999

[69] Chang S.H.-C. et al., A review of myopia studies in Taiwan in Myopia Updates II, Proceedings of the 7th International Conference on Myopia, Springer, Tokyo 2000

[70] Norton T.T., Siegwart JT. Animal models of emmetropization : matching axial length to the focal plane; J. Am Optom Assoc 1995; 66(7): 405-414

[71] Chang S H-C, Y-F Shih, Lin L L-K, A review of myopia studies in Taiwan, in Proceedings of the 7th International Conference on Myopia, Springer, Tokyo 200,0 p. 134

[72] Saw SM, Hong RZ, Zhang MZ, Fu ZF, Ye M, Tan D, Chew SJ, Near-work activity and myopia in rural and urban schoolchildren in China, J Pediatr Ophthalmol Strabismus 2001 May-Jun; 38(3): 149-55

[73] Garner LF, et al., Prevalence of myopia in Sherpa and Tibetan children in Nepal. Optom Vis Sci 1999 May;76(5):282-5

[74] Scharfblick für alle? Focus 47, 1999

[75] Lin LL-K, Shih YF, Morbidity of myopia among schoolchildren in Taiwan, in Proceedings of the 7th International Conference on Myopia, Springer, Tokyo 2000, p. 7

[76] Schultz-Zehden W, Bischof F, Auge und Psychosomatik, Deutscher Aerzte Verlag, Köln, 1986, p. 188

[77] Garner LF, Owens H, Kinnear RF, Frith MJ. Prevalence of myopia in Sherpa and Tibetan children in Nepal. Optom Vis Sci. 1999 May;76(5):282-5

[78] Young FA, Francis A, The transmission of refractive errors within Eskimo families, Am J Optom and Arch Am Acad Optom 1969; 46(9), referenced in The prevention of acquired myopia, http://members.aol.com/myopiaprev/page2.htm

[79] McCarty, CA, Livingston PM, Taylor HR, Prevalence of myopia in adults: implications for refractive surgeons, J Refract Surg 1997 May-Jun; 13(3): 229-34

[80] Chandran S, Comparative study of refractive errors in West Malaysia, J Brit Ophthalmol 1972; 56: 492-495

[81] Boniuk V, Refractive problems in native peoples, Can J. Ophthalmol 1973; 8: 229-233

[82] Wu HM, et al. Does education explain ethnic differences in myopia prevalence? A population-based study of young adult males in Singapore. Optom Vis Sci 2001;78:234-239

[83] Kleinstein RN, et al. Refractive error and ethnicity in children. Arch Ophthalmol. 2003 Aug;121(8):1141-7

[84] Grosvenor T., Goss D. A., Clinical management of myopia, Butterworth-Heinemann, Boston 1999, p. 23

[85] Yeow PT, Progression of myopia in different ethnic groups in Malaysia, Med J Malaysia 1994 Jun; 49 (2): 138-41

[86] Wong TY, Foster PJ, Hee J, Ng TP, Tielsch JM,.Chew SJ, Johnson GJ, Seah SK. Prevalence and risk factors for refractive errors in adult Chinese in Singapore, Invest Ophthalmol Vis Sci 2000 Aug; 41(9): 2486-94

[87] http://news.1chinastar.com/news.shtml?l=english&a=express&p=1233882

[88] Choo V. A look at slowing progression of myopia. Lancet. 2003 May 10;361(9369):1622-3

[89] Mavracanas TA, et al., Prevalence of myopia in a sample of Greek students. Acta Ophthalmol Scand 2000 Dec;78(6):656-9

[90] Richler A, The distribution of refraction in three isolated communities in Western Newfoundland, Am. J. Optom. Physiol. Optics 57 1980, 861 referenced in Trichtel F., Zur Enstehung und Therapie der Myopie, Enke, Stuttgart 1986, p. 56

[91] Scholz D, Die Beziehung zwischen Myopie und Schulerfolg, Wachstum und sozialen Faktoren, Öff. Ges. Wesen 26, 1972, 330, referenced in Trichtel F., Zur Enstehung und Therapie der Myopie, Enke, Stuttgart 1986, p. 59

[92] Goss DA, Rainey BB, Relation of childhood myopia progression rates to time of year, J Am Optom Assoc, 1998; 69; 262-266, referenced in Grosvenor T., Goss D. A., Clinical management of myopia, Butterworth-Heinemann, Boston 1999, p.S. 52

[93] Goss DA, Rainey BB, J Am Optom Assoc 1998 Apr; 69(4): 262-266

[94] Fulk GW, Cyert LA, Parker DA, Seasonal variation in myopia progression and ocular elongation, Optom Vis Sci 2002 Jan; 79(1): 46-51

[95] Duke E, An investigation into the effect upon the eyes of occupations involving close work, Brit J Ophthalmol 14, (1930), 609, referenced in Trichtel F., Zur Enstehung und Therapie der Myopie, Enke, Stuttgart 1986Trichtel p. 61

[96] Ponomarenko PA, Versuch einer Verhütung der Berufskurzsichtigkeit be den Fadengeberinnen und – aufnehmerinnen der Webereien Orechovo-Zuev, Vestn Oftalmol, 32,1 (1953), 42, refrenced in Trichtel F., Zur Enstehung und Therapie der Myopie, Enke, Stuttgart 1986Trichtel p. 61

[97] Cernea P, Sandulescu G, Kurzsichtigkeit und Naharbeit, Oftamologia (Bucaresti), 5, (1961), 345, referenced in Trichtel F., Zur Enstehung und Therapie der Myopie, Enke, Stuttgart 1986Trichtel p. 61

[98] Young FA, The effect of nearwork illumination level on monkey refraction, Am J Optom and Arch Am Acad Optom 1962 Feb; 39(2): 60-67

[99] Young, Francis A, unpublished study, referenced in The prevention of acquired myopia, http://members.aol.com/myopiaprev/page2.htm

[100] Clarkson PM, Sayers SP, Etiology of exercise-induced muscle damage, Can J Appl Physiol 1999 Jun; 24(3): 234-48

[101] Brown S, Day S, Donnelly A, Indirect evidence of human skeletal muscle damage and collagen breakdown after eccentric muscle damage, J Sports Sci 1999 May; 17(5): 397-402

[102] Kinge B, Midelfart A, Jacobsen G, Rystad J, The influence of near-work on development of myopia among university students. A thre—year longitudinal study among engineering students in Norway, Acta Ophthamol Scand 2000 Feb; 78(1): 26-29

[103] Chen C-C, Lin L L-K, Shih Y-F, Hsiao C-H K, Hung PT, Epidemiological studies on multiple risk factors for myopia in Taiwan: gene-environment interaction, in Proceedings of the 7th International Conference on Myopia, Springer, Tokyo 2000, p. 19

[104] Qiang M, Zhao R, A logistic regression analysis of relations between juvenile myopia and TV-watching, trace elements, and psychological characteristics, Chung Hua Yu Fang I Hsueh Tsa Chih 1991, Jul; 25(4): 222-224

[105] Saw SM, et al., Near-work activity, night lights, and myopia in the Singapore-China study. Arch Ophthalmol 2002 May;120(5):620-7

[106] Parssinen O, Lyyra AL, Myopia and myopic progression among schoolchildren: a three-year follow-up study. Invest Ophthalmol Vis Sci 1993 Aug;34(9):2794-802

[107] Cui W, Bryant MR, Sweet PM, McDonnell PJ. Changes in gene expression in response to mechanical strain in human scleral fibroblasts. Exp Eye Res. 2004 Feb; 78(2):275-284

[108] Rosenfield M, Abraham-Cohen JA, Blur sensitivity in myopes. Optom Vis Sci 1999 May;76(5):303-7

[109] Schaeffel F, Diether S, The growing eye: an autofocus system that works on very poor images. Vision Res 1999 May;39(9):1585-9

[110] Rosenfield M, Desai R, Portello JK, Do progressing myopes show reduced accommodative responses? Optom Vis Sci 2002 Apr;79(4):268-73

[111] Yap M, Garner L, Kinnear R, Frith M, Tonic accommodation and refractive change in children, in Proceedings of the 7th International Conference on Myopia, Springer, Tokyo 2000, p. 59

[112] Zadnik K, Mutti DO, Kim HS, Jones LA, Qui PH, Moeswchberger ML, Tonic accommodation, age, and refractive error in children, Invest Ophthalmol Vis Sci 1999 May; 40(6): 1050-60

[113] Woung LC, Lue YF, Shih YF, Accommodation and pupillary response in early-onset myopia among schoolchildren, Optom Vis Sci 1998 Aug; 75(8): 611-6

[114] Gwiazda J, Bauer J, Thorn F, Held R, Shifts in tonic accommodation after near work are related to refractive errors in children, Ophthalmic Physiol Opt 1995 Mar; 15(2): 93-7

[115] Kushner BJ. Does overcorrecting minus lens therapy for intermittent exotropia cause myopia? Arch Ophthalmol 1999 May;117(5):638-42

[116] Sergienko NM, Kondratenko IuN, Accommodative hyperemia of the ciliary bods as one of the pathogenetic factors in myopia, Oftalmol Zh 1989; (8): 474-6

[117] Trichtel F., Zur Enstehung und Therapie der Myopie, Enke, Stuttgart 1986, p. 47

[118] Abbot ML, Schmid KL, Strang NC, Differences in the accommodation stimulus response curves of adult myopes and emmetropes, Ophthalmic Physiol Opt 1998 Jan; 18(1): 13-20

[119] Fong DS, Is myopia related to amplitude of accommodation? Am J Ophthalmol 1997 Mar; 123(3): 416-8

[120] Schaeffel F, Zrenner E, Steuerung des Augenlaengenwachstums durch Sehen, Deutsches Aerzteblatt 1997 Apr; 94(17): A1121-A1128

[121] Gwiazda J, Grice K, Held R, Thorn F, Bauer J, Insufficient accommodation and near esophoria: Precursores or concomitants of juvenile-onset myopia? in Proceedings of the 6th International Conference on Myopia, Springer, Tokyo 1998, p. 92

[122] McBrien NA, Millodot M. Amplitude of accommodation and refractive error. Invest Ophthalmol Vis Sci. 1986 Jul;27(7):1187-90

[123] Grosvenor T., Goss D. A., Clinical management of myopia, Butterworth-Heinemann, Boston 1999, p. 88

[124] Edwards MH, Law LF, Lee CM, Leung KM, Lui WO, Clinical norms for amplitude of accommodation in Chinese. Ophthalmic Physiol Opt 1993 Apr;13(2):199-204

[125] Walker TW, Mutti DO. The effect of accommodation on ocualer shape. Optom Vis Sci 2002 Jul;79(7):424-30

[126] Ciuffreda KJ, Wallis DM, Myopes show increased susceptibility to nearwork aftereffects, Invest Ophthalmol Vis Sci 1998 Sep; 39 (10): 1797-1803

[127] Vers-Diaz F, Strang N, Winn B. Nearwork induced transient myopia during progression. Curr Eye Res 2002 Apr;24(4):289-95

[128] Ciuffreda J, Lee M. Differential refractive susceptibility to sustained nearwork. Ophthalmic Physiol Opt 2002 Sep(5):372-9

[129] O'Leary DJ, Allen PM. Facility of accommodation in myopia. Ophthalmic Physiol Opt 2001 Sep;21(5):352-5

[130] Wolffsohn JS, et al. Nearwork-induced transient myopia in preadolescent Hong Kong Chinese. Invest Ophthalmol Vis Sci 2003 May;44(5):2284-9

[131] Gwiazda J, Grice K, Thorn F, Response AC/A ratios are elevated in myopic children, Ophthalmin Physiol Opt 1999 Mar; 19(2): 173-9

[132] Schmid KL, Robert Iskander D, Li RW, Edwards MH, Lew JK. Blur detection thresholds in childhood myopia : single and dual target presentation. Vision Res. 2002 Jan;42(2):239-47

[133] Alm P, et al. Nitric oxide synthase-containing neurons in rat parasympathetic, sympathetic and sensory ganglia: a comparative study. Histochem J. 1995 Oct;27(10):819-31

[134] Fulk GW, Cyert LA, Parker DE, A randomized trial of the effect of single-vision vs. bifocal lenses on myopia progression in children with esophoria, Optom Vis Sci 2000 Aug; 77(8): 395-401

[135] Attenborough A, http://www.altguide.com/therapy/info/bates.html, Bates method for better eyesight without glasses,

[136] Eulenberg A, The case for the preventability of myopia, http://www.i-see.org/prevent_myopia.html

[137] Tippelskirch, Naturgemaesse Heilung von Augenleiden, Bruno Wilkens Verlag Hannover, 1960

[138] "Dr. Jacob Raphaelson's Story". http://chinamyopia.org/jacobenglish.htm

[139] Liberman J, Take off your Glasses and See. Crown Pub. 1996

[140] http://www.vision-training.com/Training/Myopia.htm

[141] http://www.i-see.org

[142] http://www.geocities.com/otisbrown17268/

[143] Bowan M, Toward a unified theory of ametropia: refractive error as a lesion, http://www.simplybrainy.com/Whatsadoctortodo.html

[144] Trachtman JN. Biofeedback of accommodation to reduce myopia: a review. Am J Optom Physiol Opt 1987 Aug;64(8):639-43

[145] Grosvenor T., Goss D. A., Clinical management of myopia, Butterworth-Heinemann, Boston 1999, p. 105

[146] Koslowe KC, et al. Evaluation of accommotrac biofeedback training for myopia control. Optom Vis Sci 1991 May;68(5):338-43

[147] http://www.accommotrac.com

[148] Wildsoet CF, Active emmetropization – evidence for its existence and ramifications for its existence and ramifications for clinical practice. Ophthalmic Physiol Opt 1997 Jul;17(4):279-90

[149] McBrien NA, Gentle A, Cottriall C. Optical correction of induced exial myopia in the tree shrew: implications for emmetropization. Optom Vis Sci 1999 Jun;76(6):419-27

[150] Oakley KH, Young FA. Bifocal control of myopia. Am J Optom Physiol Opt 1975 Nov;52(11):758-64

[151] Leung JT, Brown B, Progresion of myopia in Hong Kong Chinese schoolchildren is slowed by wearing progressive lenses, Optom Vis Sci 1999 Jun; 76(6): 346-54

[152] Tokoro T, Kabe S, Treatment of the myopia and the changes in optical components, Report II, Full or under-correction of myopia by glasses, Acta Soc Ophthalmol Jpn, 1965, 69, I40 – I44, referenced in Grosvenor T., Goss D. A., Clinical management of myopia, Butterworth-Heinemann, Boston 1999 Grosvenor p. 125

6 REFERENCES

[153] Lane BC, Myopia prevention and reversal: new data confirms the interaction of accommodative stress and deficit-inducing nutrition, Journal of IAPM, November 1982

[154] Brown O, http://www.i-see.org/otis_brown

[155] Colgate S, http://www.geocities.com/otisbrown17268/AboutUs.txt

[156] Grosvenor T., Goss D. A., Clinical management of myopia, Butterworth-Heinemann, Boston 1999, p. 113

[157] Edwards MH, et al. The Hong Kong progressive lens myopia control study: study design and main findings. Invest Ophthalmol Vis Sci 2002 Sep;43(9):2852-8

[158] Ong E, Grice K, Held R, Gwiazda. Effects of spectacle intervention on the progression of myopia in children. Optom Vis Sci 1999 Jun;76(6):363-9

[159] Gwiazda J, et al. A randomized clinical trial of progressive addition lenses versus single vision lenses on the progression of myopia in children. Invets Ophthalmol Vis Sci 2003 Apr;44(4):1492-500

[160] Choy CK, et al. Addition lens alleviates reading-induced ocular stress. Clin Exp Optom. 2000 Jan-Feb;83(1):12-15

[161] Eckstein AK, Fischer M, Esser J. [Normal accommodative convergence excess – long term follow-up of conservative therapy with bifocal eyeglasses]. Klin Monatsbl Augenheilkd. 1998 Apr;12(4):218-25

[162] Goss DA, Rainey BB, Irvin J. Effectiveness of Myopia Control with Bifocals as a Function of Near Phoria and Relative Accommodation Moidpoint. www.opt.indiana.edu/research/posters/myopia2001.pdf

[163] Brown B, Edwards MH, Leung JT. Is esophoria a factor in slowing of myopia by progression lenses? Optom Vis Sci 2002 Oct;79(19):638-42

[164] Grosvenor T., Goss D. A., Clinical management of myopia, Butterworth-Heinemann, Boston 1999, p. 121

[165] Fulk GW, Cyert LA, Parker DE. A randomoized clinical trial of bifocal glasses for myopic children with esophoria: results after 54 months. Optometry 2002 Aug;73(8):470-6

[166] Bowan M, personal information

[167] http://myopia.org

[168] Zhu X, Winawer JA, Wallmann J. Potency of myopic defocus in spectacle lens compensation. Invest Ophthalmol Vis Sci. 2003 Jul;44(7):2818-27

[169] Chung K, Mohidin N, O'Leary DJ. Undercorrection of myopia enhances rather than inhibits myopia progression. Vis Res 2002; 42(22):2555-2559

[170] Raviola E, Wiesel TN, An animal model on myopia. N Engl J Med 1985 Jun 20;312(25):1609-15

[171] Schaeffel F, Diether S, Feldkaemper M, Hagel G, Kaymak, Ohngemach S, Schwahn H, Myopia development as a result of visual deprivation? Systems analysis and possible biochemical correlates, in Proceedings of the 6th International Conference on Myopia, Springer, Tokyo 1998, p. 255

[172] Wallmann J, How is emmetropization controlled? Results of research on experimental myopia, in Proceedings of the 6th International Conference on Myopia, Springer, Tokyo 1998, p. 13

[173] Schaeffel F, Glasser A, Howland HC. Accommodation, refractive error and eye growth in chicken. Vision Res. 1988;28(5):639-57

[174] Wildsoet CF, Pettigrew JD, Kainic acid-induced eye emlargement in chickens: Differential effects on anterior and posterior segments, Invest Ophthalmol Vis Sci (1988), 29:311-319, referenced in Stone RA, Neural mechaniosms and eye control, in Proceedings of the 6th International Conference on Myopia, Springer, Tokyo 1998, p. 243

[175] Feldkaemper M, Diether S, Kleine G, Schaeffel F, Interactions of spatial and luminance information in the retina of chickens during myopia development; Exp Eye Res 1999 Jan; 68(1): 105-15

[176] Barutchu A, Crewther SG, Crewther DP, Effects of optical defocus and spatial contrast on anterior chamber depth in chicks. Clin Experiment Ophthalmol 2002 Jun;30(3):217-20

[177] Mei Q, Rong Z, Early signs of myopia in Chinese schoolchildren. Optom Vis Sci 1994 Jan;71(1):14-6

[178] Rohrer B, Iuvone PM, Stell WK, Stimulation of dopamineric amacrine cells by stroboscopic illumination or fibroblast growth factor (bFGF), FGF-2) injections:possible roles in prevention of form-deprivation myopia in the chick. Brain Res 1996;686:169-181

[179] Schwahn HN, Schaeffel F, Flicker parameters are different for suppression of myopia and hyperopia; Vision Res, 1997; 37(19): 2661-2673

[180] Ohngemach S, Feldkaemper M, Schaeffel F, Pineal control of the dopamine D2-receptor gene and dopamine release in the retina of the chicken and their possible relation to growth rhythms of the eye, J Pineal Res 2001; 31: 145-154

[181] Smith EL, Hung LF, Kee CS, Qiao Y, Effects of brief periods of unrestricted vision on the development of form-deprivation myopia in monkeys. Invest Ophthalmol Vis Sci 2002 Feb;43(2):291-9

[182] Napper GA, et al., The effect of an interrupted daily period of normal visual stimulation on form deprivation myopia in chicks. Vision Res 1997 Jun;37(12):1557-64

[183] McBrien N, Structural and metabolic changes associated with recovery from experimentally induced myopia: A brief review, in Proceedings of the 6th International Conference on Myopia, Springer, Tokyo 1998, p. 278

[184] Gentle A, McBrien NA, Modulation of scxleral DNA synthesis in development of and recovery from induced axial myopia in the tree shrew, Exp Eye Res 1999 Feb; 68(2): 155-63

[185] Wildsoet C, Wallman J, Choroidal and scleral mechanisms of compensation for spectacle lenses in chicks. Vision Res. 1995 May;35(9):1175-94

[186] Hung LF, Wallman J, Smith EL 3rd. Vision-dependent changes in the choroidal thickness of macaque monkeys. Invest Ophthalmol Vis Sci. 2000 May;41(6):1259-69

[187] Seko Y, Tanaka Y, Tokoro T, Amorphine inhibits the growth-stimulating effect of retinal pigment epithelium on scleral cells in vitro, Cell Biochem Funct 1997 Sep; 15(3): 191-6

[188] Schaeffel F, Feinsteuerung des Augenlaengenwachstums durch Sehen, Neuroforum 1995; 4: 12-21

[189] Whikehart DR. Biochemistry of the eye. Butterworth Heinemann, 2003

[190] Stone RA, Neural mechaniosms and eye control, in Proceedings of the 6th International Conference on Myopia, Springer, Tokyo 1998, p. 241

[191] Fischer AJ, Miethke P, Morgan IG, Stell WK. Cholinergic amacrine cells are not required for the progression and atropine-mediated suppression of form-deprivation myopia. Brain Res. 1998 May 25;794(1):48-60

[192] Fischer AJ, Morgan IG, Stell WK. Colchicine causes excessive ocular growth and myopia in chicks. Vision Res. 1999 Feb.;39(4):685-97

[193] Devadas M, Megaw P, Boelen MK, Morgan IG, LIght-driven rhythms in scleral precursor synthesis, in Proceedings of the 6th International Conference on Myopia, Springer, Tokyo 1998, p. 358

[194] Seko Y, Shimokawa H, Pang J, Tokoro T, Disturbance of electrolyte balance in vitreous of chicks with form-deprivation myopia. Jpn J Ophthalmol 2000 Jan-Feb;44(1):15-9

[195] Mertz JR, Wallmann J, Choroidal retinoic acid synthesis: a possible mediator between refractive error and compensatory eye growth, Exp Eye Res 2000 Apr; 70(4): 519-27

[196] Draeger U, Vitamin A and the developing eye, Eunice Kennedy Shriver Center, http://www.umassmed.edu/shriver/research/biomedical/projects/vitamina.cfm

[197] McBrien NA, Gentle A. Role of the sclera in the development and pathological complications of myopia. Prog Retin Eye Res. 2003 May;22(3):307-38

[198] Phillips JR, McBrien NA, Form deprivation myopia: elastic properties of sclera; Ophthalmic Physiol Opt 1995 Sep; 15(5): 357-62

[199] Funata M, Tokoro T, Scleral change in experimentally myopic monkeys, Graefes Arch Clin Exp Ophthalmol 1990; 228(2): 174-9

[200] Rada JA, Nickla DL, Troilo D, Decreased proteoglycan synthesis associated with form deprivation myopia in mature primate eyes. Invets Ophthalmol Vis Sci 2000 Jul;41(8):2050-8

6 REFERENCES

[201] Norton TT, Rada JA, Reduced extracellular matrix in mammalian sclera with induced myopia, Vision Res 1995 may; 35(9): 1271-81

[202] Rada JA, Achen VR, Rada KG, Proteoglycan turnover in the sclera of normal and experimentally myopic chick eyes, Invest Ophthalmol Vis Sci 1998 Oct; 39(11): 1990-2002

[203] Jones BE, Thompson EW, Hodos W, Waldbillig RJ, Chader GJ, Scleral matrix metalloproteinases, serine proteinase activity and hydrational capacity are increased in myopia induced by retinal image degradation, Exp Eye Res 1996 Oct; 63(4): 369-381

[204] Kusakari T, Sato T, Tokoro T. Visual deprivation stimulates the exchange of the fibrous sclera into the cartilaginous sclera in chicks. Exp Eye Res 2001 Oct;73(4):533-46

[205] Rada JA, Brenza HL, Increased latent gelatinase activity in the sclera of visually deprived chicks. Invest Ophthalmol Vis Sci 1995 Jul;36(8):1555-1565

[206] Siegwart JT, Norton TT, Increased scleral creep in tree shrews with deprivation induced myopia, Invest Ophthalmol Vis Sci 1994; 35(4): 2068 (abstract 3772), referenced in Norton TT, Siegwart JT, Animal models of emmetropization: matching exial length to the focal plane, J Am Optom Assoc 1995 Jul; 66(7): 405-14

[207] Kusakari T, Sato T, Tokoro T. Regional scleral changes in form-deprivation myopia in chicks. Exp Eye Res 1997 Mar;64(3):465-76

[208] Gentle A, Liu Y, Martin JE, Conti GL, McBrien NA. Collagen gene expression and the altered accumulation of scleral collagen during the development of high myopia. J Biol Chem 2003 Feb 26

[209] Zadnik K, Mutti DO, How applicable are animal myopia models to human juvenile onset myopia? Vision Res 1995 May; 35(9): 1283-1288

[210] Lawrence MS, Azar DT, Myopia and models and mechanisms of refractive error control. Ophthalmol Clin North Am 2002 Mar;15(1):127-33

[211] Hodos W, Revzin AM, Kuewnzel WJ. Thermal gradients in the chick eye: a contributing factor in experimental myopia. Invest Ophthalmol Vis SCI 1987 Nov;28(11):1859-66

[212] Wildsoet CF, Schmid KL, Emmetropization in chicks uses optical vergence and relative distance cues to decode defocus. Vision Res 2001 Nov;41(24):3197-204

[213] Flitcroft DI, A model of the contribution of oculomotor and optical factors to emmetropization and myopia. Vision Res 1998 Oct;38(19):2869-79

[214] Liou SW, Chiu CJ. Myopia and contrast sensitivity function. Curr Eye Res 2001 Feb;22(2):81-4

[215] Artal P, Berrio E, Guirao A, Piers P, Contribution of the cornea and internal surfaces to the change of ocular aberrations with age. J Opt Soc Am A Opt Image SCI Vis 2002 Jan;19(1):137-43

[216] Ninomiya S, et al. Changes of ocular aberration with accommodation. Am J Ophthalmol 2002 Dec;134(6):924-6

[217] He JC, et al. Monochromatic aberrations in the accommodated human eye. Vision Res 2000;40(1):41-8

[218] Hong X, Himebaugh N, Thibos LN. On-eye evaluation of optical performance of rigid and soft contact lenses. Optom Vis Sci 2001 Dec;78(12):872-80

[219] Carney LG, Mainstone JC, Henderson BA. Corneal topography and myopia. A cross-sectional study. Invest Ophthalmol Vis Sci 1997 Feb;38(2):311-20

[220] Nio YK, et al. Spherical and irregular aberratiuons are important for the optimal performance of the human eye. Ophthalmic Physiol Opt 2002 Mar;22(2):103-12

[221] Paquin MP, et al. Objective measurement of optical aberrations in myopic eyes. Optom Vis Sci 2002 May;79(5):285-91

[222] Carkeet A, Luo HD, Tong L, Saw SM, Tan DT. Refractive error and monochromatic aberrations in Singaporean children. Vision Res 2002 Jun;42(14):1809-24

[223] Cheng X, et al. Relationship between refractive error and monochromatic aberrations of the eye. Optom Vis Sci 2003 Jan;80(1):43-9

[224] Feldkamper M, Schaeffel F. Interactions of genes and environment in myopia. Dev Ophthalmol 2003;37:34-49.

[225] Grosvenor T., Goss D. A., Clinical management of myopia, Butterworth-Heinemann, Boston 1999, p. 25

[226] Chung KM, Chong E. Near esophoria is associated with high myopia. Clin Exp Optom 2000 Mar-Apr;83(2):71-75

[227] Mutti DO, Jones LA, Moeschberger ML, Zadnik K, AC/A ratio, age, and refractive error in children. Invest Ophthalmol Vis Sci 2000 Aug;41(9):2469-78

[228] Chen JC, et al. AC/A ratios in myopic and emmetropic Hong Kong children and the effect of timolol. Clin Exp Optom. 2003 Sep;86(5):323-330

[229] http://arapaho.nsuok.edu/~salmonto/VSIII/Lecture4.pdf, a lecture given by the Northeastern State University

[230] Blackie CA, Howland HC, An extension of an accommodation and convergence model of emmetropization to include the effects of illumination intensity. Ophthalmic Physiol Opt 1999 Mar;19(2):112-25

[231] Jiang BC, Gish KW, Leibowitz HW, Effect of luminance on the relation between accommodation and convergence. Optom Vis Sci 1991 Mar; 68(3): 220-5

[232] Heron G, Charman WN, Schor CM, Age changes in the interactions between the accommodation and vergence systems. Optom Vis Sci 2001 Oct;78(19):754-62

[233] Hung GK. Adaptation model of accommodation and vergence. Ophthalmic Physiol Opt. 1992 Jul;12(3):319-26

[234] Grosvenor T., Goss D. A., Clinical management of myopia, Butterworth-Heinemann, Boston 1999, p. 90

[235] Gwiazda J, Thorn F. Development of refraction and strabismus. Curr Opin Ophthalmol. 1999 Oct;10(5):293-9

[236] Paerssinen O, Astigmatism and school myopia, Acta Ophthalmol (Copenh) 1991 Dec;69(6):876-90

[237] Goss DA, Shewey WB, Rates of childhood myopia progression as a function of type of astigmatism. Clin Exp Optom 1990;73:159-163, referenced in Grosvenor T., Goss D. A., Clinical management of myopia, Butterworth-Heinemann, Boston 1999 Grosvenor, p. 25

[238] Gwiazda J, McLellan J, Grice Kenneth, Thorn F, Is astigmatism related to emmetropization and the development of myopia in children? in Proceedings of the 7th International Conference on Myopia, Springer, Tokyo 2000, p. 51

[239] http://www.unm.edu/~bioanth3/behavior/myopia.htm

[240] Maples WC, et al., An epidemiological study of the ocular and visual profiles of Oklahoma Cherokees and Minnesota Chippewas. J Am Optom Assoc 1990 Oct;61(10):784-8

[241] Reim M, Augenheilkunde, Ferdinand Enke Verlag, Stuttgart, 1990, p. 46, p. 58

[242] Mays LE, Gamlin PD, Neuronal circuitry controlling the near response, Curr Opin Neurobiol 1995 Dec; 5(6): 763-8

[243] David T, Smye S, James T, Dabbs T, Time-dependent stress and displacement of the eye wall tissue of the human eye, Med Eng Phys 1997 Mar; 19(2): 131-9

[244] Muller C, Stoll W, Schmal F. The effect of optical devices and repeated trials on the velocity of saccadic eye movements. Acta Otolaryngol. 2003 May;123(4):471-6

[245] Hennekes R, Pillunat L, Asynchronism of saccadic eye movement in young diabetics as related to HbAlc. Graefes Arch Clin Exp Ophthalmol 1985;223(1):50-2

[246] Alessandrini M, et al., Saccadic eye movement and visual pathways function in diabetic patients. An Otorrinolaringol Ibero Am 2001;28(3):269-80

[247] Kelly TS, Myopia and expansion glaucoma, In Doc Ophthalmol Proc Series 28, Third Annual conference on Myopia 1980, The Hague, referenced in Grosvenor T., Goss D. A., Clinical management of myopia, Butterworth-Heinemann, Boston 1999 , p. 40

[248] Tokoro T, Funata M, Akazawa Y, Influence of intraocular pressure on axial elongation. J Ocul Pharmacol 1990; 6(4): 285-291

[249] Jensen H, Myopia progression in young school children and intraocular pressure. Doc Ophthalmol 1992; 82(3): 249-255

[250] Quinn GE, Berlin Ja, Young TL, Ziylan S, Stone RA, Association of intraocular pressure and myopia in children. Ophthalmology 1995 feb; 102(2): 180-185

6 REFERENCES

[251] Nomura H, et al. The relationship between intraocular pressure and refractive error adjusting for age and central corneal thickness. Ophthalmic Physiol Opt. 2004 Jan;24(1):41-45

[252] Lee AJ, et al. Intraocular pressure associations with refractive error and axial length in children. Br J Ophthalmol. 2004 Jan;88(1):5-7

[253] Lin Z, et al. [Refractive error and the intraocular pressure: findings in the Chinese eyes]. Yan Ke Xue Bao. 2003 Dec; 19(4):208-10, 220

[254] Perkins ES, Morbidity from myopia, Sight Sav Rev 1979, (Spring, 49): 11-19, referenced in Grosvenor T., Goss D. A., Clinical management of myopia, Butterworth-Heinemann, Boston 1999, p. 40

[255] Mitchell P, et al., The relationship between glaucoma and myopia: the Blue Mountains Eye Study. Ophthalmology 1999 Oct;106(10):2010-5

[256] Junghans BM, Crewther SG, Liang H, Crewther DP, A role for choroidal lymphatics during recovery from form deprivation myopia? Optom Vis Sci 1999 Nov;76(11):796-803

[257] Young FA, The development and control of myopia in human and subhuman primates. Contacto 1975;19(6):16-31, referenced in Greene P, Mechanical considerations in myopia:relative effects of accommodation, convergence, intraocular pressure, and the extraocular muscles. Am J Optom Physiol Opt 1980 Dec;57(12):902-14

[258] Grosvenor T., Goss D. A., Clinical management of myopia, Butterworth-Heinemann, Boston 1999, p. 51, 53

[259] Edwards MH, Brown B, IOP in myopic children: the relationship bvetween increases in IIOP and the development of myopia. Ophthalmic Physiol Opt 1996 May; 16(3): 243-246

[260] Tiburtius H, Tiburtius K, New treatment possibilities of progressive school myopia, Klin Monatsbl Augenheilkd 1991 Aug; 199(2): 120-1

[261] Goldschmidt E, Myopia in humans: can progression be arrested? Ciba Found Symp 1990; 155: 222-9; discussion 230-4

[262] Tyler CW, Ryu S, Stamper R, The relation between visual sensitivity and intraocular pressure in normal eyes. Invest Ophthalmol Vis Sci 1984 Jan; 25(1): 103-105

[263] Stocker FW, New ways of influencing the intraocular pressure. N Y State J Med 1949; 49: 58-63

[264] Lane BC, Diet and the glaucomas. J Am Coll Nutr 1991; 10(5):536

[265] Dielemans I, de Jong PT, Stolk R, Vingerling JR, Grobbee DE, Hofman A, Primary open-angle glaucoma, intraocular pressure, and diabetes mellitus in the general elderly population. The Rotterdam study. Ophthalmology 1996 Aug; 103(8): 1271-5

[266] Lane BC, Food folate vs supplemental in myopia development & tearfil integrity. Optometry and Vision Science 1994, 71(12S), Poster # 24

[267] Schultz-Zehden W, Bischof F, Auge und Psychosomatik, Deutscher Aerzte Verlag, Köln, 1986, p. 168

[268] Lee AJ, et al. Does smoking affect intraocular pressure? Findings from the blue mountain eye study. J Glaucoma 2003 Jun;12(3):209 12

[269] Greene PR, Mechanical considerations in myopia:relative effects of accommodation, convergence, intraocular pressure, and the extraocular muscles. Am J Optom Physiol Opt 1980 Dec;57(12):902-14

[270] Robinson DA, The mechanics of human saccadic eye movement. J Physiol 1964;174:245-264

[271] Spielmann A, Nystagmus. Curr Opin Ophthalmol 1994 Oct;5(5):20-4

[272] Various references in Greene PR, Mechanical considerations in myopia:relative effects of accommodation, convergence, intraocular pressure, and the extraocular muscles. Am J Optom Physiol Opt 1980 Dec;57(12):902-14

[273] Williams RJ, Biochemical individuality, Keats Publishing Inc., New Canaan, 1998

[274] Schmid GF, Petrig BL, Riva CE, Logean E, Walti R, Measurement of eye length and eye shape by optical low coherence reflectometry. Int Ophthalmol 2001;23(4-6):317-20

[275] Zhou XD, Wang FR, Zhou SZ, Shi JS, A computed tomographic study of the relation between ocular axial biometry and refraction, in Myopia Updates, Proceedings of the 6th International Conference on Myopia, Springer, Tokyo 1998 p. 112

[276] Mutti DO, Sholtz RI, Friedman NE, Zadnik K, Peripheral refraction and ocular shape in children. Invest Ophthalmol Vis Sci 2000 Apr;41(5):1022-30

[277] Wojciechowski R, et al. Age, gender, biometry, refractive error, and the anterior chamber angle among Alaskan Eskimos. Ophthalmology 2003 Feb;110(2):365-75

[278] Nickla DL, Wildsoet C, Wallman J, The circadian rhythm in intraocular pressure and its relation to diurnal ocular growth changes in chicks. Exp Eye Res 1998 Feb;66(2):183-93

[279] Nickla DL, Wildsoet CF, Troilo D, Endogenous rhythms in axial length and choroidal thickness in chicks: implications for ocular growth regulation. Invest Ophthalmol Vis Sci 2002 Mar;42(3):584-8

[280] Quinn GE, Shin CH, Maguire MG, Stone RA, Myopia and ambient lighting at night, Nature vol. 399, pages 113-114, 1999

[281] Gwiazda J, Ong E, Held R, Thorn F, Myopia and ambient night-light lighting, Nature vol. 404, page 144, 2000

[282] Zadnik K, Jones LA, Irvin BC, Kleinstein RN, Manny RE, Shin JA, Mutti DO, Myopia and ambient night-light lighting, Nature vol. 404, pages 143-144, 2000

[283] Stone RA, Maguire MG, Quinn GE, Myopis and ambient night-light lighting, Nature, vol. 404, page 144, 2000

[284] Glickman G, Levin R, Brainard GC, Ocular input for human melatonin regulation:relevance to breat cancer. Neuroendocrinol Lett 2002 Jul;23 Suppl 2:17-22

[285] Hoffmann M, Schaeffel F, Melatonin and deprivation myopia in chickens, Neurochem Int 1996 Jan; 28(1): 95-107

[286] Reiter RR, Robinson J, Melatonin, Bantam Books, 1995, p. 58

[287] Mervyn L, Thorsons complete Guide to vitamins & minerals, Thorsons, London, 2000, p. 190

[288] Tinker D, Rucker RB, Role of selected nutrients in synthesis, accumulation, and chemical modification of connective tissue proteins. Physiological review 1985 Jul; 65(3): 607-657

[289] Woung LC, Lue YF, Shih YF, Accommodation and pupillary response in early-onset myopia among schoolchildren, Optom Vis Sci 1998 Aug; 75(8): 611-6

[290] Young, Francis A, The effect of nearwork illumination level on monkey refraction, Am J Optom and Arch Am Acad Optom 1969; 46(9), referenced in referenced in The prevention of acquired myopia, http://members.aol.com/myopiaprev/page2.htm

[291] Lang G, Augenheilkunde, Georg Thieme Verlag Stuttgart New York, 2000, p. 228

[292] Roberts JE, Visible light induced changes in the immune response through an eye-brain mechanism (photoneuroimmunology), I Photochem Photobiol B 1995 Jul; 29(1): 3-15

[293] Atchison DA, Smith G, Efron N, The effect of pupil size on visual acuity in uncorrected and corrected myopia, Am J Optom Physiol Opt 1979 May; 56(5): 315-23

[294] Paquin MP, Hamam H, Simonet P, Objective measurement of optical aberaations in myopic eyes. Optom Vis Sci 2002 May;79(5):285-91

[295] Owens, Liebowitz, Accommodation, convergence, and distance perceprtion in low illumination. Am J Optom Physiol Opt 1980 Sep;57(9):540-50

[296] Kersten D, Legge GE, Convergence accommodation. J Opt Soc Am 1983 Mar;73(3):332-8

[297] Vannas AE, et al. Myopia and natural lighting extremas: risk factors in Finnish army conscripts. Acta Ophthalmol Scand. 2003 Dec;81(6):588-95

[298] Millodot M, Stevenson RW, Electrophysiological evidence of adaptation to colored filters. Am J Optom Physiol Opt 1982 Jun;59(6):507-10

[299] Schmid KL, Wildsoet CF. Contrast and spatial-frequency requirements for emmetropization in chicks. Vision res 1997 Aug;37(15):2011-21

6 REFERENCES

[300] Kroger RH, Binder S. Use of paper selectively absorbing long wavelengths to reduce the impact of educational near work on human refractive development. Br J Ophthalmol 2000 Aug;84(8):890-3

[301] Kubena T, Kubena K, Galatik A, Neumann P. Effect of infrared rays on the eye in progressive myopia. Cesk Slov Oftalmol 1999 May;55(3):155-9

[302] Liberman J, Light: Medicine of the future, Bear & Co, 1992

[303] Dorner GT, et al. Hyperglycemia affects flicker-induced vasodilation in the retina of healthy subjects. Vision Res. 2003 Jun;43(13):1495-500

[304] Dorner GT, et al. Nitric oxide regulates retinal vascular tone in humans. Am J Physiol Heart Circ Physiol. 2003 Aug;285(2):H631-6.Epub 2003 May 15.

[305] http://www.i-see.org/vtintro.html (an introduction to vision training by F. Eisner with numerous sources for further reading)

[306] http://www.oep.org

[307] http://www.covd.org

[308] Scharfblick für alle? Focus 47, 1999, with contributions from Schaeffel F, et al.

[309] Loman J, et al., Darkness and near work: myopia and ist progression in third-year law students. Ophthalmology 2002 May;109(5):1032-8

[310] Harris ED, McGroskery PA. Influence of temperature and fibril stability on degradation of cartilage collagen by rheumatoid synovial collagenase, New Engl J Med 290 (1974), 1, referenced in Trichtel F., Zur Enstehung und Therapie der Myopie, Enke, Stuttgart 1986, p. 29

[311] Hodos W, Avian models of experimental myopia: environmental factors in the regulation of eye growth, Ciba Foundation Symposium 155, John Wiley & Sons, 1990

[312] Tokoro T, Experimental myopia in rabbits, Invest Ophthalmol 9 (1979), 926, referenced in Trichtel F., Zur Enstehung und Therapie der Myopie, Enke, Stuttgart 1986, p. 32

[313] Briese E, Emotional hyperthermia and performance in humans, Physiol Behav 1995 Sep; 58(3): 615-8

[314] Trichtel F., Zur Enstehung und Therapie der Myopie, Enke, Stuttgart 1986, p. 32

[315] Ravalico G, Pastori G, Croce M, Toffoli G, Pulsatile ocular blood flow in myopia, Ophthalmologica 1997: 211: 271-273

[316] Lam AK, Wong S, Lam CS, To CH, The effect of myopic axial elongation and posture on the pulsatile ocular blood flow in young normal subjects. Optom Vis Sci 2002 May;79(5):300-5

[317] Reiner A, Shih YF, Fitzgerald ME, The relationship of choroidal blood flow and accommodation to the control of ocular growth, Vision Res 1995 May; 35(9): 1227-45

[318] Dimitova G, Tamaki Y, Kato S, Nagahara M, Rectobulbar circulation in myopic patients with or without myopic choroidal neovascularisation. Br J Ophthalmol 2002 Jul;86(7):771-3

[319] Akyol N, et al., Choroidal and retinal blood flow changes in degenerative myopia. Can J Ophthalmol 1996 Apr;31(3):113-9

[320] Golychev VN, Morozova IV, A combination of scleroplasty with intrascleral revascularization in myopia, Oftalmol Zh 1989; 3: 160-162

[321] Chang S H-C, Shih Y-F, Lin L L-K, A review of myopia studies in Taiwan, in Proceedings of the 7th International Conference on Myopia, Springer, Tokyo 2000, p. 133

[322] Fitzgerald ME, Wildsoet CF, Reiner A, Temporal relationship of choroidal blood flow and thickness changes during recovery from form deprivation myopia in chicks. Exp Eye Res 2002 May;74(5):561-70

[323] Lazuk AV, Slepova S, Tarutta P, Antibodies to collagen in patients with progressive myopia, in Proceedings of the 6th International Conference on Myopia, Springer, Tokyo 1998, p. 120

[324] Semenova GS, Meleshko VE, Gogina IF, Velozo L, Circulating immune complexes in the blood and anterior chamber fluid in patients with glaucoma and diabetic angioretinopathy complicated by myopia and senile cataract, Vestn Oftalmol 1989 Jul-Aug; 105(4): 70-1

[325] Puchkovskaia NA, Shul'gina NS, Bushueva NN, Degtiarenko TV, Usov NI, Disorders of the immune status of the body in patients with myopia, Oftalmol Zh 1988; (3): 146-50

[326] Dolezalova V, Mottlava D, Relation between myopia and intelligence, Cesk Oftalmol 1995 Sep; 51(4): 235-9

[327] Baldwin W, A review of statistical studies of relations between myopia and ethnic, behavioral, and physiological characteristics, Am J Optometry & Physiol Optics Jul 1981; 58(7): 516-527

[328] Gardiner PA, James G, Association between maternal disease during pregnancy and myopia in the child, Br J Ophthalmol 1960; 44: 172-178, referenced in Baldwin W, A review of statistical studies of relations between myopia and ethnic, behavioral, and physiological characteristics, Am J Optometry & Physiol Optics Jul 1981; 58(7): 516-527

[329] Fledelius H, Zak M, Pedersen FK, Refraction in juvenile chronic arthritis: a lonf-term follow-up study, with emphasis on myopia, Acta Ophthalmol Scand 2001 Jun; 79(3): 237-9

[330] Trichtel F., Zur Enstehung und Therapie der Myopie, Enke, Stuttgart 1986, p. 1

[331] Markwardt KL, Magnino PE, Pang IH, Histamine induced contraction of human ciliary muscle cells. Exp Eye Res 1997 May;64(5):713-7

[332] B5 Wissenschaftsnachrichten Gesundheit 06.10.2001

[333] Xu GZ, Li WW, Tso MO. Apoptosis in human retinal degenerations. Trans Am Ophthalmol Soc 1996;94:411-30; discussion 430-1

[334] Grodzicky T, Elkon KB. Apoptosis: a case where too much or too little can lead to autoimmunity. Mt Sinai J Med 2002 Sep;69(4):208-19

[335] Janeway CA, Travers P, Immunologie, Spektrum Akademischer Verlag, Heidelberg Berlin Oxford, 1997, p. 489, 495

[336] Romero FJ, Bosch-Morell F, Romero MJ, Jareno EJ, Romero B, Marin NM, Roma J, Lipid peroxidation products and antioxidants in human disease, Environ Health Perspect 1998, Oct; 106 Suppl 5: 1229-1234

[337] Florence TM. The role of free radicals in disease. Aust N Z J Ophthalmol 1995 Feb;23(1):3-7

[338] Simonelli F, et al., Lipid peroxidation and human cataractogenesis in diabetes and severe myopia. Wxp Eye Res 1989 Aug;49(2):181-7

[339] Bosch-Morell F, et al. Lipid peroxidation products in human subretinal fluid. Free Radic Biol Med 1996;20(7):899-903

[340] Vinetskaia MI, et al. Significance of lacrimal fluid peroxidation and anti-radical defense parameters for prediction and treatment of complicated myopia. Vestn Oftalmol 2000 Sep-Oct;116(5):54-6

[341] Garcia M, Vecino E. Intracellular pathways leading to apoptosis of retinal cells. Arch Soc Esp Oftalmol 2003 Jul;78(7):351-64

[342] Nunes VA, et al. Antioxidant deficiency induces caspase activation in chick skeletal muscle cells. Braz J Biol Res. 2003 Aug;36(8):1047-53

[343] Behndig A, et al. Superoxide dismutase isoenzymes in the human eye. Invest Ophthalmol Vis Sci. 1998 Mar;39(3):471-5

[344] Romero FJ, Bosch-Morell F, Romero MJ, Jareno EJ, Romero B, Marin N, Roma J, Lipid peroxidation products and antioxidants in human disease, Environ Health Perspect 1998 Oct; 106 Suppl 5: 1229-34

[345] Kolosov VI, Kurochkin VN, Activity of biological oxidation enzymes in the blood of children at different stages of development and with different dynamics of myopia. Oftalmol Zh 1985; (5): 293-6

[346] http://www.books.md/B/dic/bloodretinalbarrier.php

[347] Rizzolo LJ. Polarity and the development of the outer blood-retinal barrier. Histol Histopathol. 1997 Oct;12(4):1057-67

6 REFERENCES

[348] Kitaya N, et al. Changes in blood-retinal barrier permeability in form deprivation myopia in tree shrews. Vision Res. 2000;40(17):2369-77

[349] Schneck ME, Fortune B, Adams AJ. The fast oscillation of the electrooculogram reveals sensitivits of the human outer retina/retinal pigment epithelium to glucose level. Vision Res 2000;40(24):3447-53

[350] Shih YF, et al. The blood-aqueous barrier in anisometria and high myopia. Ophthalmic Res. 1996;28(2):137-40

[351] Bishop PN. Structural Macromelecules and supramolecular organization of the vitreous gel. Progress Ret Eye Res 2000;19:323-344

[352] Morita H, Funata M, Tokoro T. A clinical study of the development of posterior vitreous detachment in high myopia. Retina 1995;15(2):117-24

[353] Chiou GCY, Review: Effects of nitric oxide on eye diseases and their treatment, Journal of Ocular Pharmacology and their Therapeutics 2001; 17(2): 189-98

[354] Kamikawatoko S, et al. Nitric oxide relaxes bovine ciliary muscle contracted by carbachol through elevation of cyclic GMP. Exp Eye Res 1998 Jan;66(1):1-7

[355] Beauregard C, Liu Q, Chiou GC, Effects of nitric oxide donors and nitric oxide synthase substrates on ciliary muscle contracted by carbachol and endothelin for possible use in myopia prevention, J Ocul Pharmacol Ther 2001 feb; 17(1): 1-9

[356] Tokoro T, Developmental mechanism of low myopia and its treatment, in Proceedings of the 7th International Conference on Myopia, Springer, Tokyo 2000, p. 73

[357] Xu H, Huang K, Gao Q, Gao Z, Han X, A study on the prevention and treatment of myopia with nacre on chicks, Pharmacological Research 2001; 44(1): 1-6

[358] Fujikado T, Kawasaki Y, Fujii J, Taniguchi N, Okada M, Suzuki A, Ohmi G, Tano Y, The effect of nitric oxide synthase inhibitor of form-deprivation myopia. Curr Eye Res 1997 Oct; 16(10): 992-6

[359] Fujikado T, Tsujikawa K, Tamura M, Hosohata J, Kawasaki Y, Tano Y, Effect of a nitric oxide synthase inhibitor on lens-induced myopia, Ophthalmic Res 2001 Mar-Apr; 33(2): 75-9

[360] Hu D-N, Roberts JE, McCormick SA, Role of uveal melanocytes in the development of myopia, in Proceedings of the 7th International Conference on Myopia, Springer, Tokyo 2000, p. 125

[361] Honda Y. Cellular and molecular biology of ischemic retina. Nippon Ganka Gakkai Zasshi 1996 Dec;100(12):937-55

[362] Fujii S, Honda S, Sekiya Y, Yamasaki M, Yamamoto M, Saijoh K, Differential expression of nitric oxide synthase isoforms in form-deprived chick eyes, Curr Eye Res 1998 Jun; 17(6): 586-93

[363] Kiel JW, et al. Effects of nitric oxide synthays inhibition on ciliary blood fow, aqueous production and intraocular pressure. Exp Eye Res 2001 Sep;73(3):355-64

[364] Doganay S, et al. Decreased nitric oxide production in primary open-angle glaucoma. Eur J Ophthalmol 2002 Jan-Feb;12(1):44-8

[365] Chuman, et al. The effect of L-arginine on intraocular pressure in the human eye. Curr Eye Res 2000 Jun;20(6):511-6

[366] Bugnon O, Schaad NC, Schorderet M. Nitric oxide modulates andogenoud dopamine release in bovine retina. Neuroreport 1994 Jan 12;5(4):401-4

[367] Neal MJ, Cunningham JR. Release of endogenous ascorbic acid preserves extracellular dopamine in the mammalian retina. Invest Ophthalmol Vis Sci 1999 Nov;40(12):2983-7

[368] Haamedi SN, Djamgoz MB, Dopamine and nitric oxide control both flickering and steady-light-induced cone contraction and horizontal cell spinule formation in the teleost (carp) retina:Serial interaction of dopamine and nitric oxide. J Comp Neurol 2002 Jul 22;449(2):120-8

[369] Tamm ER, et al. Nerve cells in the human ciliary muscle: ultrastructural and immunocytochemical characterization. Invest Ophthalmol Vis Sci 1995 Feb;36(2):414-26

[370] Ando A, et al. Blockade of nitric-oxide synthase reduces choroidal neovascularization. Mol Pharmacol 2002 Sep;62(3):539-44

[371] Scheerer R, A short observation on the cause of myopia, Klin Monatsbl Augenheilkd 1976 Dec; 169(6): 787-788

[372] Avetisov ES, Savitskaya NF, Vinetskaya MI, Iomdina EN, A study of biochemical qualities of normal and myopic eye sclera in humans of different age groups, Metab Pediatr Syst Ophthalmol 1983; 7(4): 183-8

[373] Chang SW, et al., The cornea in young myopic adults. Br J Ophthalmol 2001 Aug;85(8):916-20

[374] Balacco-Gabrieli C, Aetiopathogenesis of myopia: a new neuroendocrine-genetic theory, Recenti Progressi in Medicina 1989 Apr; 80(4): 197-200

[375] Modern nutrition in health and disease, editors Shils ME, Olson JA, Shike M, Ross AC, Lippincott Williams & Wilkins, 1998, p. 245

[376] Bowan MD, Stress and eye: new speculations on refractive error, J Behavioral Opotometry 1996; 7(5)

[377] Balacco-Gabrieli C, Tundo R, A study on the effect of some steroid hormones in degenerative myopia, Doc Ophthalmol Proc Ser 28: 129-134, referenced in Proceedings of the 7th International Conference on Myopia, Springer, Tokyo 2000, p.95

[378] Balacco-Gabrieli C, Moramarco A, Regine F, Abdolrahimzadeh B, Correlation between steroid hormone balance and etiopathology of high myopia: Clinical trial, in Proceedings of the 6th International Conference on Myopia, Springer, Tokyo 1998, p. 379

[379] Ojha, Singh R, Maurya O, Agrawal JK, Myopia and plasma cortisol, Indian J Ophthalmol 1989 Apr; 37(2): 91-93

[380] Rosmond R, Bjorntorp P, Low cortisol production in chronic stress, Lakartidningen 2000 Sep 20; 97(38): 4120-4

[381] Trichtel F., Zur Enstehung und Therapie der Myopie, Enke, Stuttgart 1986, p. 39

[382] Schultz-Zehden W, Bischof F, Auge und Psychosomatik, Deutscher Aerzte Verlag, Köln, 1986, p. 167

[383] Elmadfa I, Leitzmann C, Ernaehrung des Menschen, Verlag Eugen Ulmer Stuttgart, 1990, p.329

[384] Anderson RA, Bryden NA, Polansky MM, Thorp JW, Effects of carbohydrate loading and underwater exercise on circulating cortisol, insulin and urinary losses of chromium and zinc. Eur J Appl Physiol 1991; 63(2): 146-150

[385] Schultz-Zehden W, Bischof F, Auge und Psychosomatik, Deutscher Aerzte Verlag, Köln, 1986, p. 190

[386] Avetisov ES, Gundorova RA, Shakarian AA, Oganesian AA, Effects of acute psychogenic stress on the state of several functions of the visual analyzer, Vestn Oftalmol 1991 Jan-Feb; 107(1): 17-9

[387] Grosvenor T, Why is there an epidemic of myopia? Clin Exp Optom. 2003 Sep;86(5):273-5

[388] Wolffsohn JS, et al. Refractive error, cognitive demand and nearwork-induced transient myopia. Curr Eye Res. 2003 Dec;27(6):363-70

[389] Peckham CS, Gardiner PA, Goldstein H, Acquired myopia in 11-year-old-children, Brit Med J I (1977), 542, referenced in Trichtel F., Zur Enstehung und Therapie der Myopie, Enke, Stuttgart 1986, p. 70

[390] Sofaer JA, Emery AE, Genes for super-intelligence? J Med Genet 1981 Dec; 18(6): 410-3

[391] Benbow CP, Physiological correlates of extreme intellectual precocity, Neuropsychologia 1986; 24(5): 719-25

[392] Beedle SL, Young FA, Values, personality, physical characteristics, and refractive error, Am J Optom Physiol Opt 1976 Nov; 53(11): 735-9

[393] Miller EM, On the correlation of myopia and intelligence, Genet Soc Gen Psychol Monogr 1992 Nov; 118(4): 361-83

[394] http://www.nb.net/~sparrow/vision.html

[395] Qureshi IA, Effects of mild, moderate and severe exercise on intraocular pressure of sedentary subjects. Ann Hum Biol 1995 Nov-Dec;22(6):545-53

[396] Pizzarello LD. Refractive changes in pregnancy. Graefes Arch Clin Exp Ophthalmol 2003 May 8

[397] Furushima M, et al., Changes in refraction caused by induction of acute hyperglycemia in healthy volunteers. Jpn J Ophthalmol 1999 Sep-Oct;43(5):398-403

6 REFERENCES

[398] Grosvenor T., Goss D. A., Clinical management of myopia, Butterworth-Heinemann, Boston 1999, p. 94

[399] Okamoto F, et al., Refractive changes in diabetic patients during intensive glycaemic control. Br J Ophthalmol 2000 Oct;84(10):1097-102

[400] Tabandeh H, Ranganath L, Marks V, Visual function during acute hypoglycaemia. Eur J Ophthalmol 1996 Jan-Mar;6(1):81-6

[401] Fledelius HC, Diabetes, thyroid disease, and rheumatoid arthritis: an association with myopia? Proceedings of the 7th International Conference on Myopia, Springer, Tokyo 2000, p. 97

[402] Kovalenko VV, Diabetes mellitus and the state of ocular accommodation in schoolchildren. Probl Endokrinol (Mosk) 1978 Jul;24(4):17-19

[403] Du Y, Miller CM, Kern TS. Hyperglycemia increases mitochondrial superoxide in retina and retinal cells. Free Radic Biol Med. 2003 Dec 1;35(11):1491-9

[404] Cleave TL, The saccharine disease. John Wright & Sons Ltd. Bristol, UK, 6-27,

[405] Cordain L, Eaton SB, Brand Miller J, Lindeberg S, Jensen C, An evolutionary analysis of the aetiology and pathogenesis of juvenile-onset myopia. Acta Ophthalmol Scand 2002 Apr;80(2):125-35

[406] Cordain L, Eades MR, Eades MD. Hyperinsulinemic diseases of civilization: more than just Syndrome X. Comp Biochem Physiol A Mol Integr Physiol. 2003 Sep;136(1):95-112

[407] Garner LF et al., Acta Ophthalmol (Copenh) 1985 Jun;63(3):323-6

[408] Wong L, et al., Education, reading, and familial tendency as risk factors for myopia in Hong Kong fishermen. J Epidemiol Community Health 1993 Feb;47(1):50-3

[409] Jansson L, Naeser P. An increased number of mast cells in the sclera of alloxan-diabetic mice. Acta Ophthalmol (Copenh). 1987 Apr;65(2):203-5

[410] Perrott RL, North RV, Drasdo N, Ahmed KA, Owens DR, The influence of plasma glucose upon pulsatile ocular blood flow in subjects with type II diabetes mellitus. Diabetologia 2001 Jun;44(6):700-5

[411] Various books by Michel Montignac about diet and nutrition

[412] Dumesnil JG, et al., Effect of a low-glycaemic index-low-fat-high protein diet on the atherogenic metabolic risk profile of abdominally obese men, Br J Nutr 2001 Nov;86(5):557-68

[413] Knapp AA, Blindness: forty years of original research, J Intl Acad. Prev Med 1977; 4(1), 50-73

[414] Gardiner PA, Dietary treatment of myopia in children, The Lancet, 31 May 1958, 1152-1155

[415] Juchheim JK, Haaranalyse, Mineralstoffe und Ernaehrung, Karl F. Haug Verlag, Heidelberg, 1991, p. 34

[416] Pohlandt F, Hypothesis: myopia of prematurity is caused by postnatal bone mineral deficiency. Eur J Pediatr 1994 Apr;153(4):234-236

[417] Price WA, Nutrition and physical degeneration, Keats Publishing Inc., New Canaan, 1997, p. 275

[418] Torralbo A, Pina E, Portoles J, Sanchez-Fructuoso A, Barrientos A, Renal magnesium wasting with hypercalciuria, nephrocalcinosis and ocular disorders, Nephron 1995; 69(4): 472-475

[419] Rodriguez-Soriano J, Vallo A, Garcia-Fuentes M, Hypomagnesaemia of hereditary renal origin, Pediatr Nephrol 1987 Jul; 1(3): 465-472

[420] Geven WB, Monnens LA, Willems JL, Magnesium metabolism in childhood, Miner Electrolyte Metab 1993; 19(4-5): 308-313

[421] Thalasselis A. Thalasselis syndrome and genetic theories on keratokonus. J Am Optom Assoc 1995 Aug;66(8):495-9

[422] Appel A, et al. Cell-free synthesis of hyaluronic acid in Marfan syndrome. J Biol Chem 1979 Dec 10;254(23):12199-203

[423] Vinetskaia MI, Iomdina EN, Study of lacrimal fluid trace elements in several eye diseases, Vestn Oftalmol 1994 Oct; 110(4): 24-26

[424] Shiue C, Ko LS, Study on serum copper and zinc levels in high myopia, Acta Ophthalmologica 1988, Supplement 185, 141-142

[425] Avetisov ES, Vinetskaia, Iomdina EN, Makhmudova FR, Boltaeva ZK, Tarutta EP, Copper metabolism in scleral tissue and possibilities of its correction in myopia, Vestn Oftalmol 1991 Sep-Oct; 107(5): 31-4

[426] Avetisov E, Tarutta EP, Iomdina E, Vinetskaya M, Andreyeva L, A new composition for the treatment of progressive myopia and its efficiency, in Proceedings of the 6th International Conference on Myopia, Springer, Tokyo 1998, p.220

[427] Huibi X, Kaixun H, Quihua G, Yushan Z, Xiuxian H, Prevention of axial elongation in myopia by the trace element zinc, Biol Trace Elem Res 2001 Jan; 79(1): 39-47

[428] Srinivas C, Simple myopia with an indigenous drug (clinical study), in Proceedings of the 6th International Conference on Myopia, Springer, Tokyo 1998, p. 201

[429] Puri RN, Thakur V, Nema HV. Role of zinc (Yashad Bhasma) in arrest of myopia. Indian J Ophthalmol 1983;31 Suppl:816-22

[430] Lane BC, Aggarwala KR. High myopes are biochemically different from hyperopes. Myopia 2000: Proceedings of the VIII International Conference on Myopia, p. 232

[431] Ueda Y, et al., The retinal pigment epithelium of Cr-deficient rats. Life Sci 2002 Aug 16;71(13):1569-77

[432] Amemiya T, The eye and nutrition. Jpn J Ophthalmol 2000 May;44(3):320

[433] Gong H, Amemiya T, Ultrastructure of retina of manganese-deficient rats. Invest Ophthalmol Vis Sci 1996 Sep;37(10):1967-74

[434] Trichtel F., Zur Enstehung und Therapie der Myopie, Enke, Stuttgart 1986, p. 77

[435] DeVreis D, The statistical relationship between the occurrence of myopia and struma in school children, Tid. Soc. Genneskd. Delft, 1950; 28(5): 79-80 referenced in Baldwin W, A review of statistical studies of relations between myopia and ethnic, behavioral, and physiological characteristics, Am J Optometry & Physiol Optics Jul 1981; 58(7): 516-527

[436] Bothman L, The relation of the basal metabolic rate to progressive axial myopia, Am J Ophthalmol 1931; 14: 918-924 referenced in Baldwin W, A review of statistical studies of relations between myopia and ethnic, behavioral, and physiological characteristics, Am J Optometry & Physiol Optics Jul 1981; 58(7): 516-527

[437] Kohrle J, The trace element selenium and the thyroid gland. Biochemie 1999 May;81(5):527-33

[438] Lane BC, Calcium, chromium, protein, sugar and accommodation in myopia, Doc Ophthal Proc Series, vol 28, 141-148 (Third International Conference on Myopia Copenhagen, 1980)

[439] Langohr HD, Petruch F, Schroth G, Vitamin B 1, B 2 and B 6 deficiency in neurological disorders. J Neurol 1981;225(2):95-108

[440] Omura H, Yokota Y. [Methods of treatment of juvenile myopia. 1. Use of massive doses of thiamine propyl disulfide and thiamine tetrahydrofuryl disulfide]. J Clin Pathol 1963 Jan;17:79-84

[441] Iomdina EN, Kushnarevich NY, Vinetskaya MI, Tarutta EP, Lazuk AV, Antioxidant therapy of progressive and complicated myopia in children, in Proceedings of the 7th International Conference on Myopia, Springer, Tokyo 2000, p. 171

[442] Eckhert CD, Lockwood MK, Shen B. Influence of selenium on the microvasculature of the retina. Microvasc Res 1993 Jan;45(1):74-82

[443] Margadant D, http://www.fly.to.tardigrada

[444] Amemiya T. Retinal changes in the selenium deficient rat. Int J Vitam Nutr Res. 1985;55(3):233-7

[445] Miskulin M, Godeau G, Tixier AM, Robert AM, Experimental study of the effects of cyanoside chloride on collagen, and its potential value in ophthalmology, J Fr Ophtalmol 1984; 7(11): 737-743

[446] Sole P, Rigal D, Peyresblanques J, Effects of cyaninoside chloride and Heleniene on mesopic and scotopic vision in myopia and night blindness, J Fr Ophtalmol 1984; 7(1): 35-39

6 REFERENCES

[447] Algan B, The treatment of progressive malignant myopia with magnesium chelates of flavones. A propos of 400 cases, Bull Soc Belge Ophtalmol 1981; 192: 103-12

[448] Politzer, Zur medikamentösen Therapie bei der progredienten Myopie, Klin Mbl Augenheilk 1977; 171:616-619

[449] Hosaka A, Eine Analyse unter Anwendung der Glaskörper-Fluorophotometrie und Computersimulation. Acta Ophthalmologica 185: 95-99

[450] Stache-Schenk I, Der Augenspiegel 1982, 5: 2-8

[451] Bhutto IA, Amemiya T. Retinal vascular architecture is maintained in retinal degeneration: corrosion cast and electron microscope study. Eye 2002 Aug;15(Pt 4):531-8

[452] Eckert G, Die Behandlung der tetinalen Durchblutungsstoerungen mit Trioxyaethylrutin, Der Augenarzt 1980; (3):180-184

[453] Leuenberger S, Faulborn J, Sturrock G, Gloor B, Rehorek R, Baumgartner R, Vascular and ocular complications in a child with homocystinuria, Schweiz Med Wochenschr 1984 Jun 2; 114(22): 793-798

[454] Juszko J, Kubalska J, Kanigowska K, Ocular problems in children with homocysteinuria, Klin Oczna 1994 Jun; 96(6-7): 212-215

[455] Cruysberg JR, Boers GH, Trijbels JM, Deutman AF, Delay in diagnosis of homocytinuria: retrospective study of consecutive patients, BMJ 1996 Oct 26; 313(7064): 1037-1040

[456] Mulvihill A, Yap S, O'Keefe M, Howard PM, Naughten ER, Ocular findings among patients with late-diagnosed or poorly controlled homocyteinuria compared with a screened, well controlled population, J AAPOS 2001 Oct; 5(5): 311-5

[457] Wuu JA, Wen LY, Chuang TY, Chang GG, Amino acid concentrations in serum and aqueous humor from subjects with extreme myopia or senile cataract, Clin Chem 1988 Aug; 34(8): 1610-1613

[458] Mulvihill A, et al., Ocular findings among patients with late-diagnosed or poorly controlled homocystinuria compared with a screened, well-controlled population. J AAPPOS 2001 Oct ;5(5):311-5

[459] Chaitow L, Thorsons guide to amino acids, Thorsons, 1991, p. 51

[460] Frankel P, The methylation miracle, St. Martin's Paperbacks, 1999, p. 124

[461] Biesalski HK et al., Ernaehrungsmedizin, Georg Thieme Verlag Stuttgart New York 1999

[462] Josephson E, Nearsightedness is preventable, New York Chedney Press, 139, referenced in Eulenberg A, The case for the preventability of myopia, http://www.i-see.org/prevent_myopia.html

[463] Edwards MH, Leung SSF, Lee WTK, Do variations in normal nutrition play a role in the development of myopia? Optom Vis Sci. 1996 Oct;73(10):638-43

[464] Spanheimer R, et al., Collagen production in fasted and food-restricted rats:response to duration and severety of food deprivation. J Nutr 1991 Apr;121(4):518-24

[465] http://www.medicaltribune.net/dispserchcontent.cfm?pg=1&id=10173

[466] Grosvenor T., Goss D. A., Clinical management of myopia, Butterworth-Heinemann, Boston 1999, p. 130

[467] Schwahn HN, Kaymak H, Schaeffel F. Effects of atropine on refractive development, dopamine release and slow retinal potentials in the chick. Vis Neurosci 2000 Mar-Apr;17(2):165-76

[468] Grosvenor T., Goss D. A., Clinical management of myopia, Butterworth-Heinemann, Boston 1999, p. 133

[469] Williams RM, Bienenstock J, Stead RH, Mast cells: the neuroimmune connection. Chem Immunol. Basel, Karger, 1995, vol 61: 208-235

[470] Saw SM, Gazzard G, Au Eong KG, Tan DT. Myopia: attempts to arrest progression. Br J Ophthalmol 2002 Nov;86(11):1306-11

[471] Barclay L. Myopia may be pharmacologically controlled. Medscape Medical News, www.medscape.com/viewarticle/453554

[472] Ouyang CH, Chu RY, Hu WZ. [Effects of pirenzipine on lens induced myopia in the guinea-pig]. Zhonghua Yan Ke Za Zhi. 2003 Jun;39(6):348-51

[473] Bartlett JD, et al. A tolerrability study of pirenzipine ophthalmic gel in myopic children. J Ocul Pharmacol Ther. 2003 Jun;19(3):271-9

[474] http://www.fehlsichtig.de/PIRENZIPINE.htm

[475] Winn B, et al. Effect of beta-adrenoceptor antagonists on autonomic control of ciliary smooth muscle. Ophthalmic Physiol Opt. 2002 Sep;22(5):359-65

[476] Trier K, et al. Biochemical and ultrastructural changes in rabbit sclera after treatment with 7-methyxanthine, theobromine, acetazolamide, or L-ornithine. Br J Ophthalmol. 1999 Dec;83(12):1370-5

[477] Chew S-J, Hoh S-T, Tan J, Cheng H-M, Muscarinic antagonists for myopia control, in Proceedings of the 6th International Conference on Myopia, Springer, Tokyo 1998, p. 155

[478] Cottriall CL, Brew J, Vessey KA, McBrien NA, Diisopropylfluorophoshate alters retinal neurotransmitter levels and reduces experimentally-induced myopia, Naunyn Schmiedebergs Arch Pharmacol 2001 Oct; 364(4): 372-82

[479] Houchin B, http://www.sticklers.org/sip/def.html

[480] Snead MP, Yates JR. Clinical and molecular genetics of Stickler syndrome. J Med Genet 1999 May;36(5):353-9

[481] Traboulsi EI, et al. Ocular findings in mitral valve prolapse syndrome. Ann Ophthalmol 1987 Sep;19(9):354-7, 359

[482] Seckin U, et al. The prevalence of joint hypermobility among high school students. Rheumatol Int. 2004 Jan 24

[483] Khoo CY, Chong J, Rajan U, A 3-year study on the effect of RGP contact lenses on myopic children. Singapore Med J 1999 Apr; 40(4): 230-7

[484] Perregrin J, Perregrin D, Quintero S, Grosvenor T, Silicone acrylate contact lenses for myopia control: 3-year results, Optom Vis Sci 1990, 67, 765-769, referenced in Grosvenor T., Goss D. A., Clinical management of myopia, Butterworth-Heinemann, Boston 1999, p. 157

[485] Schelle H, Kontaktlinsen, Trias Verlag, Stuttgart, 2000

[486] Katz J, et al. A randomized trial of rigid gas permeable contact lenses to reduce progression of children's myopia. Am J Ophthalmol. 2003 Jul;136(1):82-90

[487] Andreo LK, Long-term effects of hydrophilic contact lenses on myopia. Ann Ophthalmol 1990 Jun; 22(6): 224-7, 229

[488] Fulk GW, Cyert LA, Parker DE, West RW. The effect of changing from glasses to soft contact lenses on myopia progression in adolescents. Ophthalmol Physiol Opt 2003 Jan;23(1):71-7

[489] Grosvenor T, Perrigin D, Perrigin J, Quintero S, Rigid gas-permeable contact lenses for myopia control: effects of discontinuation of lens wear. Optom Vis Sci 1991 May; 68(5): 385-389

[490] PerriginJ, Perrigin D, Quintero S, Grosvenor T, Silicone-acrylate contact lenses for myopia control: 3-year results. Optom Vis Sci 1990 Oct; 67(19): 764-9

[491] Tarutta EP, Andreeva LD, Markosian GA, Iomdina EN, Lazuk AV, Kruzhkova GV, Reinforcement of the sclera with new synthetic materials in progressive myopia, Vestn Oftalmol 1999 Sep-Oct; 115(5): 8-10

[492] Zhang J, Wu N, Retinal detachment-severe complicatio after posterior scleral reinforcement operation, Chung Hua Ko Tsa Chih 1997 May; 33(3): 210-2

[493] Li B, Lng L, Chen J, Chen L, Xu W, Gao R, Yang B, Li W, Wu B, Observation on the relation between propagated sensation along meridians and the therapeutic effect of acupuncture on myopia of youngsters, Zhen Ci Yan Jiu 1993; 18(2): 154-8

[494] Liu H, Lu Y, Dong Q, Zhong X, Treatment of adolescent myopia by pressure plaster of semen implantis on otoacupoints, J Tradit Chin Med 1994 Dec; 14(4): 283-6

[495] Tsikova TD, Laser puncture in the combined treatment of a weak degree of myopia in schoolchildren, Oftalmol Zh 1990; (1): 39-42

[496] Gray B. Homeopathy science of myth? North Atlantic Books, Berkeley 2000

[497] Okovitov VV. Transconjunctival electrostimulation of eye in pathogenic therapy of progressive myopia. Vestn Oftalmol 1997 Sep-Oct;113(5):24-6

6 REFERENCES

[498] Grosvenor T., Goss D. A., Clinical management of myopia, Butterworth-Heinemann, Boston 1999, p. 163

[499] Hom MM, Manual of contact lens prescribing and fitting, Butterworth-Heinemann, 1997, p. 381

[500] Young AL et al. Orthokeratology lens–related corneal ulcers in children. Ophthalmology. 2004;111:590-595

[501] Alharbi A, Swarbrick HA. The effects of overnight orthokeratology lens wear on corneal thickness. Invest Ophthalmol Vis Sci. 2003 Jun;44(6):2518-23

[502] Grosvenor T., Goss D. A., Clinical management of myopia, Butterworth-Heinemann, Boston 1999, p. 181

[503] Lam DSC, Poon ASY, Leal JV, In search of excellence: From radial keratotomy to laser-assisted in situ keratomileusis, in Proceedings of the 6th International Conference on Myopia, Springer, Tokyo 1998, p. 163

[504] Grosvenor T., Goss D. A., Clinical management of myopia, Butterworth-Heinemann, Boston 1999, p. 187

[505] Ditzen K, Huschka H, Laser in situ keratomileusis (LASIK) for myopia, in Proceedings of the 6th International Conference on Myopia, Springer, Tokyo 1998, p. 169

[506] Report on vision research trends from ARVO 2001, http://optistock.com/spotlight8.htm

[507] Machet JJ, LASIK overview: the good, the bad, and the ugly. Ocular Surg News 1997a, (Suppl): 38-39, referenced in Grosvenor T., Goss D. A., Clinical management of myopia, Butterworth-Heinemann, Boston 1999, p. 199

[508] Grosvenor T., Goss D. A., Clinical management of myopia, Butterworth-Heinemann, Boston 1999, p. 200

[509] Xie RZ, Stretton S, Sweeney DF. Artificial Cornea: Towards a synthetic onlay for correction of refractive error. Biosci Rep. 2001 Aug;21(4):513-36

[510] Grosvenor T., Goss D. A., Clinical management of myopia, Butterworth-Heinemann, Boston 1999, p. 207

[511] Jiminez-Alfaro I, Benitez del Castillo JM, Garcia-Feijoo J, Gil de Bernabe JG, Serrano de La Iglesia JM, Safety of posterior chamber phakic intraocular lenses for the correction of high myopia: anterior segment changes after posterior chamber intraocular lens implantation, Ophthalmology 2001 Jan; 108(1): 90-9

[512] "Myopic Haste", Forbes Magazine, May 6, 1985, referenced in Grosvenor T., Goss D. A., Clinical management of myopia, Butterworth-Heinemann, Boston 1999, p. 207

[513] Dick HB, et al. Refractive lens exchange with an array multifocal intraocular lens. J Refract Surg 2002 Sep-Oct;18(5):509-18

[514] Biedenkopf A, Auffahrt GU, Becker KA, Martin M, Voelcker HE, Multifocale Intraocularlinsen in der refraktiven Chirurgie, Klin Monatsbl Augenheilkd 2002: IV. Wissenschaftliche Sitzung Multifocale Intraocularlinsen, 44P

[515] Implantable contact lens effective for myopics, Reuters Medical News, Nov 13, 2001

[516] Sanders DR, et al. U.S. Food and Drug Administration clinical trial of the Implantable Contact Lens for moderate to high myopia. Ophthalmology 2003 Feb;110(2):255-266

[517] Sanders DR. Actual and theoretical risks for visual loss following use of the implantable contact lens for moderate to high myopia. J Cataract Refract Surg 2003 Jul;29(7):1323-32

[518] Lleo Perez A, et al. [Comparative clinical study of visual results between two different types of bifocal intraocular lenses. Arch Soc Esp Oftalmol. 2003 Dec;78(12)665-74

[519] http://www.optometry.co.uk/articles/20010504/lavin.pdf

[520] Celorio JM, PruettRC. Prevalence of lattice degeneration and its relation to axial length in severe myopia. Am J Ophthalmol. 1991 Jan 15;111(1):20-3

[521] Modern nutrition in health and disease, editors Shils ME, Olson JA, Shike M, Ross AC, Lippincott Williams & Wilkins, 1998, p. 1003

[522] Ames BN, Elson-Schwab H, Silver E, High-dose vitamin therapy stimulates variant enzymes with decreased coenzyme binding affinity: relevance to genetic disease and polymorphismus. Am J Clin Nutr 2002; 75:616-58

[523] Rosenberg LE, Vitamin-responsive inherited metabolic disorders. Adv Hum Genet 1976; 6:1-74

[524] Tischendorf, Meyer, Spraul, Auge und innere Medizin. Schattauer, 2004

[525] Price WA, Nutrition and physical degeneration, Keats Publishing Inc., New Canaan, 1997

[526] Couzy F, Aubree E, Magliola C, Mareschi JP, Average mineral and trace element content in daily adjusted menus of French adults. J Trace Elem Electrlytes Health Dis 1988; 2:79-83

[527] Dart AM, Qi XL. Determinants of arterial stiffness in Chinese migrants to Australia. Atheriosclerosis 1995 Oct;117(2):263-72

[528] Bergner P, The healing power of minerals, special nutrients and trace elements. Prima Publishing, 1997

[529] Eaton SB, Eaton SB III, Konner MJ, Paleolithic nutrition revisited: a twelve-year retrospective on its nature and implications. Eur J Clin Nutr 1997 Apr;51(4):207-16

[530] Eckhardt RB. Genetic research and nutritional individuality. J Nutr 2001 Feb;131(2):336S-9S

[531] Bland JS, Genetic Nutritioneering, Keats Publishing, Los Angeles 1999

[532] Bland J, ediotor, Medical applications of clinical nutrition, Keats Publishing, referenced in Chaitow L, Thorsons guide to amino acids, Thorsons, 1991, p. 48

[533] Independent.co.uk, Connor S., Glaxo chief: Our drugs do not work on most patients. http://news.independent.co.uk/world/science_medical/storyjsp?story=471139

[534] Biesalski HK et al., Ernaehrungsmedizin, Georg Thieme Verlag Stuttgart New York 1999, p. 88

[535] Modern nutrition in health and disease, editors Shils ME, Olson JA, Shike M, Ross AC, Lippincott Williams & Wilkins, 1998, p. 441

[536] Berg RA, Kerr JS, Nutritional aspects of collagen metabolism. Annu Rev Nutr 1992; 12:369-90

[537] Junqueira LC, Carneiro J, Kelley RO, Basic histology, Appleton & Lange, Stamford, 1998

[538] University of Florida PA Program, Organization of human tissues, http://www.medinfo.ufl.edu/pa/chuck/summer/handouts/connect.htm

[539] Connective Tissue Disorder Site: http://www.ctds.info/index.html

[540] Volk E, Connective tissue. http://www.mesomirphosis.com/exclusive/volk/connective01-print.htm

[541] Shingleton WD, Hodges DJ, Brick P, Cawsto TE, Collagenase: a key enzyme in collagen turnover. Biochem Cell Biol 1996;74(6):759-75

[542] Cimpean A, Caloianu M, Matrix metalloproteinases with role in collagen biodegradation. Romanian J Biol Sci 1997; 1-2:1-14

[543] Rehnberg M, Ammitzboll T, Tengroth B, Collagen distribution in the lamina cribrosa and the trabecular meshwork of the human eye. Br J Ophthamol 1987 Dec;71(12):886-92

[544] Moses RA, et al., Elastin content of the scleral spur, trabecular mesh, and sclera. Invest Ophthalmol Vis Sci 1978;17(8):817-8

[545] University of Florida PA Program, Introduction to medicine I, Immunity basics, http://www.medinfo.ufl.edu/pa/chuck/fall/handouts/immune1.htm

[546] Janeway CA, Travers P, Immunologie, Sprektrum akademischer Verlag, 1997

[547] Bramley AM, Roberts CR, Schellenberg RR, Collagenase increases shortening of human bronchial smooth muscle in vitro. Am J Respir Care Med 1995 Nov;152(5 Pt 1):1513-7

[548] Roche Lexikon Medizin, Urban & Schwarzenberg, 1998, p. 757

[549] Wojtecka-lukasik E, Maslinski S, Histamine, 5-hydroxytryptamine and compound 48/80 activate PMN-leucocyte collagenase of the rat. Agents Actions 1984 Apr;14(3-4):451-3

[550] Wojtecka-lukasik E, Maslinski S, Is histamine involved in ethanol-induced inflammation? Agents Actiona 1988 Apr;23(3-4):321-3

[551] Takeda T, et al., Effect of histamine on human fibroblast in vitro. Arzneimittelforschung 1997 Oct;47(19):1152-5

[552] Lane IW, Baxter S, Immune power, Avery Publishing Group, 1999, p. 87

[553] Stralin P, Marklund SL. Multiple cytokines regulate the expression of extracellular superoxide dismutase in human vascular smooth muscle cells. Atheriosclerosis 2000 Aug;151(2):433-41

6 REFERENCES

[554] Spellberg B, Edwards JE, Type1/Type 2 immunity in infectious diseases. Clin Infect Dis 2001 Jan; 32(1): 76-102

[555] Sprietsma JE, Modern diets and diseases: NO-zinc balance. Med Hypotheses 1999; 53(1):6-16

[556] Greene LS, Asthma, oxidant stress, and diet. Nutrition 1999 Nov-Dec;15(11-12):899-907

[557] Sueddeutsche Zeitung Online – Gesundheit, Impfprogramme unter Beschuss, 23. Jan 2001

[558] Marshall GD, Agarwal SK, Stress, immune regulation, and immunity: applications for asthma. Allergy Asthma Proc 2000 Jul-Aug;21(4):241-6

[559] Maestroni GJ, The immunotherapeutic potential of melatonin. Expert Opin Investig Drugs 2001 Mar; 10(3): 467-76

[560] Panajotova V, The effect of dopaminergic agents on cell-mediated immune response in mice. Physiol Res 1997;46(2):113-8

[561] Gottwald T, et al., The mast cell-nerve axis in wound healing: a hypothesis. Wound Repair and Regeneration 1998 Jan-Feb;6(1):8-19

[562] Basu S, Dasgupta PS, Dopamine, a neurotransmitter, influences the immune system. J Neuroimmunol 2000 Jan;102(2):113-24

[563] Dringenberg HC, De Souza-Silva MA, Schwarting RK, Huston JP, Increased levels of extracellular dopamine in neostriatum and nucleus accumbens after histamine H1 receptor blockade. Naunyn Schmiedebergs Arch Pharmacol 1998Oct;358(4):423-9

[564] Esch T, Stefano G, Fricchione G, Benson H, Stress-related diseases – a potential role for nitric oxide. Med Sci Monit 2002 Jun;8(6):RA103-18

[565] Quan N, Avitsur R, Stark JL, He L, Shah M, Caliguri M, Padgett DA, Marucha PT, Sheridan JF, Social stress increases the susceptibility to endotoxic shock. J Neuroimmunol 2001 Apr 2;115(1-2):36-45

[566] Kalandarov S, Frenkel' ID, Nekrasova LI, Human histamine and serotonin levels during neuro-emotional stress. Kosm Biol Aviakosm Med 1980 Nov-Dec;14(6):29-32

[567] Fuck LM, Die Auswirkung von Examansstress auf den immunologischen Verlauf einer experimentellen gingivitis. http://www.ulb.uni-duesseldorf.de/diss/med/2001/fuck.html

[568] Van Amsterdam JGC, Opperhuizen A, Nitric oxide and biopterin in depression and stress. Psychiatry Research 1999, 85:33-38

[569] Madrigal JL, et al. The increase in TNF-alpha levels is implicated in NF-kappaS activation and inducible oxide synthase expression in brain cortex after immobilization stress. Neuropsychopharmacology 2002 Feb;26(2):155-63

[570] Oishi K, et al., Oxidative stress and haematological changes in immobilized rats. Acta Physiol Scand 1999;165:65-69

[571] Work pressures help strengthe the immune system, gory videos do the opposite, Ohio State Research10/28/01, http://www.acs.ohio-state.edu/researchnews/archive/acustrs.htm

[572] Poon AMS, Liu ZM, Pang SF, Cross-talk between the pineal gland and the immune system. Chinese Medical Journal 1998; 111(1):7-11

[573] Pierpaoli W, Regelson W, Colman C, Melatonin miracle, Simon & Schuster, 1995

[574] Liaw SJ, et al., Beneficial role of melatonin on microcirculation in endotoxin-induced gastropathy in rats: possible implication in nitrogen oxide reduction. J Formos Med Assoc 2002 Feb;101(2):129-35

[575] Balch JF, The Super Antioxidants, M. Evans and Company, 1998

[576] Henrotin YE, Bruckner P, Pujol JP. The role of reactive oxygen species in homeostasis and degradation of cartilage. Osteoarthritis Cartilage. 2003 Oct;11(10):747-55

[577] Thomas SR, Chen K, Keaney JF Jr. Oxidative stress and endothelial nitric oxide bioactivity. Antioxid Redox Signal. 2003 Apr;5(2):181-94

[578] Junqueira LC, Carneiro J, Kelley RO, Basic histology, Appleton & Lange, Stamford, 1998, p. 119

[579] Weber CE, Copper response to rheumatoid arthritis. Med Hypotheses 1984;15:333-348

[580] Oxlund H, Sims T, Light ND, Changes in mechanical properties, thermal stability, reducible cross-links and glycosyl-lysines in rat skin induced by corticosteroid treatment. Acta Endocrinol (Copenh) 1982 Oct;101(2):312-20

[581] Siegel RC, Collagen cross-linking. Synthesis of collagen cross-links in vitro with highly purified lysyl oxidase. J Biol Chem 1976 Sep 25;251(18):5786-92

[582] Jarvelainen H, et al. Effect of cortisol on the proliferation and protein synthesis of human aortic smooth muscle cells in culture. Acta Med Scand Suppl 1982;660:114-22

[583] Lovallo WR, Stress & health, Sage Publications, 1997

[584] Modern nutrition in health and disease, editors Shils ME, Olson JA, Shike M, Ross AC, Lippincott Williams & Wilkins, 1998, p. 245

[585] Apresto E, Nitric oxide. http://www.science.mcmaster.ca/Biology/4S03/NO.html

[586] Wu G, Meininger CJ. Regulation of nitric oxide synthesis by dietary factors. Annu Rev Nutr 2002;22:61-86

[587] Chaitow L, Thorsons guide to amino acids, Thorsons, 1991

[588] Riedel W. Role of nitric oxide in the control of the hypothalamic-pituitary-adrenocortical axis. Z Rheumatol 59(suppl 2):II/36-II/42

[589] Nakamura M, et al. Glutathione reverses endothelial damage from peroxynitrite, the byproduct of nitric oxide degradation, in crystalloid cardioplegia. Circulation 2000 Nov 7;102(19 Suppl 3):III332-8

[590] Sies H, Arteel GE. Interaction of peroxynitrite with selenoproteins and glutathione peroxidase mimics. Free Radic Biol Med 2000 May 15;28(19):1451-5

[591] Chow CK, Hong CB. Dietary vitamin E and selenium and toxicity of nitrite and nitrate. Toxicology. 2002 Nov 15;180(2):195-207

[592] Aldini G, et al. Procyanidins from grape seeds protect endothelial cells from peroxynitrite damage and enhance endothelium-dependent relaxation in human artery: new evidences for cardioprotection. Life Sci. 2003 Oct 17;73(22):2883-98

[593] Brophy CM. Stress and vascular disease at the cellular and molecular levels. World J Surg 2002 Jul;26(7):779-82

[594] Prast H, et al., Nitric oxide influences the release of histamine and glutamate in the rat hypothalamus. Naunyn Schmiedebergs Arch Pharmacol 1996 Dec;354(6):731-5

[595] Coleman JW, Nitric oxide: a regulator of mast cell activation and mast cell mediated inflammation. Clin Exp Immunol 2002 Jul;129(1):4-10

[596] Bogdan C, Nitric oxide and the immune response. Nat Immunol 2001 Oct;2(10):907-16

[597] Coleman JW. Nitric oxide in imunity and inflammation. Int Immunopharmacol 2001 Aug;1(8):1397-408

[598] Lopez_figueroa MO, Day HE, Akil H, Watson SJ. Histol Histopathol 1998 Oct;13(4):1243-52

[599] Stefano GB, et al., Morphine- and anandamide-stimulated nitric oxide production inhibits presynaptic dopamine release. Brain Res 1997 Jul 18;763(1):63-8

[600] Grammatikopoulos G, et al., Inhibition of neural nitric oxide synthesis by 7-nitroindazole reduces hyperactivity and increases non-selective attention in the naples high excitability rat moedl of Adhd: an evidence in favour of an hyperfunctioning dopamine system. INABIS 2000, 6th Internet World Congress for Biomedical Sciences, presentation # 112

[601] Berendji D, et al., Nitric oxide mediates intracytoplasmic and intranuclear zinc release. FEBS Lett 1997 Mar 17;405(1):37-41

[602] Yamaoka J, et al., Suppressive effect of zinc ion on iNOS expression induced by interferon-gamma or tumor necrosis factor-alpha in murine keratinocytes. J Dermatol Sci 2000 May;23(1):27-35

[603] Blute TA, Lee MR, Eldred WD, Direct imaging of NMDA-stimulated nitric oxide production in the retina. Vis Neurosci 2000 Jul-Aug; 17(4): 557-66

6 REFERENCES

[604] Riedel W. Temperature homeostasis and redox homeostasis. Paper in Kosaka M et al. (eds.), Thermotherapy for neoplasia, inflammation, and pain. Springer-Verlag Tokyo 2001

[605] Schmid HA, Riedel W, Simon E. Role of nitric oxide in temperature regulation. Prog Brain Res 1998;115:87-110

[606] Miles D, et al. Association between biosynthesis of nitric oxide and changes in immunological and vascular parameters in patients treated with interleukin-2. Eur J Clin Invest. 1994 Apr;24(4):287-90

[607] Blantz RC, Munger K. Role of nitric oxide in inflammatory conditions. Nephron 2002 Apr;90(4):373-8

[608] Drexler H, Hornig B. Endothelial dysfunction in human disease. J Mol Cell Cardiol. 1999 Jan;31(1):51-60

[609] Komatsu S, et al. Dietary vitamin B6 suppresses colon tumorgenesis, 8-hydroxyguanosine, 4-hydroxynonenal, and inducible nitric oxide synthase protein in azoxymethane-treated mice. J Nutr Sci Vitaminol (Tokyo) 2002 Feb;48(1):65-8

[610] Prabhu KS, et al. Selenium deficiency increases the expression of inducible nitric oxide synthase in RAW 264.7 macrophages: role of nuclear factor-kappaB in up-regulation. Biochem J 2002 Aug 15;366(Pt 1):203-9

[611] Southan GJ, Salzman AL, Szabo C. Potent inhibition of the inducible isoform of nitric oxide synthase by aminoethylisoselenourea and related compounds. Life Sci 1996;58(14):1139-48

[612] Morihara N, et al. Aged garlic extract enhances production of niric oxide. Life Sci 2002 Jun 21;71(5):509-17

[613] Mazzio E, et al. Characterization of neurotransmitters and dopamine attenuation of inducible nitric oxide synthase in glioma cells. J Neuroimmunol 2002 Oct;131(1-2):70-82

[614] Mershon JL, et al. Estrogen increases iNOS expression in the ovine coronary artery. Am J Physiol Heart Circ Physiol 2002 Sep;283(3):H1169-80 c718

[615] Mathew SJ, Coplan JD, Gorman JM, Neurobiological mechanisms of social anxiety disorder. Am J Psychiatry 2001 Oct; 158(10):1558-1567

[616] Madras B, et al., Brain Imaging of the dopamine transporter in ADHD. INABIS 2000, 6th Internet World Congress for Biomedical Sciences, presentation # 113

[617] Papageorgiou, et al., Association of serum nitric oxide levels with depressive symptoms: a study with endstage renal failure patients. Psychother Psychosom 2001 Jul-Aug;70(4):216-20

[618] Pani L, Porcella A, Gessa, The role of stress in the pathophysiology of the dopaminergic system. Molecular Psychiatry 2000: 5:14-21

[619] Ghiadoni L, et al. Mental stress induces transient endothelial dysfunction in humans. Circulation. 2000 Nov 14;102(29):2473-8

[620] Frankel P, The methylation miracle, St. Martin's Paperbacks, 1999, p. 49

[621] Krajcovicova-Kudlackova M, et al. Homocysteine and vitamin C. Bratisl Lek Listy 2002;103(4-5):171-3

[622] Frankel P, The methylation miracle, St. Martin's Paperbacks, 1999, p. 104

[623] McCully KS, McCully M, The heart revolution, Perennial, 1999

[624] Frankel P, The methylation miracle, St. Martin's Paperbacks, 1999

[625] Brown JC, Strain JJ, Effect of dietary homocysteine on copper status in rats. J Nutr 1990 Sep;120(9):1068-74

[626] Schlussel E, Preibisch G, Putter S, Elstner EF, Homocysteine-induced oxidative damage: mechanisms and possible roles in neurogegenerative and atherogenic processes. Z Naturforsch [C] 1995 Sep;50(9-10):699-707

[627] Cortelezzi A, et al. Hyperhomocysteinemia in myelodysplasic syndromes: specific association with autoimmunity and cardiovascular disease. Leuk Lymphoma 2001 Mar;41(1-2):147-50

[628] McCully KS, McCully M, The heart revolution, Perennial, 1999, p. 185

[629] Lubec B, Evidence for McKusnick's hypothesis of deficient collagen cross-linking in patients with homocysteinuria. Biochim Biophys Acta 1996 Apr 12;1315(3):159-62

[630] Liu G, Nellaiappan K, Kagan HM, Irreversible inhibition of lysyl oxidase by homocysteine thialactone and its selenium and oxygen analogues. J Biol Chem 1997 Dec 19; 272(51):32370-32377

[631] Griffiths R, Tudball N, Thomas J, Efect of induced elevated plasma levels of homocysteine and methionine in rats on collagenand elastin structures. Connect Tissue Res 1976;4(2):101-6

[632] Krumdieck CL, Prince CW, Mechanisms of homocysteine toxicity on connective tissues: implications for the morbidity of aging. J Nutr 2000 Feb;130(2S Suppl):365S-368S

[633] Holven KB, et al., Effect of folic acid treatment on endothelium-dependent vasodilation and nitric oxide-derived and products in hyperhomocysteinemic subjects. Am J Med 2001 May;110(7):536-42

[634] Weiss N, et al., Overexpression of cellular glutathione peroxidase rescues homocysteine-induced endothelial dysfunction. Proc Natl Acad Sci USA 2001 Oct 23;98(22):12503-8

[635] Fu WY, et al., Homocysteine attenuates hemodynamic responses to nitric oxide in vivo. Atheriosclerosis 2002 Mar;161(1):169-76

[636] Bottiglieri T, Laundy M, Crellin R, Toone BK, Carney MWP, Reynolds EH, Homocysteine, folate, methylation, and monoamine metabolism in depression. J Neurol Neurosurg Psychiatry 2000 Aug;69:228-232

[637] Reiter R, Robinson J, Melatonin, Bantam Books, 1995

[638] Reiter RJ, Maestroni GJ, Melatonin in relation to the antioxidative defense and immune systems: possible implications for cell and organ transplantation. J Mol Med 1999 Jan;77(1):36-9

[639] Cutolo M, et al., Melatonin influences interleukin-12 and nitric oxide production by primary cultures of rheumatoid synovial macrophages and THP-1 cells. Ann N Y Acad Sci 1999 Jun 22;876:246-54

[640] Mocchegiani E, Bulian D, Santarelli L, Tibaldi A, Muzzioli M, Pierpaoli W, Fabris N, The immuno-reconstituting effect of melatonin or pineal grafting and its relation to zinc pool in aging mice. J Neuroimmunol 1994 Sep;53(2):189-201

[641] Roth JA, Kim BG, Lin WL, Cho MI, Melatonin promotes oseoblast differentiation and bone formation. J Biol Chem Jul 30;274(31):22041-7

[642] Nakade O, Koyama H, Ariji H, Yajima A, Kaku T, Melatonin stimulates proliferation and type I collagen synthesis in human bone cells in vitro. J Pineal Res 1999 Sep;27(2):106-10

[643] Bubenik GA, et al., Prospects of the clinical utilization of melatonin. Biol Signals Recept 1998 Jul-Aug;7(4):195-219

[644] Iacovitti L, Stull ND, Johnston K, Malatonin rescues dopamine neurons from cell death in tissue culture models of oxidative stress. Brain Res 1997 Sep 12;768(1-2):317-326

[645] Saenz DA, Physiological concentrations of melatonin inhibit the nitrideric pathway in the Syrian hamster retina. J Pineal Res 2002 Aug;33(1):31-6

[646] Uludag O, et al. Temporal variation in serum nitrite levels in rats and mice. Chronobiol Int 1999 Jul;16(4):527-32

[647] Gryz EA, et al., Etiopathogenesis of diabetic neuropathy. Przegl Lek 2000;57(12):727-31

[648] Duckworth WC, Hyperglycemia and cardiovasular disease. Curr Atheroscler Rep 2001 Sep;3(5):383-91

[649] Yamada S, Ohkubo C, The influence of frequent and excessive intake of glucose on microvascular aging in healthy mice. Microcirculation 1999 Mar;6(1):55-62

[650] Spanheimer RG, Inhibition of collagen productin by diabetic rat serum: response to insulin and insulin-like growth factor-I added in vitro. Endocrinology 1991 Dec;129(6):3018-26

[651] Lien YH, Stern R, Fu JC, Siegel RC. Inhibition of collagen formation in vitro and subsequent cross-linking by glucose. Science 1984 Sep 28;225(4669):1489-91

[652] Maritim AC, et al. Diabetes, oxidative stress, and antioxidants: a review. J Biochem Mol Toxicol. 2003;17(1):24-38

[653] Catherwood MA, et al., Glucose-induced oxidative stress in mesangial cells. Kidney Int 2002 Feb;61(2):599-608

[654] Manuel y Keenoy B, et at., Divergent effects of different oxidants on glutathione homeostasis and protein damage in erythrocytes from diabetic patients: effects of high glucose. Mol Cell Biochem 2001 Sep;225(1-):59-73

[655] Koska J, et al., Insulin, catecholamines, glucose and antioxidant enzymes in oxidative damage during different loads in healthy humans, Physiol Res 2000;49 Suppl 1:S95-100

6 REFERENCES

[656] Powell LA, et al., Restoration of glutathione levels in vascular smooth muscle cells exposed to high glucose conditions. Free Radic Biol Med 2001 Nov 15;31(10):1149-55

[657] Faure PF, et al., Vitamin E improves the free radical defense system potential and insulin sensitivity of rats fed high fructose diets. http://www.faseb.org/asns/journal/tocs/jnjan97.html

[658] Koska J, et al., Insulin, catecholamines, glucose and antioxidant enzymes in oxidative damage during different loads in healthy humans. Physiol Res 2000;49 Suppl 1:S95-100

[659] Kersten JR, et al., Hyperglycemia reduces coronary collateral blood flow through a nitric oxide-mediated mechanism. Am J Physiol Heart Circ Physiol 2001 Nov;281(5):H2097-104

[660] Ishii N, et al., Nitric oxide synthesis and oxidative stress in the renal cortex of rats with diabetes mellitus. J Am Soc Nephrol 2001 Aug;12(8):1630-9

[661] Lash JM, et al., Acute hyperglycemia depresses arteriolar NO formation in skeletal muscle. Am J Physiol 1999 Oct;277(4Pt2):H1513-20

[662] Federici M, et al., Insulin-dependent activation of endothelial nitric oxide synthase is impaired by O-linked glycosylation modification of signaling proteins in human coronary endothelial cells. Circulation 2002 Jul 23;106(4):466-72

[663] Booth G, et al., Elevated ambient glucose induces acute inflammatory events in the microvasulature:efects of insulin. Am J Physiol Endocrinol Metab 2001 Jun;280(6):E848-56

[664] Gleeson M, Bishop NC, Special feature for the Olympics: effects of exercise on the immune system: modification of immune responses to exercise by carbohydrate, glutamine and anti-oxidant supplements. Immunol Cell Biol 2000 Oct; 78(5):554-61

[665] Nieman DC, Nutrition, exercise, and immune system function. Clin Sports Med 1999 Jul; 18(3):537-48

[666] Figlewicz DP, Endocrine regulation of neurotransmitter transporters. Epilepsy Res 1999 Dec;37(3):203-10

[667] Schaffer MR, et al., Diabetes-impaired healing and reduced wound nitric oxide synthesis: a posible pathophysiologic correlation. Surgery 1997 May;121(5):513-9

[668] Bailey AJ, et al., Chemistry of collagen cross-links:glucose-mediated covalent cross-linking of type-IV collagen in lens capsules. Biochem J 1993 Dec 1;296 (Pt 2):489-96

[669] Zhang Z, et al., High glucose inhibits glucose-6-phosphate dehydrogenase via cAMP in aortic endothelial cells. J Biol Chem 2000 Dec 22;275(51):40042-7

[670] Gaskin RS, et al., G6PD deficiency:irs role in the high prevalence of hypertension and diabetes mellitus. Ethn Dis 2001 Fall;11(4):749-54

[671] Price KD, et al., Hyperglycemia-induced ascorbic acid deficiency promotes endothelial dysfunction and the development of atheriosclerosis. Atheriosclerosis 2001 Sep;158(1):1-12

[672] Fisher E et al., Interaction of ascorbic acid and glucose on production of collagen and proteoglycan by fibroblasts. Diabetes 1991 Mar;40(3):371-6

[673] Modern nutrition in health and disease, editors Shils ME, Olson JA, Shike M, Ross AC, Lippincott Williams & Wilkins, 1998, p. 243

[674] Kenney MA, McCoy JH, Magnesium deficiency in the rat: effects of fructose, boron and copper. Magnes res 2000 Mar;13(1):19-27

[675] McCarty MF, Insulin secretion as a potential determinant of homocysteine levels. Med Hypotheses 2000 Nov;55(5):454-5

[676] Chipkin SR, et al., Exercise and diabetes. Cardiol Clin 2001 Aug;19(3):489-505

[677] Smorawinski J, et al., Comparison of changes in glucose tolerance and insulin secretion induced by three-day bed rest in sedentary subjects and endurance or strength trained athletes. J Gravit Physiol 1998 Jul;5(1):P103-4

[678] Valero G, et al., High prevalence of stress hyperglycemia in children with febrile seizures and traumatic injuries. Acta Paediatr 2001 Jun;90(6):618-22

[679] Thibault L, Roberge AG, Dietary protein and carbohydrate effects on blood parameters related to stress in cat. Physiol Behav 1988;42(1):1-5

[680] http://www.cspinet.org/new/sugar_limit.html

[681] Zhou MS, et al. Potassium augments vascular relaxation mediated by nitric oxide in the carotid arteries of hypertensive Dahl rats. Am J Hypertens. 2000 Jun;13(6 Pt 1):666-72

[682] Sofola OA, et al. Change in endothelial function in mesenteric arteries of Sprague-Dawley rats fed a high salt diet. J Physiol. 2002 Aug 15;543(Pt 1):255-60

[683] Bayorh MA, et al. The role of oxidative stress in salt-induced hypertension. Am J Hypertens. 2004 Jan;17(1):31-6

[684] Houben AJ, et al., Microvascular effects of atrial natriuretic peptide (ANP) in man: studies during high and low salt diet. Cardiovasc Res 1998 Aug;39(2):442-50

[685] Lenda DM, Boegehold MA, Effect of a high salt diet on microvascular antioxidant enzymes. J Vasc Res 2002 Jan-Feb;39(1):41-50

[686] Frisbee JC, Lombard JH, Development and reversibility of altered skeletal muscle arteriolar structure and reactivity with high salt diet and reduced renal mass hypertension. Microcirculation 1999 Sep;6(3):215-25

[687] Ogihara T, et al., High-salt diet enhances insulin signaling and induces insulin resistance in Dahl salt-sensitive rats. Hypertension 2002 Jul;40(1):83-9

[688] McCarty MF, Up-regulation of endothelial nitric oxide activity as a central strategy for prevention of ischemic stroke – Just say NO to stroke! Med Hypotheses 2000 Nov;55(5):386-403

[689] http://www.sacn.gov.uk/salt-health-draft-rep-sacn.pdf Scientific Advisory Committee on Nutrition: Salt and Health

[690] Fenster BE, Tsao PS, Rockson SG. Endothelial dysfunction: clinical strategies for treating oxidant stress. Am Heart J. 2003 Aug;146(2):218-26

[691] Kuiper JI, et al. Physical workload of student nurses and serum markers of collagen metabolism. Scand J Work Environ Health 2002 Jun;28(3):168-75

[692] Sen CK, Antioxidants in exercise nutrition. Sports Med 2001;31(13):891-908

[693] Ho HY, et al. Enhanced oxidative stress and accelerated cellular senescence in glucose-6-phosphate dehydrogenase (G6PD)-deficient human fibroblasts. Free Radic Biol Med 2000 Jul 15;29(2):156-69

[694] Leopold JA, et al. Glucose-6-phosphate dehydrogenase deficiency promotes endothelial oxidant stress and decreases endothelial nitric oxide bioavailability. FASEB J 2001 Aug;15(10):1771-3

[695] Cheng ML, Ho HY, Liang CM, Chou YH, Stern A, Lu FJ, Chiu DT, Cellular glucose-6-phosphate dehydrogenase (G6PD) status modulates the effects of nitric oxide (NO) on human fibroblasts. FEBS Lett 2000 Jun 23;475(3):257-62

[696] Garcia-Nogales P, et al. Peroxinitrite protects neurons against nitric-oxide-mediated apoptosis: A key role for glucose-6-phsophate dehydrogenase activity in neuroprotection. J Biol Chem 2002 Oct 31;

[697] Garcia-Nogales P, et al. Induction of glucose-6-phosphate dehydrogenase by lipopolysaccharide contributes to preventing nitric oxide –mediated glutathione depletion in cultured rat astrocytes. J Neurochem 1999 Apr;72(4):1750-8

[698] Leopold JA, Cao A, Scribner AW, Stanton RC, Loscalzo J, Glucose-6-phosphate dehydrogenase deficiency promotes endothelial oxidant stress and decreases endothelial nitric oxide bioavailability. FASEB J 2001 Aug;15(10):1771-3

[699] Hussein L, Arafah A, Yamamah G, The vitamin B1 status among young Egyptians from the oasis in relation to glucose-6 phosphate dehydrogenase deficiency. Int J Vitamin res 1989;59(1):52-54

[700] Taniguchi M, Hara T, Effects of riboflavin and selenium deficiencies on glutathione and its relating enzyme activities with respect to lipid peroxide content of rat livers. J Nutr Sci Vitaminol (Tokyo) 1983 Jun;29(3):283-92

[701] Anderson BB; et al., Glutathione reductase activity and its relationship to pyridoxine phosphate activity in G6PD deficiency. Eur J Haematol 1987 Jan;38(1):12-20

6 REFERENCES

[702] Dutta P, et al., Acute ethanol exposure alters hepatic glutathione metaboislm in riboflavin deficiency. Alcohol 1995 Jan-Feb;12(1):43-7

[703] Dodds RA, et al., Abnormalities in fracture healing induced by vitamin B6-deficiency in rats. Bone 1986;7(6):489-495

[704] Ribaya JD, Gershoff SN, Interrelationships in rats among dietary vitamin B6, glycine and hydroxyproline. Effects of oxalate, glyoxylate, and glycine on liver enzymes. J Nutr 1979 Jan;109(1):171-183

[705] Dodds RA, et al., Putrescine may be a natural stimulator of glucose-6-phosphate dehydrogenase. FEBS Lett 1986 May 26;201(1):105-8

[706] Hunter JE, Harper AE, Stability of some pyridoxal phosphate-dependent enzymes in vitamin B-6 deficient rats. J Nutr 1976 May;106(5):653-64

[707] Sardar S, et al., Comparative effectiveness of vitamin D3 and dietary vitamin E on peroxidation of lipids and enzymes of the hepatic antioxidant system in Sprague-Dawley rats. Int J Vitam Res 1996;66(1):39-45

[708] Nasr LB, et al., Vitamin D3 and glucose-6-phosphate dehydrogenase in rat duodenal epithelial cells. Am J Physiol 1989 Nov;257(5 Pt 1):G760-G765

[709] Williams WJ, Beutler E, Erslev AJ, Lichtman MA, Hematology, McGraw-Hill Publishing Comp., 1990, p. 600

[710] Uche-Nwachi EO, Caxton-Martins AE, Effects of folic acid deficiency in pregnant Wistar rats on the activities of D5-3 beta hydoxysteroid dehydrogenase and glucose-6 phosphate dehydrogenase in the ovaries of their litters. Kaibogaku Zasshi 1997 Jun;72(3):195-8

[711] Karunanithy R, Saha N, Ng SE, Serum and red blood cell magnesium, copper, and zinc content in G6PD deficiency. Am J Hematol 1990;35:136-138

[712] Hafez, et al., Improved erythrocyte survival with combined vitamin E and selenium therapy in children with glucose-6-phosphate dehydrogenase deficiency and mild chronic hemolysis. J Pediatr 1986 Apr;108(4):558-61

[713] Stabile LP, et a.., Posttranscriptional regulation of glucose-6-phosphate dehydrogenase by dietary polyunsaturated fat. Arch Biochem Biophys 1996 Aug 15;332(2):269-279

[714] Wold LE, et al. Isolated ventricular myocytes from copper-deficient hearts exhibit enhanced contractile function. Am J Physiol Heart Circ Physiol 2001 Aug;281(2):H476-81

[715] Vadlamudi RK, et al. Copper deficiency alters collagen types and covalent crosslinking in swine myocardium and cardiac valves. Am J Physiol 1993 Jun;264(Pt2):H2154-61

[716] Medeiros DM, et al. Myofibrillar, mitochondrial and valvular morphological alterations in cardiac hypertrophy among copper-deficient rats. J Nutr 1991 Jun;121(6):815-24

[717] Saari JT, Schuschke DA. Cardiovascular effects of dietary copper deficiency. Biofactors 1999;10(4):359-75

[718] Shiry LJ, et al. Heart murmurs, valvular regurgitation and electrical disturbances in copper-deficient genetically hypertensive, hypertropic cardiomyopathic rats. J Am Coll Nutr 1999 Feb;18(1):51-60

[719] Heller LJ, et al. Decreased passive stiffness of cardiac myocytes and cardiac tissue from copper-deficient rat hearts. Am J Physiol Heart Circ Physiol 2000 Jun;278(6):H1840-7

[720] Wildman RE, et al. Marginal copper-restricted diets produce altered cardiac ultrastructure in the rat. Proc Soc Exp Biol Med 1995 Oct;210(1):43-9

[721] Lewis CG, et al. Effect of coenzyme Q10 supplementation on cardiac hypertrophy of male rats consuming a high-fructose, low-copper diet. Biol Trace Elem Res 1993 May-Jun;37(2-3):137-49

[722] Kremer JM, Bigaouette J. Nutrient intake of patients with rheumatoid arthritis is deficient in pyridoxine, zinc, copper, and magnesium. J Rheumatol 1996 Jun;23(6):990-4

[723] Deluca HF, Cantorna MT. Vitamin D: its role and uses in immunology. FASEB J 2001 Dec;15(14):2579-85

[724] Modern nutrition in health and disease, editors Shils ME, Olson JA, Shike M, Ross AC, Lippincott Williams & Wilkins, 1998

[725] Elmadfa I, Leitzmann C, Ernaehrung des Menschen, Verlag Eugen Ulmer Stuttgart, 1990

[726] Biesalski HK et al., Ernaehrungsmedizin, Georg Thieme Verlag Stuttgart New York 1999, p. 320

[727] Rao CN, Rao VH, Steinmann B, Bioflavonoid-mediated stabilization of collagen in adjuvant-induced arthritis. Scand J Rheumatol 1983;12(1):39-42

[728] Klimova OA, Sokol'nikov AA, Kodensatova VM, Glinka ELu, Arkhapchev IuP, Sergeev IN, Vitamin D and calcium metabolism in relation to different levels of vitamins B6 and D. Vopr Pitan 1991Jul;4:56-59

[729] Kaul P, Sidhu H, Sharma SK, Nath R, Calculogenic potential of galactose and fructose in relation to urinary excretion of lithogenic substances in vitamin B6 deficient and control rats. J Am Coll Nutr 1996 Jun;15(3):295-302

[730] Masse PG, Weiser H, Pritzker KP, Effects of modifying dietary protein in the presence and absence of vitamin B6, on the regulation of plasm calcium and phosphorus levels-positive impact of yeast Saccharomyces cerevisiae. Int J Vitam Res 1994;64(1):47-55

[731] Modern nutrition in health and disease, editors Shils ME, Olson JA, Shike M, Ross AC, Lippincott Williams & Wilkins, 1998, p. 147

[732] Ho SC, et al. Sodium is the leading dietary factor associated with urinary calcium excretion in Hong Kong Chinese adults. Osteoporos Int. 2001;12(9):723-31

[733] Wang XB, Zhao XH, The effect of dietary sulfur-containing amino acids on calcium excretion, Adv Exp Med Biol 1998;442:495-499

[734] Koenig W, Baron M, Ehring F, Effect of calcium mineral solutions on the histamine release from human peripheral leukocytes. Arzneim.-Forsch./Drug Res 1984, 34(I), 1, 52-54

[735] Kies C, Harms JM, Copper absorption as affected by supplemental calcium, magnesium, manganese, selenium and potassium. Adv Exp Med Biol 1989;258:45-58

[736] Koshimura K, et al., Involvement of nitric oxide in glucose toxicity on differentiated PC12 cells: prevention of glucose toxicity by tetrahydrobiopterin, a cofactor for nitric oxide synthase. Neurosci Res 2002 May;43(1):31-8

[737] Juchheim JK, Haaranalyse, Mineralstoffe und Ernaehrung, Karl F. Haug Verlag, Heidelberg, 1991

[738] Katz ML, Stone WL, Dratz EA, Fluorescent pigment accumulation in retinal pigment epithelium of antioxidant-deficient rats. Invest Ophthalmol Vis Sci 1978 Nov;17(11):1049-1058

[739] Jain SK, Kannan K. Chromium chloride inhibits oxidative stress and TNF-alpha secretion caused by exposure to high glucose in cultured U937 monocytes. Biochem Biophys Res Commun. 2001 Dec 7;289(3):687-91

[740] Shrivastava R, et al. Effects of chromium on the immune system. FEMS Immunol Med Microbiol 2002 Sep 6;34(1):1

[741] Moore JW, Maher MA, Banz WJ, Zemel MB, Chromium picolinate modulates rat vascular smooth muscle cell intracellular calcium metabolism. J Nutr 1998 Feb;128(2):180-4

[742] Xi X, et al. Retinal dopamine transporter in experimental myopia. Chin Med J (Engl) 2002 Jul;115(7):1027-30

[743] Wapnir RA, Copper absorption and bioavailability, Am J Clin Nutr 1998;67(suppl.):1054S-60S

[744] Modern nutrition in health and disease, editors Shils ME, Olson JA, Shike M, Ross AC, Lippincott Williams & Wilkins, 1998, p. 241

[745] Reiser S, et al. Indices of copper status in humans consuming a typical American diet containing either fructose or starch. Am J Clin Nutr 1985 Aug;42(2):242-51

[746] Turnlund JR, et al., A stable-isotope study of zinc, copper, and iron absorption and retention by young women fed vitamin B-6-deficient diets. Am J Clin Nutr 1991 Dec;54(6):1059-64

[747] Rucker RB, Kosonen T, Clegg MS, Mitchell AE, Rucker BR, Uriu-Hare JY, Keen CL. Copper, lysyl oxidase, and extracellular matrix protein cross-linking. Am J Clin Nutr 1998May;67(5 Suppl):996S-1002S

[748] Schuschke DA, Dietary copper in the physiology of the microcirculation. J Nutr. 1997 Dec;127(12):2274-81

[749] Heller LJ, et al., Decreased passive stiffness of cardiac myocytes and cardiac tissue from copper-deficient rat hearts. Am J Physiol Heart Circ Physiol 2000 Jun;278(6):H1840-7

6 REFERENCES

[750] Heraud F, Savineau C, Harmand MF. Copper modulation of extracellular matrix synthesis by human articular chondrocytes. Scand J Rheumatol 2002;31(5):279-84

[751] Trivedy C, et al. Copper stimulates human fibroblasts in vitro: a role in the pathogenesis of dral submucous fibrosis. J Oral Pathol Med 2001 Sep;30(8):465-70

[752] Sharma SC, Jande MB, Inhibition of mast cell histamine release by copper. Arch Int Pharmacol Ther May-Jun;299:254-68

[753] Schuschke DA, et al. Relationship between dietary copper concentration and acetylcholine-induced vasodilation in the microcirculation of rats. Biofactors 1999;10(4):321-7

[754] Schuschke DA, Falcone JC, Saari JT, Fleming JT, Percival SS, Young SA, Pass JM, Miller FN, Endothelial cell calcium mobilization to acetylcholine is attenuated in copper-deficient rats. Endothelium 2000;7(2):83-92

[755] Lynch SM, Strain JJ, Dietary saturated or polyunsaturated fat and copper deficiency in the rat. Biol Trace Elem Res 1989 Nov;22(2):131-9

[756] Sukalski KA, LaBerge TP, Johnson WT, In vivo oxidative modification of erythrocyte membrane prteins in copper deficiency. Fre Radic Biol Med 1997;22(5):835-42

[757] O'Dell BL, Roles of zinc and copper in the nervous system. Prog Clin Biol Res 1993;380:147-62

[758] Klevay LM, Cardiovasculare diesease from copper deficiency – a history. J Nutr 2000 Feb;130(2S Suppl):489S-492S

[759] Klevay LM, Lack of a recommended dietary allowance for copper may be hazardous to your health. J Am Coll Nutr 1998 Aug;17(4):322-9

[760] Miesel R, Zuber M. Copper-dependent antioxidase defenses in inflammatory and autoimmune rheumatic diseases. Inflammation 1993 Jun;17(3):283-94

[761] Lamb DJ, et al. Effect of dietary copper supplementation on cell composition and apoptosis in atheriosclerotic lesions of cholesterol-fed rabbits. Atheriosclerosis 2002 Oct;164(2):229-36

[762] Wildman RE, Hopkins R, Failla ML, Medeiros DM. Marginal copper-restricted diets produce altered cardiac ultrastructure in the rat. Proc Soc Exp Biol Med 1995 Oct;210(1):43-9

[763] Hamilton IM, Gilmore WS, Strain JJ. Marginal copper deficiency and atheriosclerosis. Biol Trace Elem Res 2000 Winter;78(1-3):179-89

[764] Uauy R, Olivares M, Gonzalez M, Essentiality of copper in humans. Am J Clin Nutr 1998 May;67(5 Suppl):952S-959S

[765] Milne DB, Copper intake and assessment of copper status. Am J Clin Nutr 1998;67(suppl):1041S-5S

[766] Milanino R, et al. Copper and zinc status during acute inflammation: studies on blood, liver and kidneys metal levels in normal and inflamed rats. Agents Actions 1986 Nov;19(3-4):215-23

[767] Bannister JV, Rotilio G, Aspects of the structure, function, and applications of superoxide dismutase. CRC Critical Reviews in Biochemistry 1987; 22(2):111-180

[768] Mervyn L, Thorsons complete Guide to vitamins & minerals, Thorsons, London, 2000

[769] Galland LD et al., Magnesium deficiency in the pathogenesis of mitral valve prolapse. Magnesium 1986;5(3-4):165-74

[770] Planells E, Effect of magnesium deficiency on vitamin B2 and B6 status in the rat. J Am Coll Nutr 1997 Aug;16(4):352-6

[771] Modern nutrition in health and disease, editors Shils ME, Olson JA, Shike M, Ross AC, Lippincott Williams & Wilkins, 1998, p. 741

[772] McCoy H, Kenney MA, Interactions between magnesium and vitamin D: possible implications in the immune system. Magnesium Research 1996;9(3):185-203

[773] Johnson S, The possible role of gradual accumulation of copper copper, cadmium, lead and iron and gradual depletion of zinc, magnesium, selenium, Vitamisn B2, B6, D, and E and essential fatty acids in multiple sclerosis. Med Hypotheses 2000 Sep;55(3):239-241

[774] Biesalski HK et al., Ernaehrungsmedizin, Georg Thieme Verlag Stuttgart New York 1999, p. 171
[775] Dimai HP et al., Daily oral magnesium supplementation suppresses bone turnover in young adult males. J Clin Endocrinol Metab 1998 Aug;83(8):2742-8
[776] Modern nutrition in health and disease, editors Shils ME, Olson JA, Shike M, Ross AC, Lippincott Williams & Wilkins, 1998, p. 116
[777] Johnson S, The multifaceted and widespread pathology of magnesium deficiency. Med Hypotheses 2001 Feb; 56(2):163-70
[778] Modern nutrition in health and disease, editors Shils ME, Olson JA, Shike M, Ross AC, Lippincott Williams & Wilkins, 1998, p. 1334
[779] Kuo S, et al., In vivo architecture of the manganese superoxide dismutase promotor. J Biol Chem 1999 Feb 5;274(6):3345-54
[780] Wedler FC, Biological significance of manganese in mammalian systems. Prog Med Chem 1993; 30:89-133
[781] Biesalski HK et al., Ernaehrungsmedizin, Georg Thieme Verlag Stuttgart New York 1999, p. 180
[782] Cotzias GC, et al., Interactions between manganese and brain dopamine. Med Clin North America 1976; 60(4):729-738
[783] Bonilla E, The regional distribution of manganese in the normal human brain. Neurochem Res 1982 Feb;7(2):221-7
[784] Gong H, Amemiya T, Corneal changes in manganese-deficient rats. Cornea 1999 Jul;18(4):472-82
[785] Modern nutrition in health and disease, editors Shils ME, Olson JA, Shike M, Ross AC, Lippincott Williams & Wilkins, 1998, p. 291
[786] Lehninger AL, Nelson DL, Cox MM, Prinzipien der Biochemie. Spektrum Akademischer Verlag, 1998, p. 815
[787] Warkentin O, Geschichte von Paracetamol. http://www.hschickor.de/parac.htm
[788] Rayman MP, The importance of selenium to human health. Lancet 2000 Jul 15;356(9225):233-41
[789] Modern nutrition in health and disease, editors Shils ME, Olson JA, Shike M, Ross AC, Lippincott Williams & Wilkins, 1998, p. 269
[790] McCarty MF, Oxidants downstream from superoxide inhibit nitric oxide production by vascular endothelium – a key role for selenium-dependent enzymes in vascular health. Med Hypotheses 1999 Oct;53(4):315-25
[791] Gomez RM, et al. Reduced inotropic heart response in selenium-deficient mice relates with inducible nitric oxide. Am J Physiol Heart Circ Physiol. 2003 Feb;284(2):H442-8
[792] Turan B, Zaloglu N, Koc E, Saran Y, Akkas N, Dietary selenium- and vitamin E-induced alterations in some rabbit tissues. Biol Trace Elem Res 1997 Sep;58(3):237-253
[793] Sweeny PR, Brown RG, Ultrastructural studies of the myotendonous junction of selenium-deficient ducklings. Am J Pathol 1980 Aug;100(2):481-96
[794] Castano A, et al., Low selenium diet increases the dopamine turnover in prefrontal cortex of the rat. Neurochem Int 1997 Jun;30(6):549-55
[795] McCarty MF, Russell AL, Niacinamide therapy for oseoarthritis – does it inhibit nitric oxide synthase induction by interleukin 1 in chondrocytes. Med Hypotheses 1999 Oct;53(4):350-60
[796] Deutsche Gesellschaft für Ernaehrung et al., Referenzwerte für die Naehrstoffzufuhr. Umschau Braus Verlagsges., 2000, p. 196
[797] Reinhold U, Specific application of single nutrients as a basic treatment in immunostimulating therapy. Med Hypotheses 1987;22:159-169
[798] Skripchenko ND, et al. [Effect of selenium enriched diet on lipied peroxidation in patients with diabetes mellitus type 2]. Vopr Pitan. 2003;72(1):14-7
[799] Lockwood MK, Eckhert CD. Sucrose-induced lipid, glucose, and insulin elevations, microvascular injury, and selenium. Am J Physiol. 1992 Jan;262(1 Pt 2):R144-9

6 REFERENCES

[800] Djujic IS, et al. Bioavailability and possible benefits of wheat intake naturally enriched with selenium and its products. Biol Trace Elem Res 2000 Dec;77(3):273-85

[801] Modern nutrition in health and disease, editors Shils ME, Olson JA, Shike M, Ross AC, Lippincott Williams & Wilkins, 1998, p. 271

[802] Mehta U, et al. Studies of apoptosis and bcl-2 in experimental atheriosclerosis in rabbit and influence of selenium supplementation. Gen Physiol Biophys 2002 Mar;21(1):15-29

[803] Selak I, Skaper SD, Varon S. Age-dependent requirements of sympathetic neurons in serum-free culture. Brain res. 1983 Apr;283(2-3):171-9

[804] Seaborn CD, Nielsen FH. Dietary silicon and arginine affect mineral element composition of rat femur and vertebra. Biol Trace Elem Res 2002 Dec;89(3):239-50

[805] Seaborn CD, Nielsen FH. Silicon deprivation decreases collagen formation in wounds and bone, and ornithine transaminase enzyme activity in liver. Biol Trace Elem Res 2002 Dec;89(3):251-61

[806] Refitt DM, et al. Orthosilic acid stimulates collagen type 1 synthesis and osteoblastic differentiation in human osteoblast-like cells in vitro. Bone 2003 feb;32(2):127-35

[807] Rodriguez JP, Rosselot G, Effects of cell proliferation and proteoglycan characteristics of epiphyseal chondrocytes. J Cell Biochem 2001;82(3):501-11

[808] Agren MS, Franzen L, Influence of zinc deficieny on breaking strength of 3-week-old skin incisions in the rat. Acta Chir Scand 1990 Oct;156(10):667-70

[809] Turnlund JR, et al. Copper absorption in young men fed adequate and low zinc diets. Biol Trace Elem Rews 1988 Sep-Dec;17:31-41

[810] Roughead ZK, et al. Dietary copper primarily affects antioxidant capacity and dietary iron mainly affects iron status in a surface response study of female rats fed varying concentrations of iron, zinc and copper. J Nutr 1999 Jul;129(7):1368-76

[811] Sugawara T, et al. Overexpression of copper/zinc superoxide dismutase in transgenic rats protects vulnerable neurons against ischemic damage by blocking the mitochondrial pathway of caspase activation. J Neurosci. 2002 Jan 1;22(1):209-17

[812] Yousef MI, et al. Dietary zinc deficiency induced changes in the activity of enzymes and the levels of free radicals, lipids and protein electrophoretic behaviour in growing rats. Toxicology 2002 Jun 14;175(1-3):223-34

[813] Anderson RA, et al. Potential antioxidant effects of zinc and chromium supplementation in people with type 2 diabetes mellitus. J Am Coll Nutr 2001 Jun;20(3):212-8

[814] Modern nutrition in health and disease, editors Shils ME, Olson JA, Shike M, Ross AC, Lippincott Williams & Wilkins, 1998, p. 742

[815] Frankel P, The methylation miracle, St. Martin's Paperbacks, 1999, p. 195

[816] Hanck A, Spektrum Vitamine, Aesopus Verlag, 1986, p.17

[817] Bamji MS, Vitamin deficiencies in rice-eating populations. Effects of B-vitamin supplements. Experientia Suppl 1983;44:245-63

[818] Dutta P, Rivlin RS, Pinto J, Enhanced depletion of lens reduced gluathione Adriamycin in riboflavin-deficient rats. Biochem Pharmacol 1990 Sep 1;40(5):1111-5

[819] Luan Eng LI, Ng T, Wan WP, Ganesan J, Stimulation of erythrocyte reductase activity by flavin adenine dinucleotide (FAD) in Malaysian adults and newborns and their parents. Br J Haematol 1975 Nov;31(3):337-42

[820] Prasad R, Lakshmi AV, Bamji MS, Impaired collagen maturity in vitamins B2 and B6 deficiency – probable molecular basis of skin lesions. Biochem Med 1983 Dec;30(3):333-41

[821] Spoerl E, Seiler T, Techniques for stiffening the cornea. J Refract Surg 1999 Nov-Dec;15(6):711-3

[822] Grimble RF, Effect of antioxidative vitamins on immune function with clinical applications. Int J Vitam Nutr Res 1997;67(5):312-20

[823] Miyamoto Y, Sancar A, Vitamin B2-based blue-light photoreceptors in the retinohypothalamic tract as the photoactive pigments for setting the circadian clock in mammals. Proc Natl Acad Sci USA 1998 May 26;95(11):6097-102

[824] Modern nutrition in health and disease, editors Shils ME, Olson JA, Shike M, Ross AC, Lippincott Williams & Wilkins, 1998, p. 396

[825] McCully KS, McCully M, The heart revolution, Perennial, 1999, p. 172

[826] Agte VV, Paknikar KM, Chiplonkar SA, Effect of reiboflavin supplementation on zinc and iron absorption and growth performance in mice. Biol Trace Elem Res 1998 Nov;65(2):109-15

[827] Lakshmi AV, Riboblavin metabolism – relevance to human nutrition. Indian J Med Res 1998 Nov;108:182-90

[828] Sauberlich HE, Interactions of thiamin, riboflavin, and other B-vitamins. Ann N Y Acad Sci 1980;355:80-97

[829] Modern nutrition in health and disease, editors Shils ME, Olson JA, Shike M, Ross AC, Lippincott Williams & Wilkins, 1998, p. 397

[830] Eckhert CD, Hsu MH, Pang N, Photoreceptor damage following exposure to excess riboflavin. Experientia 1993 Dec 15;49(12):1084-7

[831] Vaxman F, et al. Can the wound healing process be improved by vitamin supplementation? Experimental study on humans. Eur Surg Res. 1996 Jul-Aug;28(4):306-14

[832] Biesalski HK et al., Ernaehrungsmedizin, Georg Thieme Verlag Stuttgart New York 1999, p. 139

[833] Gregory JF, Bioavailability of vitamin B-6. Europ J Clin Nutr 1997; 51 Suppl. 1:S43-S48

[834] Cabrini L, et al., Vitamin B6 deficiency affects antioxidant defences in rat liver and heart. Biochem Mol Biol Int 1998 Nov;46(4):689-97

[835] Benderitter M, et al., Effects of exhaustive exercise and vitamin B6 deficiency on free radical oxidative process in male trained rats. Free Radic Biol Med 1996;21(4):541-9

[836] Grimble RF, Effect of antioxidative vitamins on immune function with clinical applications. Int J Vitam Nutr Res 1997;67(5):312-20

[837] Garcia M, Gonzalez R, Effect of pyridoxine on histamine liberation and degranulation of rat mast cells. Allergol Immunopathol (Madr) 1979 Nov-Dec;7(6):427-32

[838] Jarisch R, Wantke F, Wine and headache. Int Arch Allergy Immunol 1996 May;110(1):7-12

[839] Doke S, Inagaki N, Hayakawa T, Tsuge H, Effect of vitamin B6 deficiency on an antibody production in mice. Biosci Biotechnol Biochem 1997 Aug;61(8):1331-6

[840] Cassel S, Robson L, Rosse C, The effects of vitamin B6 deficiency on the bone marrow of the rat. Anat Rec 1978 May;191(1):47-53

[841] Boehles H, Ernaehrungsstoerungen im Kindesalter. Wissenschaftliche Verlagsgesellschaft Stuttgart, 1991, p. 194

[842] Modern nutrition in health and disease, editors Shils ME, Olson JA, Shike M, Ross AC, Lippincott Williams & Wilkins, 1998, p. 146

[843] Guilarte TR, Effect of vitamin B-6 nutrition on the levels of dopamine, dopamine metabolites, dopa decarboxylase activity, tyrosine, and GABA in the developing rat corpus striatum. Neurochem Res 1989 Jun;14(6):571-8

[844] Gerster H, The importance of vitamin B 6 for development of the infant. Human medical and animal experiment studies. Z Ernaehrungswiss 1996 Dec;35(4):309-17

[845] Munoz_hoyos A, Pineal response after pyridoxine test in children. J Neural Transm Gen Sect 1996;103(7):833-42

[846] Dakshinamurti K, et al., Neuroendocrinology of pyridoxine deficiency. Neurosci Biobehav Rev 1988 Fall-Winter;12(3-4):189-93

[847] Reiter RR, Robinson J, Melatonin. Bantam Books, 1995, p. 196

[848] Dakshinamurti K, et al., Neurobiology of pyridoxine. Ann N Y Acad Sci. 1990;585:128-44

[849] Elmadfa I, Leitzmann C, Ernaehrung des Menschen, Verlag Eugen Ulmer Stuttgart, 1990, p. 291

6 REFERENCES

[850] Okada M, et al., Dietary protein as a factor affecting vitamin B6 requirement. J Nutr Sci Vitaminol (Tokyo) 1998 Feb;44(1):37-45

[851] Lakshmi AV, Riboflavin metabolism – relevance to human nutrition. Indian J Med Res 1998 Nov;108:182-90

[852] Zinc and the regulation of vitamin B6 metabolism. Nutr rev 1990 Jun;48(6):255-8

[853] Hanck A, Spektrum Vitamine, Aesopus Verlag, 1986, p. 78

[854] Dreon DM, Butterfield GE, Vitamin B6 utilization in active and inactive young men. Am J Clin Nutr 1986 May;43(5):816-824

[855] Ellis JM, Vitamin B6 Therapy. Avery Publishing Group, 1999, p. 22

[856] Hanck A, Spektrum Vitamine, Aesopus Verlag, 1986, p. 76

[857] Honma K, Kohsaka M, Fukuda N, Morita N, Honma S, Effects of vitamin B12 on plasma melatonin rhythm in humans: increased light sensitivity phase – advances the circadian clock? Experientia 1992 Aug 15;48(8):716-20

[858] Tamura J, et al., Immunomodulation by vitamin B12. Clin Exp Immunol 1999 Apr;116(1):28-32

[859] Modern nutrition in health and disease, editors Shils ME, Olson JA, Shike M, Ross AC, Lippincott Williams & Wilkins, 1998, p. 439

[860] Nosova IM, Zaidenberg MA, Korotkina RN, Effect of folic acid on metabolic processes in wounds. Farmakol Toksikol 1979 Jan-Feb;42(1):63-8

[861] Kamen B, Folate and antifolate pharmacology. Semin Oncol 1997 Oct;24(5 Suppl 18):S18-30-S18-39

[862] Gospe SM et al., Behavioral and neurochemical changes in folate-deficient mice. Physiol Behav 1995 Nov;58(5):935-41

[863] Gospe SM et al., Behavioral and neurochemical changes in folate-deficient mice. Physiol Behav 1995 Nov;58(5):935-41

[864] Fournier I, et al. Folate deficiency alters melatonin secretion in rats. J Nutr 2002 Sep;132(9):2781-4

[865] Mayer O, et al., The effects of folate supplementation on some coagulation parameters and oxidative status surrogates. Eur J Clin Pharmacol 2002 Apr;58(1):1-5

[866] Forgione MA, et al., Cellular glutathione peroxidase deficiency and endothelial dysfunction. Am J Physiol Heart Circ Physiol 2002 Apr;282(4):H1255-61

[867] Gu L, et al. Involvement of DNA mismatch repair in folate deficieny-induced apoptosis small star, filled. J Nutr Biochem 2002 Jun;13(6):355-363

[868] Vitamin D supplement in early chilshood and risk for type I (insulin-dependent) diabeted mellitus. Diabetologia 1999 Jan;42(1):51-4

[869] Giovannucci E, Epidemiologic studies of folate and colorectal neoplasia: a review. J Nutr 2002 Aug;132(8 Suppl):2350S-2355S

[870] Baggott JE, et al. Inhibition of folate-dependent enzymes by non-steroidal anti-inflammatory drugs. Biochem J. 1992 Feb 15;282(Pt1):197-202

[871] Modern nutrition in health and disease, editors Shils ME, Olson JA, Shike M, Ross AC, Lippincott Williams & Wilkins, 1998, p. 442

[872] Berkson B, All about B vitamins. Avery Publishing Group, 1998, p. 46

[873] Bonke D, Nickel B, Improvement of fine motoric movement control by elevated dosages of vitamin B1, B6, and B12 in target shooting. Int J Vitam Nutr Suppl 1989;30:198-204

[874] Vitamin D supplement in early chilshood and risk for type I (insulin-dependent) diabeted mellitus. Diabetologia 1999 Jan;42(1):51-4

[875] DeLuca HF, Zierold C, Mechanisms and functions of vitamin D. Nutr Rev 1998 Feb;56(2 Pt 2):S4-10; discussions S54-75

[876] Amento EP, Vitamin D and the immune system. Steroids 1987 Jan-Mar;49(1-3):55-72

[877] Cantorna MT, Vitamin D and autoimmunity:is vitamin D status an environmental factor affecting autoimmune disease prevalence? Proc Soc Exp Biol Med 2000 Mar;223(3):230-3

[878] Thomasset M, Vitamin D and the immune system. Pathol Biol (Paris) 1994 Feb;42(2):163-72

[879] Ponsonby AL, et al. Ultraviolet radiation and autoimmune disease: insights from epidemiological research. Toxicology 2002 Dec 27;181-182:71-8

[880] Cade C, Norman AW, Vitamin D3 improves impaired glucose tolerance and insulin secretion in the vitamin D-deficient rat in vivo. Endocrinology 1986 Jul;119(1):84-90

[881] Holick MF, McCollum Award Lecture, 1994: vitamin D – new horizons for the 21st century. Am J Clin Nutr 1994 Oct;60(4):619-30

[882] Glerup H, et al., Commonly recommended daily intake of vitamin D is not sufficient if sunlight exposure is limited. J Intern Med 2000 Feb;247(2):260-8

[883] Carnevale V, et al., Longitudinal evaluation of vitamin D status in healthy subjects from southern Italy:seasonal and gender differences. Osteoporos Int 2001 Dec;12(!"):1026-30

[884] Vieth R, et al., Wintertime vitamin D insufficiency is common in young Canadian women, and their vitamin D intake does not prevent it. Eur J Clin Nutr 2001 Dec;55(12):1091-7

[885] Modern nutrition in health and disease, editors Shils ME, Olson JA, Shike M, Ross AC, Lippincott Williams & Wilkins, 1998, p. 335

[886] Jablonski NG, Chaplin G, The evolution of human skin coloration. J Hum Evol 2000 Jul;39(1):57-106

[887] Fogarty A, Dietary vitamin E, IgE concentrations, and atopy. The Lancet 2000;356:1573-74

[888] Martin A et al., Effect of vitamin E intake on levels of vitamins E and C in the central nervous system and peripheral tissues: implications for health recommendations. Brain Res 1999 Oct 16;845(1):50-9

[889] Mervyn L, Thorsons complete Guide to vitamins & minerals, Thorsons, London, 2000, p. 321

[890] Biesalski HK et al., Ernaehrungsmedizin, Georg Thieme Verlag Stuttgart New York 1999, p. 126

[891] Hattori S, et al., Pentamethyl-hydroxychromane, vitamin E derivative, inhibits induction of nitric oxide synthase by bacterial lipopolysaccharide. Biochem Mol Biol Int Jan;35(1):177-83

[892] Davidge ST, Vascular function in the vitamin E-deprived rat: an interaction between nitric oxide and superoxide anions. Hypertension 1998 Mar;31(3):830-5

[893] Boehm H, et al., Flavonole, Flavone und Anthocane als natuerliche Antioxidantien der Nahrung und ihre moegliche Rolle bei der Praevention chronischer Erkrankungen. Z Ernaehrungswiss 1998; 37:147-163

[894] Kuttan R, et al., Collagen treated with (+)-catechin becomes resistant to the action of mammalian collagenase. Experientia 1981 Mar 15;37(3):221-3

[895] Biesalski HK et al., Ernaehrungsmedizin, Georg Thieme Verlag Stuttgart New York 1999, p. 393

[896] Modern nutrition in health and disease, editors Shils ME, Olson JA, Shike M, Ross AC, Lippincott Williams & Wilkins, 1998, p. 1276

[897] Packer L, Rimbach G, Virgili F, Antioxidant activity and biologic properties of a procyanidin-rich extract from pine (pinus maritima) bark, pycnogenol. Free Radic Biol Med 1999 Sep;27(5-6):704-24

[898] Bagchi D et al., Free radicals and grape seed proanthocyanidin extract: importance in human health and disease prevention. Toxicology 2000 Aug 7;148(2-3):187-97

[899] Ueda T, Armstron D, Preventive effect of natural and synthetic antioxidants on lipid peroxidation in the mammalian eye. Ophthalmic Res 1996;28(3):184-92

[900] Berg PA, Daniel PT, Effects of flavonoid compounds on the immune response. Prog Clin Biol Res. 1988;280:157-71

[901] Romero J, Marak GE, Rao NA, Pharmacologic modulation of acute ocular inflammation with quercetin. Ophthalmic Res 1989;21(2):112-7

[902] Middleton E, Effect of plant flavonoids on immune and inflammatory cell function. Adv Exp Med Biol 1998;439:175-82

[903] Ishiwa J et a., A citrus flavonoid, nobiletin, suppresses production and gene expression of matrix metalloproteinase 9/gelatinase B in rabbit synovial fibroblasts. J Rheumatol 2000 Jan;27(1):20-5

[904] Kimata M et al., Effects of luteolin and other flavonoids on IgE.mediated allergic reactions. Planta Med 2000 Feb;66(1):25-9

[905] Bronner C, Landry Y, Kinetics of the inhibitory effect of flavonoids on histamine secretion from mast cells. Agents Actions 1985 Apr;16(3-4):147-51

[906] Jaffar ZH, Pearce FL, Some characteristics of the ATP-induced histamine trlease from and permeabilization of rat mast cells. Agents Actions 1993 Sep;40(1-2):18-27

[907] Formica JV, Regelson W, Review of the biology of mquercetin and related bioflavonoid. Food Chem Toxicol 1995 Dec;33(12):1061-80

[908] Wang ZR, et al., Effect of total flavonoids of hippophae rhamnoides on contarctile mechanics and calcium transfer in stretched myocyte. Space Med Med Eng (Beijing) 2000 Feb;13(1):6-9

[909] McCully KS, McCully M, The heart revolution, Perennial, 1999, p. 165

[910] Rohdewald P, A review of the French maritime pine bark extract (Pycnogenol), a herbal medication with a diverse clinical pharmacology. Int J Clin Pharmacol Ther 2002 Apr;40(4):158-68

[911] Packer team findes pine bark extract a potent antioxidant, http://www.berkeley.edu/news/berkeleyan/1998/0304/packer.html

[912] Sakata K, et al. Inhibition if inducible isoforms of cyclooxygenase and nitric oxide synthase by flavonoid hesperidin in mous macrophage cell line. Cancer Lett. 2003 Sep 25;199(2):139-45

[913] Duffy SJ, Vita JA. Effects of phenolics on vascular endothelial function. Curr Opin Lipidol. 2003 Feb;14(1):21-7

[914] Sarkar A, Bhaduri A, Black tea is a powerful chemopreventor of reactive oxygen and nitrogen species: comparison with its individual catechin constituents and green tea. Biochem Biophys Res Commun 2001 Jun 1;284(1):173-8

[915] Paquay JB, et al., Protection against nitric oxide toxicity by tea. J Agric Food Chem 2000 Nov;48(11):5768-72

[916] Freedman JE, et al., Select flavonoids and whole juice from purple grapes inhibit platelet function and enhance nitric oxide release. Circulation 2001 Jun 12;103(23):2792-8

[917] Shen SC, et al., In vitro and in vivo inhibitory activities of rutin, wogonin, and quercetin on lipopolysaccharide-induced nitric oxide and prostaglandin (E(2) production. Eur J Pharmacol 2002 Jun 20;446(1-3):187-194

[918] Kim JS, et al., Inhibition of alpha-glucosidase and amylase by luteolin, a flavonoid. Biosci Biotechnol Biochem 2000 Nov;64(11):2458-61

[919] Valikangas L, et al. The effects of high levels of glucose and insulin on type I collagen synthesis in mature human odontoblasts and pulp tissue in vitro. Adv Dent Res 2001 Aug;15:72-5

[920] http://www.ultranet.com/~jkimball/BiologyPages/F/Fats.html

[921] Biesalski HK et al., Ernaehrungsmedizin, Georg Thieme Verlag Stuttgart New York 1999, p. 75 ff

[922] Yaqoob P, Monounsaturated fats and immune function. Braz J Med Biol Res 1998 April;31(4):453-465

[923] Fernandes G, Jolly C, Nutrition and autoimmune disease. Nutr Rev 1998 Jan; 56(1):S161-S169

[924] Fernandes G, Dietary lipids and risk of autoimmune disease. Clin Immunol Immunopathol 1994 Aug;72(2):193-7

[925] Harbige LS, Dietary n-6 and n-3 fatty acids in immunity and autoimmune disease. Proc Nutr Soc 1998 Nov;57(4):555-62

[926] Modern nutrition in health and disease, editors Shils ME, Olson JA, Shike M, Ross AC, Lippincott Williams & Wilkins, 1998, p. 744

[927] de Pablo MA et al., The effect of dietary fatty acid manipulation on phagocytic activity and cytokine production by peritoneal cells from Balb/c mice. J Nutr Sci Vitaminol (Tokyo) 1998 Feb;44(1):57-67

[928] Kankaanpaa P et al., Dietary fatty acids and allergy. Ann Med 1999 Aug;31(4):282-7
[929] Fang YZ, et al. Free radicals, antioxidants, and nutrition. Nutrition 2002 Oct;18(10):872-9
[930] Chaitow L, Thorsons guide to amino acids, Thorsons, 1991, p. 47
[931] Modern nutrition in health and disease, editors Shils ME, Olson JA, Shike M, Ross AC, Lippincott Williams & Wilkins, 1998, p. 525
[932] Vanderhaeghe LR, Bouic PJD, The immune system cure, Kensington Books, 1999
[933] Bouic PJ, Lamprecht JH, Plant sterols and sterolins: a review of their immune-modulating properties. Altern Med Rev 1999 Jun;4(3):170-7
[934] Benedict H.. Plant sterols and sterolins in human health. http://www.naturleaf.com/research/clinicalstudies1.htm
[935] Okuno T, et al., Effects of caffeine on microcirculation of the human ocular fundus. Jpn J Ophthalmol 2002 Mar-Apr;46(2):170-6
[936] Kojima S, et al., Effect of the consumption of ethanol on the microcirculation of the human optic nerve head in the acute phase. Jpn J Ophthalmol 2000 May;44(3):318-9
[937] Yen GC, Lai HH. Inhibition of reactive nitrogen species effects in vitro and in vivo by isoflavones and soy-based extracts. J Agric Food Chem. 2003 Dec 31;51(27):7892-900
[938] Suzuki K, et al. Relationship between serum carotenoids and hyperglycemia: a population-based cross-sectional study. J Epidemiol. 2002 Sep;12(5):357-66
[939] http://www.ciel.ch/nep2.html
[940] Schmidt E, Schmidt N. Leitfaden der Mikronährstoffe. Urban & Fischer/Elsevier, München 2004
[941] Der kleine "Souci Fachmann Kraut, Lebensmitteltabelle für die Praxis, Wissenschaftliche Verlagsgesellschaft mbH Stuttgart, 1991
[942] Biesalski HK et al., Ernaehrungsmedizin, Georg Thieme Verlag Stuttgart New York 1999, p. 320
[943] Modern nutrition in health and disease, Lippincott Williams & Wilkins, Baltimore 1999
[944] Deutsche Gesellschaft für Ernaehrung et al., Referenzwerte für die Naehrstoffzufuhr. Umschau Braus Verlagsges., 2000
[945] United States Recommended Dietary Allowances (RDA), http://daily-vitamins.com/rda.html
[946] Hathcock JN, Vitamins and minerals: efficacy and safety. Am J Clin Nutr Aug;66(2):427-37 and http://www.crnusa.org/ben_full.htm http://.lifescript.com/resources/research/ben_fullPart_III.asp
[947] McKenna MJ, Differences in vitamin D status between countries in young alults and the elderly. Am J Med 1992;93(1):69-77
[948] Biesalski HK et al., Ernaehrungsmedizin, Georg Thieme Verlag Stuttgart New York 1999, p. 135
[949] Chen J, Gao J, The Chinese total diet study in 1990. Part II. Nutrients. J AOAC Int 1993 Nov-Dec;76(6):1206-13
[950] Elmadfa I, Leitzmann C, Ernaehrung des Menschen, Verlag Eugen Ulmer Stuttgart, 1990, p. 284
[951] Bender DA, Vitamin B6 requirements and recommendations. Eur J Clin Nutr 1989 May;43(5):289-309
[952] Hansen CM, Leklem JE, Miller LT, Changes in vitamin B-6 status indicators of women fed a constant protein diet with varying levels of vitamin B-6. Am J Clin Nutr 1997 Dec;66(6):1379-87
[953] Ronnenberg AG, et al., Anemia and deficiencies of folate and vitamin B-6 are common and vary with season in Chinese women of childbearing age. J Nutr 2000 Nov;130(11):2703-10
[954] Seshadri S, Prevalence of micronutrient deficiency particularly of iron, zinc, and folic acid in pregnant women in South East Asia. Br J Nutr 2001 May;85 Suppl 2:S87-92
[955] Pizzorno J, Total Wellness. Prima Publishing 1996, referenced in Bergner P, The Healing Power of Minerals, Special Nutrients and Trace Elements. Prima Publishing 1997

6 REFERENCES

[956] Dollhite J, et al., Problems encountered in meeting the Recommended Dietary Allowances for menues designed according to the Dietary Guidelines for Americans. J Am Diet Assoc 1995 Mar;95(3):341-4, ;

[957] http://www.emory.edu/COLLEGE/HYBRIDVIGOR/issue2/eons.htm

[958] Dunne LJ, Nutrition almanac. McGraw-Hill Publishing Company, 1990

[959] Hom MM, Manual of contact lens prescribing and fitting, Butterworth-Heinemann, 1997

[960] Fletcher R, Lupelli L, Rossi A, Contact lens practoce. Blackwell Scientific Publications, 1994

[961] Buerki E, Augenaerztliche Kontaktlinsenanpassung. Ferdinand Enke Verlag, 1991

[962] Buerki E, Augenaerztliche Kontaktlinsenanpassung. Ferdinand Enke Verlag, 1991, p. 58

[963] Cheng KH, et al., Incidence of contact-lens-associated microbial keratitis and its related morbidity. Lancet 1999 Jul 17;354(9174):181-5

[964] Hamano H, Ruben M, Kontaktlinsen. Orac Verlag, 1985, p. 75

[965] Raeburn P, To your health:new contact lenses may be disposable, but risk isn't. http://detnews.com/menu/stories/20350.htm

[966] Sweeney DF, Keay L, Carnt N, Holden BA. Practitioner guidelines for continuous wear with high Dk silicone hydrogel contact lenses. Clin Exp Optom 2002;85(3):161-167

[967] Trends in contact lenses & lens care. The Bausch & Lomb annual report to vision care professionals, Dec 2001

[968] Cavanagh HD, et al. Effects of daily and overnight wear of hyper-oxygen transmissible rigid and silicone hydrogel lenses on bacterial binding to the corneal epithelium: 13-month clinical trials. Eye Contact Lens. 2003 Jan;29(1 Suppl):S14-6;

[969] Sweeney DF. Clinical signs of hypoxia with high-Dk soft lens extended wear: Is the cornea convinced? Eye Contact Lens. 2003 Jan;29(Suppl):S22-5

[970] Morgan PB, Efron N. In vivo dehydration of silicone hydrogel contact lenses. Eye Contact Lens. 2003 Jul;29(3):173-6

[971] Gurdal C, et al. Effects of extended-wear soft contact lenses on the ocular surface and central corneal thickness. Ophthalmologica. 2003 Sep-Oct;217(5):329-36

[972] Harvitt DM, Bonanno JA, Re-evaluation of the oxygen diffusion model for predicting minimum contact lens Dk/t values needed to avoid corneal anoxia. Optom Vis Sci 1999 Oct;76(10):712-9

[973] Buerki E, Augenaerztliche Kontaktlinsenanpassung. Ferdinand Enke Verlag, 1991, p. 24

[974] Ichijima H, et al., Effects of RGP lens extended wear on glucose-lactate metabolism and stromal swelling in the rabbit cornea. CLAO J 2000 Jan;26(1):30-6

[975] Ichijima H, et al., Determination of axygen tension on rabbit corneas under contact lenses. CLAO J 1998 Oct;24(4):220-6

[976] Iskeleli G, et al., Changes in corneal radius radius and thickness in response to extended wear of rigid gas permeable contact lenses. CLAO J 1996 Apr;22(2):133-5

[977] Jones L, et al., Life expectancy of rigid gas permeable and high water content contact lenses. CLAO J 1996 Oct;22(4):258-61

[978] Sweeney DF. Clinical signs of hypoxia with high-Dk soft lens extended wear: is the cornea convinced? Eye Contact Lens. 2003 Jan;29(1 Suppl):S22-5; discussion S26-9, S192-4

[979] Perez JG, Meijome JMG, Jalbert I, Sweeney DF, Ericsson P. Corneal epithelial thinning profile induced by long-term wear of hydrogel lenses. Cornea 2003;22(4):304-307

[980] Gonzalez-Meijome JM, et al. Changes in corneal structure with continuous wear of high-Dk soft contact lenses: a pilot study. Optom Vis Sci. 2003 Jun;80(6):440-6

[981] Cornish R, Sulaiman S, Do thinner rigid gas permeable contact lenses provide superior initial comfort? Optom Vis Sci 1996 Mar;73(3):139-43

[982] Carney LG, et al., The influence of center of gravity and lens mass on rigid lens dynamics. CLAO J 1996 Jul;22(3):195-204
[983] Rakow PL, Managing decentration in rigid lens wearers. J Ophthalmic Nurs Technol 1998 Sep-Oct;17(5):199-202
[984] Williams-Lyn, et al., The effect of rigid lens back optic zone radius and diameter changes on comfort. ICLC 1993 Nov/Dec;20:223-229
[985] Fink BA, Carney LG, Hill RM, Rigid lens tear pump efficiency:effects of overall diameter/base curve combinations. Optom Vis Sci 1991 Apr;68(4):309-313
[986] Sorbara L, et al., Centrally fitted versus upper lid-attached rigid gas permeable lenses. Part II. A comparison of the clinical performance. ICLC 1996 Jul/Aug;23:121-127
[987] Rengstorff RH, Corneal rehabilitation. In ES Bennet, BA Weissman (eds.), Clinical Contact Lens Practice. Lippincott, 1991, referenced in Hom MM, Manual of contact lens prescribing and fitting, Butterworth-Heinemann, 1997, p. 78
[988] Keeven J, et al., Evaluating the preservative effectiveness of RGP lens care solutions. CLAO J 1995;21(4):238-241
[989] Lin CP, Boehnke M, Influence of rigid gas permeable contact lens solutions on corneal epithelial wound healing. Kao Hsiung / Hsueh Ko Hsueh Tsa Chih 1997 Sep;13(9):562-565
[990] Begley CG, et al., Effects of rigid gas permeable contact lens solutions on the human corneal epithelium. Optom Vis Sci May;69(5):347-353
[991] Chowhan MA, et al., In vitro comparison of soaking solutions for rigid gas-permeable contact lenses. Clin Ther 1995 Mar;17(2):290-295
[992] Johannsdottir KR, Stelmach LB, Optom Vis Sci 2001 Sep;78(9):646-51
[993] Goldberg DB, Laser in situ keratomileusis monovision. J Cataract Refract Surg 2001 Sep;27(9):1449-55
[994] http://www.medscape.com/viewarticle/455878_print
[995] Patel S, Plaskow J, Ferrier C, The influence of vitamins and trace element supplements on the stability of the pre-corneal tear film. Acta Ophthamol (copenh) 1993 Dec;71(6):825-829
[996] Spotlight on 1999 refractive surgery volumes. http://www.optistock.com/spotlight2.htm
[997] http:drmcdonald.eyemdlink.com/EyeProcedure.asp?EyeProcedureID=14
[998] Augenwischerei bei der Augen-OP. Sueddeutsche Zeitung, Jan 11, 2000
[999] http://www.aao.org/aao/news/release/20030408.cfm
[1000] Slade SG, The complete book of laser surgery. Bantam Books, 2002
[1001] Barclay L. Age >40 increases risk of retreatment after LASIK. Ophthalmology 2003;110:748-754
[1002] Barclay L. Superior hinge flap causes more complications from LASIK. Ophthalmology 2003;110(5):1023-1029
[1003] Parade Magazine May 16, 1999
[1004] Cassel GH, Billig MD, Randall HG, The eye book. The Johns Hopkins University Press, 1998, p. 118
[1005] Tewes F, http://www.augen-laser-klinik.de/note.html
[1006] Vetrugno M, et al., A randomised, double masked, clinical trial of high dose vitamin A and vitamin E supplementation after photorefractive keratectomy. Br J Ophthalmol 2001 May;85(5):537-9
[1007] Parker JN, et al. The 2002 official patients sourcebook on myopia, ICON Health Publications, San Diego 2002
[1008] Parker JN, et al. The 2002 official patients sourcebook on laser eye surgery, ICON Health Publications, San Diego 2002

Printed in the United States
125202LV00003B/135/A